Heart Disease and Erectile Dysfunction

CONTEMPORARY CARDIOLOGY

CHRISTOPHER P. CANNON, MD
SERIES EDITOR

CT of the Heart: Principles and Applications, edited by *U. Joseph Schoepf, MD, 2004*

Cardiac Transplantation: The Columbia University Medical Center/New York-Presbyterian Hospital Manual, edited by *Niloo M. Edwards, MD, Jonathan M. Chen, MD, and Pamela A. Mazzeo, 2004*

Heart Disease and Erectile Dysfunction, edited by *Robert A. Kloner, MD, PhD, 2004*

Coronary Disease in Women: Evidence-Based Diagnosis and Treatment, edited by *Leslee J. Shaw, PhD, and Rita F. Redberg, MD, FACC, 2004*

Complementary and Alternate Cardiovascular Medicine, edited by *Richard A. Stein, MD and Mehmet C. Oz, MD, 2004*

Nuclear Cardiology, The Basics: How to Set Up and Maintain a Laboratory, by *Frans J. Th. Wackers, MD, PhD, Wendy Bruni, BS, CNMT, and Barry L. Zaret, MD, 2004*

Minimally Invasive Cardiac Surgery, Second Edition, edited by *Daniel J. Goldstein, MD, and Mehmet C. Oz, MD, 2004*

Cardiovascular Health Care Economics, edited by *William S. Weintraub, MD, 2003*

Platelet Glycoprotein IIb/IIIa Inhibitors in Cardiovascular Disease, Second Edition, edited by *A. Michael Lincoff, MD, 2003*

Heart Failure: A Clinician's Guide to Ambulatory Diagnosis and Treatment, edited by *Mariell L. Jessup, MD, and Evan Loh, MD, 2003*

Management of Acute Coronary Syndromes, Second Edition, edited by *Christopher P. Cannon, MD, 2003*

Aging, Heart Disease, and Its Management: Facts and Controversies, edited by *Niloo M. Edwards, MD, Mathew S. Maurer, MD, and Rachel B. Wellner, MPH, 2003*

Peripheral Arterial Disease: Diagnosis and Treatment, edited by *Jay D. Coffman, MD, and Robert T. Eberhardt, MD, 2003*

Cardiac Repolarization: Bridging Basic and Clinical Science, edited by *Ihor Gussak, MD, PhD, Charles Antzelevitch, PhD, Stephen C. Hammill, MD, Win K. Shen, MD, and Preben Bjerregaard, MD, DMSc, 2003*

Essentials of Bedside Cardiology: With a Complete Course in Heart Sounds and Murmurs on CD, Second Edition, by *Jules Constant, MD, 2003*

Primary Angioplasty in Acute Myocardial Infarction, edited by *James E. Tcheng, MD, 2002*

HEART DISEASE AND ERECTILE DYSFUNCTION

Edited by

ROBERT A. KLONER, MD, PhD

*Good Samaritan Hospital,
University of Southern California,
Los Angeles, CA*

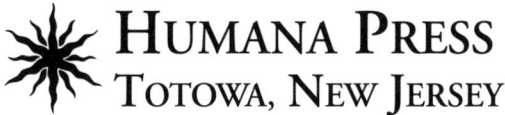

© 2004 Humana Press Inc.
999 Riverview Drive, Suite 208
Totowa, New Jersey 07512

humanapress.com

For additional copies, pricing for bulk purchases, and/or information about other Humana titles, contact Humana at the above address or at any of the following numbers: Tel.: 973-256-1699; Fax: 973-256-8341, E-mail: humana@humanapr.com; or visit our website: www.humanapress.com

All rights reserved.

No part of this book may be reproduced, stored in a retrieval system, or transmitted in any form or by any means, electronic, mechanical, photocopying, microfilming, recording, or otherwise without written permission from the Publisher.

All articles, comments, opinions, conclusions, or recommendations are those of the author(s), and do not necessarily reflect the views of the publisher.

Due diligence has been taken by the publishers, editors, and authors of this book to assure the accuracy of the information published and to describe generally accepted practices. The contributors herein have carefully checked to ensure that the drug selections and dosages set forth in this text are accurate and in accord with the standards accepted at the time of publication. Notwithstanding, as new research, changes in government regulations, and knowledge from clinical experience relating to drug therapy and drug reactions constantly occurs, the reader is advised to check the product information provided by the manufacturer of each drug for any change in dosages or for additional warnings and contraindications. This is of utmost importance when the recommended drug herein is a new or infrequently used drug. It is the responsibility of the treating physician to determine dosages and treatment strategies for individual patients. Further it is the responsibility of the health care provider to ascertain the Food and Drug Administration status of each drug or device used in their clinical practice. The publisher, editors, and authors are not responsible for errors or omissions or for any consequences from the application of the information presented in this book and make no warranty, express or implied, with respect to the contents in this publication.

Production Editor: Mark J. Breaugh.

Cover design by Patricia F. Cleary.

This publication is printed on acid-free paper. ∞
ANSI Z39.48-1984 (American National Standards Institute) Permanence of Paper for Printed Library Materials.

Photocopy Authorization Policy:
Authorization to photocopy items for internal or personal use, or the internal or personal use of specific clients, is granted by Humana Press Inc., provided that the base fee of US $25.00 per copy is paid directly to the Copyright Clearance Center at 222 Rosewood Drive, Danvers, MA 01923. For those organizations that have been granted a photocopy license from the CCC, a separate system of payment has been arranged and is acceptable to Humana Press Inc. The fee code for users of the Transactional Reporting Service is: [1-58829-216-9/04 $25.00].

E-ISBN: 1-59259-748-3

Printed in the United States of America.   10 9 8 7 6 5 4 3 2 1

Library of Congress Cataloging-in-Publication Data

Heart disease and erectile dysfunction / edited by Robert A. Kloner.
    p. ; cm. -- (Contemporary cardiology)
 Includes bibliographical references and index.
  ISBN 1-58829-216-9 (alk. paper)
 1. Impotence--Etiology. 2. Coronary heart disease. 3. Sexual
disorders--Etiology. 4. Heart--Diseases.
  [DNLM: 1. Impotence--etiology. 2. Cardiovascular
Diseases--complications. 3. Impotence--therapy. WJ 709 H435 2004]   I.
Kloner, Robert A. II. Contemporary cardiology (Totowa, N.J. :
Unnumbered)
RC889.H33 2004
616.6'922071--dc22
                            2003018237

Preface

Only a short time ago, if a man went to see his physician for erectile dysfunction (ED) he was often told that the problem was psychological. In the last 10–15 years there has been a growing appreciation of the concept that in men over the age of 50, one of the most common causes of ED is vascular. Vascular causes include endothelial dysfunction (the other ED, which is one of the earliest abnormalities in the spectrum of atherosclerosis) to full-blown obstructing atherosclerotic plaque.

Since the key component of an erection is vasodilatation, if blood vessels cannot dilate normally owing to endothelial dysfunction, then a normal erection will not occur. Endothelial dysfunction will occur when the blood vessel is exposed to certain risk factors—hypertension, lipid abnormalities, cigaret smoking, diabetes, and others. It is therefore no surprise that these same risk factors for atherosclerotic cardiovascular disease are also risk factors for erectile dysfunction.

Erectile dysfunction is a common problem in the cardiac patient. The purpose of *Heart Disease and Erectile Dysfunction* is to review the problem of erectile dysfunction from a cardiac standpoint. Chapters have been written by cardiologists, urologists, psychologists, pharmacologists, and basic scientists alike to synthesize the problem of erectile dysfunction as it relates to heart disease, review the physiology of ED, review the current therapies for ED and how they may interact with the cardiac system, review the potential application of the phosphodiesterase-5 inhibitors to cardiovascular disease, and review guidelines for dealing with the cardiac patient seeking help for ED. We hope that this is the first of many books that might help define a new subspecialty of "uro-cardiology" or "cardio-urology."

I would like to thank Chris Cannon, MD, and Paul Dolgert for their encouragement in editing this text. I would also like to thank all of the contributing authors as well as my administrative assistant, Cathy Davisson, for help with typing and organizing the chapters.

The drugs, indications for drugs, and drug dosages may or may not be approved for general use by the Food and Drug Administration. Physicians should consult the package inserts and/or Physicians' Desk Reference for drug indications, contraindications, side effects, precautions, warnings, and dosages as recommended.

Robert A. Kloner, MD, PhD

Contents

Preface v
Contributors ix

1 Physiology of Erection and Causes
 of Erectile Dysfunction 1
 *Aristotelis G. Anastasiadis, Dmitry Droggin,
 Martin Burchardt, and Ridwan Shabsigh*

2 Erectile Dysfunction: *The Scope of the Problem* 19
 Culley C. Carson

3 Erectile Dysfunction
 and Cardiovascular Risk Factors 39
 Robert A. Kloner

4 Psychologic Aspects of Erectile Dysfunction
 in Heart Patients 51
 Raymond C. Rosen

5 Management of Erectile Dysfunction: *An Overview* 65
 Harin Padma-Nathan

6 Sildenafil Citrate
 and the Nitric Oxide/Cyclic Guanosine
 Monophosphate Signaling Pathway 89
 Ian H. Osterloh and Stephen C. Phillips

7 Phosphodiesterase-5 Inhibition:
 Importance to the Cardiovascular System 117
 *Jackie D. Corbin, Stephen R. Rannels,
 and Sharron H. Francis*

8 The Hemodynamics of Phosphodiesterase-PDE5
 Inhibitors 131
 Graham Jackson

9 Cardiovascular Safety of Phosphodiesterase-5
 Inhibitors 139
 Robert A. Kloner

10	Effect of Phosphodiesterase-5 Inhibition on Coronary Blood Flow in Experimental Animals .... 163 *YingJie Chen, Jay H. Traverse, and Robert J. Bache*	
11	Safety and Hemodynamic Effects of Sildenafil in Patients With Coronary Artery Disease .... 179 *Sameer Rohatgi and Howard C. Herrmann*	
12	Cardiovascular Effects of Nonphosphodiesterase-5 Inhibitor Erectile Dysfunction Therapies .... 195 *Harin Padma-Nathan*	
13	Potential Cardiac Applications of Phosphodiesterase Type-5 Inhibition .... 207 *Michael Sweeney and Richard L. Siegel*	
14	The Physiologic Cost of Sexual Activity .... 239 *Robert F. DeBusk*	
15	Sexual Activity As a Trigger of Myocardial Infarction/Ischemia: *Implications for Treating Erectile Dysfunction* .... 251 *Robert A. Kloner*	
16	Sex After Cardiac Events and Procedures: *Counseling From the Cardiovascular Specialist's Perspective* .... 261 *Herman A. Taylor, Jr.*	
17	American College of Cardiology/American Heart Association Guidelines on the Use of Sildenafil in Patients With Cardiovascular Disease .... 271 *Adolph M. Hutter, Jr.*	
18	Risk of Heart Attack After Sexual Activity: *The Princeton Guidelines and Their Rationale* .... 279 *Robert F. DeBusk*	

Index 289

CONTRIBUTORS

ARISTOTELIS G. ANASTASIADIS, MD, *Department of Urology, College of Physicians and Surgeons, Columbia University, New York, NY*

ROBERT J. BACHE, MD, *Cardiovascular Division, Department of Medicine, University of Minnesota Medical School, Minneapolis, MN*

MARTIN BURCHARDT, MD, *Department of Urology, University of Düsseldorf, Düsseldorf, Germany*

CULLEY C. CARSON, MD, *Division of Urology, University of North Carolina School of Medicine, Chapel Hill, NC*

YINGJIE CHEN, MD, PhD, *Division of Cardiology, Department of Medicine, University of Minnesota Medical School, Minneapolis, MN*

JACKIE D. CORBIN, PhD, *Department of Molecular Physiology and Biophysics, Vanderbilt University School of Medicine, Nashville, TN*

ROBERT F. DEBUSK, MD, *Department of Medicine, Stanford University School of Medicine, Stanford, CA*

DMITRY DROGGIN, MD, *Department of Urology, College of Physicians and Surgeons, Columbia University, New York, NY*

SHARRON H. FRANCIS, PhD, *Department of Molecular Physiology and Biophysics, Vanderbilt University School of Medicine, Nashville, TN*

HOWARD C. HERRMANN, MD, *Cardiovascular Division, Hospital of the University of Pennsylvania, University of Pennsylvania School of Medicine, Philadelphia, PA*

ADOLPH M. HUTTER, JR., MD, MACC, *Department of Medicine, Massachusetts General Hospital, Harvard Medical School, Boston, MA*

GRAHAM JACKSON, FRCP, FESC, FACC, FAHA, *Cardiac Department, St. Thomas Hospital, London, UK*

ROBERT A. KLONER, MD, PhD, *The Heart Institute, Good Samaritan Hospital, Division of Cardiovascular Medicine, Keck School of Medicine, University of Southern California, Los Angeles, CA*

IAN H. OSTERLOH, MRCP, *Pfizer Global Research and Development, Pfizer Ltd., Sandwich, Kent, UK*

HARIN PADMA-NATHAN, MD, *The Male Clinic, Beverly Hills, CA; Division of Urology, Keck School of Medicine, University of Southern California, Los Angeles, CA*

STEPHEN C. PHILLIPS, PhD, *Pfizer Global Research and Development, Pfizer Ltd., Sandwich, Kent, UK*

STEPHEN R. RANNELS, PhD, *Department of Cell and Molecular Physiology, Pennsylvania State University College of Medicine, Hershey, PA*

SAMEER ROHATGI, MD, *Cardiovascular Division, Hospital of the University of Pennsylvania, Philadelphia, PA*

RAYMOND C. ROSEN, PhD, *Departments of Psychiatry and Medicine, UMDNJ-Robert Wood Johnson Medical School, New Brunswick, NJ*

RIDWAN SHABSIGH, MD, *Department of Urology, College of Physicians and Surgeons, Columbia University, New York, NY*

RICHARD L. SIEGEL, MD, *US Pharmaceuticals Group, Pfizer Inc., New York, NY*

MICHAEL SWEENEY, MD, *US Pharmaceuticals Group, Pfizer Inc., New York, NY*

HERMAN A. TAYLOR, JR., MD, FACC, FAHA, *Department of Medicine, Jackson State University, University of Mississippi Medical Center, Jackson, MS*

JAY H. TRAVERSE, MD, *Division of Cardiology, Department of Medicine, University of Minnesota Medical School, Minneapolis, MN*

1 Physiology of Erection and Causes of Erectile Dysfunction

Aristotelis G. Anastasiadis, MD,
Dmitry Droggin, MD,
Martin Burchardt, MD,
and Ridwan Shabsigh, MD

CONTENTS

INTRODUCTION
PHYSIOLOGY OF ERECTION
PATHOPHYSIOLOGY OF ED
CONCLUSION
REFERENCES

INTRODUCTION

Erectile dysfunction (ED), defined as "the persistent inability to achieve or maintain an erection sufficient for satisfactory sexual performance" *(1)*, is a highly prevalent condition. It is estimated that currently approximately 30 million men in the United States are affected *(2)*. This number is expected to at least double by 2025 as a result of the aging of the male population as well as increased awareness of the problem *(3)*. ED can have emotional, physical, and iatrogenic causes. Mixed forms are common, and ED may also be a symptom of chronic diseases.

From: *Contemporary Cardiology: Heart Disease and Erectile Dysfunction*
Edited by: R. A. Kloner © Humana Press Inc., Totowa, NJ

During the last 5 years, the understanding of the erectile process and causes of ED have improved dramatically. Major breakthroughs include, but are not limited to, the identification of nitric oxide (NO) as a major transmitter involved in erection, the role of smooth muscle in regulating arterial and venous blood flow, and changes in anatomical penile structures responsible for impairment of erectile function *(4)*. In this chapter, the complex physiological interactions responsible for erection, as well as the multiple causes for ED, are addressed.

PHYSIOLOGY OF ERECTION

Neuroanatomy

In animal studies, several brain regions have been identified as being important to penile erection. The medial preoptic area (MPOA) of the hypothalamus may be the integration point for the central control of erection. It receives sensory impulses from the amygdala that have been gathered at cortical association areas. These include norepinephrine-mediated inhibitory signals and dopamine-mediated proerectile stimuli *(5)* (Fig. 1A).

The paraventricular nucleus of the hypothalamus, which receives neural input from the MPOA, may have a proerectile action through oxytocin-mediated descending pathways.

Periaqueductal gray matter, which provides neural connections between the MPOA and the brain stem, may also have proerectile activity; neurons from the paraventricular nucleus are known to project through it to thoracic and lumbosacral nuclei concerned with erection *(5)*. Reflex erections occur in the erection-generating center of the spinal cord (T12–S3; ref. *6*). The penis is innervated by the sympathetic (T11–L2), parasympathetic (S2–S4), and somatic (S2–S4) nervous systems.

Sympathetic input is antierectile, whereas parasympathetic and somatic input is proerectile.

Both sympathetic and parasympathetic fibers reach the pelvic or inferior hypogastric plexus where autonomic input to the penis is integrated; the cavernous nerves originate from this plexus *(5)*.

The sacral reflex arc, another pathway, conveys stimuli from the perineum and the lower urinary tract mucosa.

The lesser cavernous nerves originate from the pelvic plexus and travel along the penis to supply the penile urethra and the erectile tissue of the corpus spongiosum.

Chapter 1 / Erectile Physiology and Pathophysiology

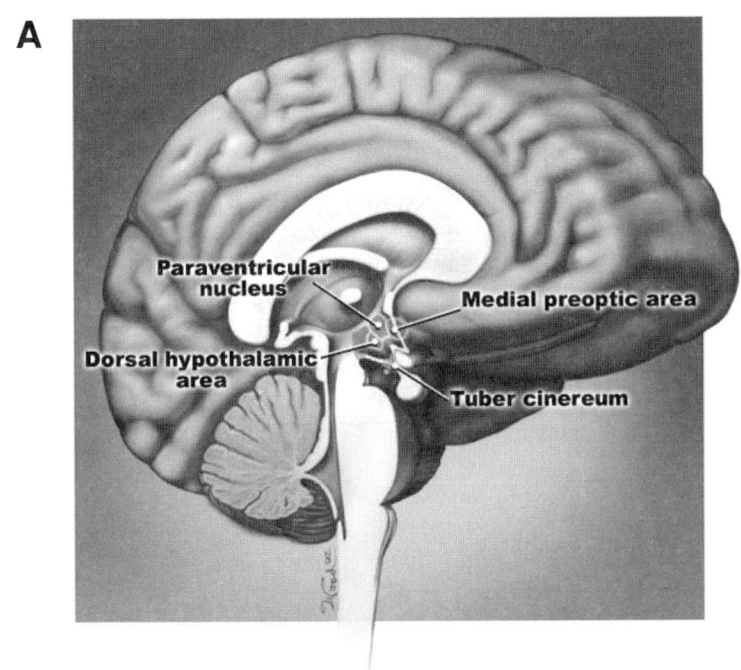

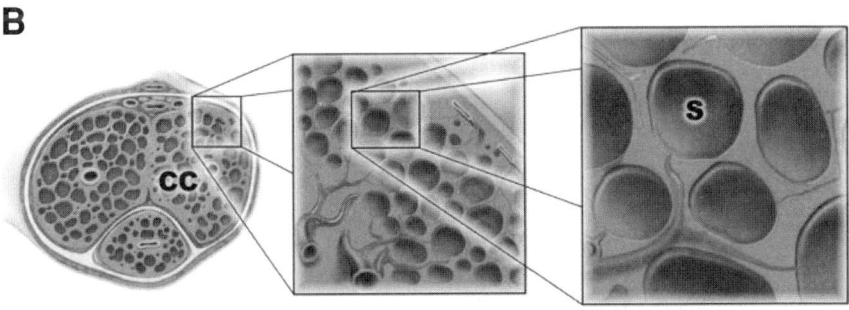

Fig. 1. Schematic depiction of anatomical, neural, and vascular structures relevant for erection. **(A)** Medial preoptic area and paraventricular nucleus of the hypothalamus. **(B)** Frontal section of the penis showing the sinuses (S) of the corpora cavernosa (CC). From *(59)*.

The greater cavernous nerves also originate in the pelvic plexus. They innervate the helicine arteries and the erectile tissue.

Intracavernous nerves are encased in fibrous tissue, which prevents their compression during an erection.

Their branches travel with prostatovesicular artery branches, which provide a visual landmark during nerve-sparing radical prostatectomy.

The dorsal penile nerves, branches of the pudendal nerves, and the ilioinguinal nerve also innervate the penis. These nerves provide sensory input from the glans penis and skin, and penile root, respectively *(5,6)*.

Penile Anatomy

The penis contains three cylindrical structures, the corpus spongiosum, which surrounds the urethra, and the two erectile bodies, the corpora cavernosa *(4)*. The tunica affords great flexibility, rigidity, and tissue strength to the penis. The tunical covering of the corpora cavernosa is a bilayered structure that has multiple sublayers. The elastic fibers of the tunica form an irregular network, on which collagen fibers rest *(4)*. The corpora cavernosa comprise two spongy-paired cylinders contained in the thick envelope of the tunica albuginea. The crura, their proximal ends, originate at the undersurface of the puboischial rami as two separate structures but merge under the pubic arch and remain attached up to the glans. The septum between the two corpora cavernosa is incomplete in humans *(4)*. Each corpus cavernosum contains sinusoids, which are larger in the center and smaller in the periphery (Fig. 1B). The structure of the corpus spongiosum and the glans is similar to that in the corpora cavernosa except that the sinusoids are larger. The tunica is thinner in the spongiosum and is absent in the glans *(4)*.

Arterial supply for the penis is usually the internal pudendal artery, a branch of the internal iliac artery. In many instances, however, accessory arteries from the external iliac, obturator, vesical, and femoral arteries exist *(7)*. Damage to these arteries during pelvic surgery may result in vasculogenic ED postoperatively *(4)*. The internal pudendal artery becomes the common penile artery, which then divides into the dorsal, the bulbourethral, and the cavernous arteries. Along its course, the cavernous artery gives off many helicine arteries, which supply the trabecular erectile tissue and the sinusoids.

The venous drainage from the three corpora originates in small venules leading from the peripheral sinusoids immediately beneath the tunica albuginea. These venules travel between the tunica and the peripheral sinusoids to form the subtunical venular plexus before exiting as the emissary veins.

Biochemistry and Hemodynamics of Erection and Detumescence

An erection is a hemodynamic event that is determined by the contractile state of penile smooth muscle.

When a penis is in its flaccid state, sympathetic neural activity predominates; this minimizes blood flow into the sinuses of the corpora cavernosa.

With sexual stimulation, parasympathetic neural activity predominates; this leads to increased blood flow into the sinuses and achievement of erection caused by smooth muscle relaxation in the corpora cavernosa.

The maintenance of the intracorporeal smooth muscle in a semi-contracted state during flaccidity results from intrinsic myogenic activity, adrenergic neurotransmission, and endothelium-derived contracting factors, such as prostaglandin $F_{2\alpha}$ and endothelins *(8)*.

Several factors are required for penile smooth muscle cells to contract, including adequate local levels of neurotransmitters, adequate expression of receptors, the integrity of the transduction mechanism, ion channel homeostasis, interactions between contractile proteins, and effective communication between smooth muscle cells over gap junctions *(5)*.

The main neurotransmitter mediating penile erection is NO, which is released from the endothelium of the corpora cavernosa during nonadrenergic, noncholinergic (NANC) neurotransmission *(9)* (Fig. 2). Within the muscle cell, NO activates a soluble guanylyl cyclase, which raises the intracellular concentration of cyclic guanosine monophosphate. In turn, cyclic guanosine monophosphate activates a specific protein kinase, which phosphorylates certain proteins and ion channels, resulting in the opening of potassium channels and hyperpolarization of the muscle cell membrane, sequestration of intracellular calcium by the endoplasmic reticulum, and blocking of calcium influx by calcium channel inhibition. The consequence is a drop in cytosolic calcium concentration and relaxation of the smooth muscle, resulting in dilation of arterial vessels and increased blood flow into the sinuses of the corpora cavernosa in both the diastolic and systolic phases *(8,9)* (Fig. 3).

Arginase, a binuclear manganese metalloenzyme that catalyzes the hydrolysis of L-arginine to form L-ornithine plus urea, regulates NO synthase activity—and, therefore, attenuates NO-dependent physiological processes—by depleting the substrate pool of L-arginine *(10)*. In the internal anal sphincter muscle, arginase suppresses NANC nerve-mediated relaxation by depleting intracellular L-arginine concentrations that would otherwise be used by NO synthase.

With the discovery of arginase activity in corpus cavernosum tissue extracts prepared from rabbit penis and human penis, Cox et al. probed the physiological relationship between arginase and NO synthase in

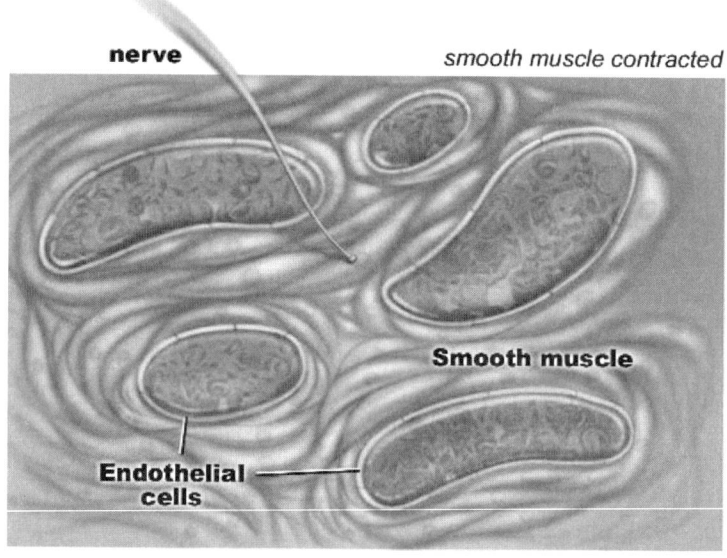
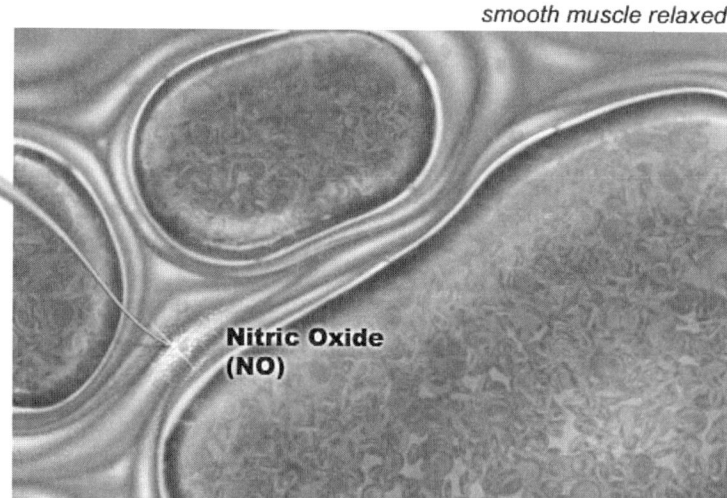

Fig. 2. Intracellular mechanisms of nitric oxide, the main neurotransmitter in penile erection. From *(59)*.

penile corpus cavernosum. They studied the effects of the arginase inhibitor 2(S)-amino-6-boronohexanoic acid (ABH) on smooth muscle contractility using organ bath preparations of rabbit penile corpus cavernosum. Tissue strips were procured and prepared, and NANC nerve-mediated responses were elicited by electrical field stimulation at

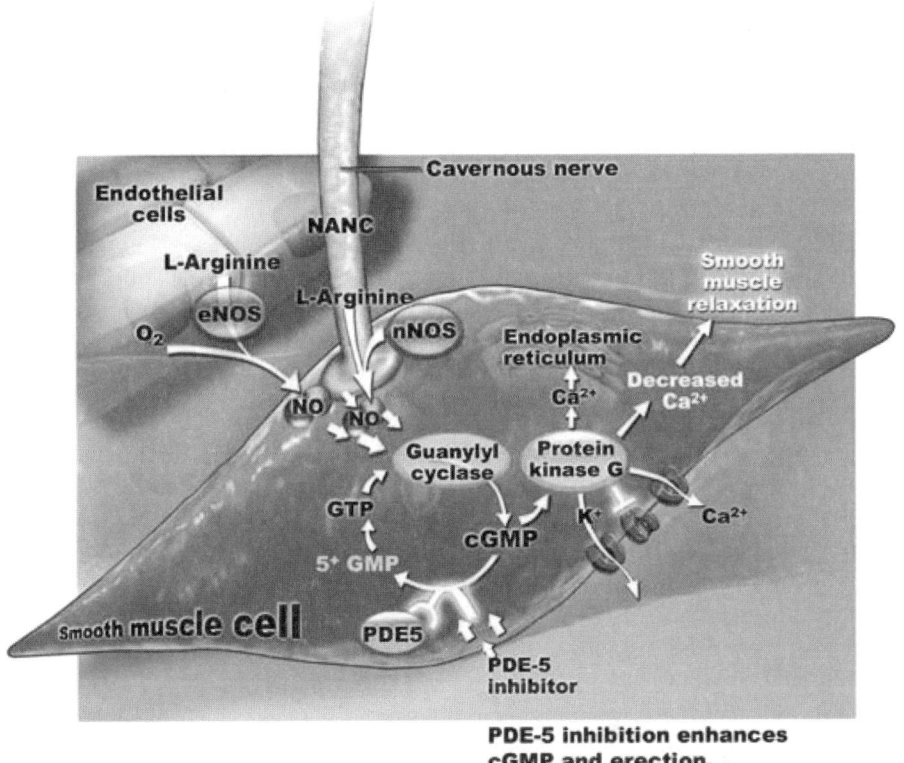

Fig. 3. Mechanism of action of PDE5 inhibitors. From *(59)*.

varying frequencies. Electrical stimulation caused frequency-dependent relaxation. The addition of ABH in the absence of electrical stimulation caused moderate relaxation as a result of the basal activity of NO synthase. ABH significantly enhanced relaxation to electrical stimulation in a dose-dependent manner *(10)*.

Recently, Bivalacqua et al. compared arginase gene expression, protein levels, and enzyme activity in diabetic human cavernosal tissue. When compared with normal human cavernosal tissue, diabetic corpus cavernosum from humans with ED had higher levels of arginase II protein, gene expression, and enzyme activity. In contrast, gene expression and protein levels of arginase I were not significantly different in diabetic cavernosal tissue when compared with control tissue. The reduced ability of diabetic tissue to convert L-arginine to L-citrulline via NO synthase was reversed by the selective inhibition of arginase ABH. These data suggest that the increased expression of arginase II in diabetic cavernosal tissue may contribute to the ED associated with this common disease process and may play a role in other manifestations of diabetic disease in which NO production is decreased *(11)*.

Recently, the inhibition of vasoconstrictors, that is, norepinephrine and endothelin-1, has also been proposed as a potential regulating mechanism in the erectile process *(12)*. The calcium-sensitizing rho A/Rho kinase pathway may play a synergistic role in cavernosal vasoconstriction to maintain penile flaccidity. Rho-kinase is known to inhibit myosin light-chain phosphatase and to directly phosphorylate myosin light-chain (in solution), altogether resulting in a net increase in activated myosin and the promotion of cellular contraction. Although Rho kinase protein and mRNA have been detected in cavernosal tissue, the role of Rho kinase in the regulation of cavernosal tone is unknown. However, using pharmacologic antagonism (Y-27632), Chitaley et al. examined the role of Rho kinase in cavernosal tone, based on the hypothesis that antagonism of Rho kinase results in increased corpus cavernosum pressure, initiating the erectile response independently of NO. Indeed, Rho kinase antagonism was able to stimulate rat penile erection independently of NO *(12,13)*.

As a result of smooth muscle relaxation in the corpora, the following events occur: (a) the incoming blood is trapped by the expanding sinusoids, (b) the subtunical venular plexuses between the tunica albuginea and the peripheral sinusoids are compressed, reducing venous outflow, (c) the tunica stretches further and decreases venous outflow to a minimum, (d) intracavernous pressure increases, raising the penis to its erect state, and (e) pressure increases further, leading to the contraction of the ischiocavernosus muscles (rigid erection phase; ref. *4*).

Penile detumescence occurs in three phases: The first phase entails a transient increase of intracorpreal pressure, indicating the beginning of smooth muscle contraction against a closed venous system. The second phase involves a slow pressure decrease, suggesting a slow reopening of the venous channels with resumption of the basal level of arterial flow. In the third phase, there is a fast pressure decrease, and venous capacity is fully restored *(4)*.

PATHOPHYSIOLOGY OF ED

Major Risk Factors for ED

Major risk factors for ED include advancing age; the presence of chronic illness, such as heart disease, hypertension, diabetes mellitus, or depression; smoking; stress; alcohol and drug abuse; and sedentary lifestyle *(14)*. The main causes of ED are organic (e.g., vascular, neurogenic, hormonal, anatomical/structural, drug induced), psychogenic, or mixed *(8)*. The mixed form is the most common. Causes can be acquired or congenital; psychogenic causes can be either generalized or situational. Aging constitutes an independent risk factor for ED *(15)*. Numerous changes occur as men age, and there is a progressive decline in sexual function as the result of various physiologic changes *(8)*. The incidence of chronic diseases also increases with age. In addition, psychological and relationship issues may contribute to ED *(14,16)*. ED can be considered a marker of serious medical conditions, such as hypertension, diabetes mellitus, cardiovascular disease, or depression, therefore playing an important role in men's health *(17,18)*. The role of androgens in erectile function remains controversial. Psychogenic causes of ED include depression, performance anxiety, relationship problems, psychosocial problems, and psychosocial distress *(19–22)*. Although in the past ED was thought to be primarily the result of psychogenic factors, it is now generally acknowledged that organic causes are present in most patients *(8)*. Organic causes are subdivided into vascular, neurogenic, hormonal, penile injury or disease, drug-induced, or those related to other systemic diseases *(6,8)*. A combination of factors is not uncommon.

Organic Causes of ED

Organic causes of ED can be subdivided into vascular causes (40%), diabetes mellitus (30%), drug-induced ED (15%), neurogenic ED, penile injury, or disease (6%), endocrine problems (3%), or those related to other neurologic or systemic diseases *(8)*.

ENDOTHELIAL DYSFUNCTION AS A CAUSE OF ED

Penile erection, being greatly dependent on adequate inflow of blood to the erectile tissue, requires coordinated arterial endothelium-dependent vasodilatation and sinusoidal endothelium-dependent corporal smooth muscle relaxation *(23)*. Therefore, any factors interfering with the arterial inflow of blood to the corpora cavernosal or the synthesis/release of NO within the corpora cavernosal are prime suspects involved in the pathophysiology of ED. This endothelial dysfunction can occur physiologically with aging but is common in pathologic conditions like diabetes and atherosclerosis. The earliest vascular modifications in atherosclerosis occur with the alteration of arterial endothelium-dependent relaxations, followed by the impairment of smooth muscle reactivity *(24)*. In this context, it has been shown that hypercholesterolemia in men and rabbits causes (a) a reduced inflow of blood to the penis by the vascular narrowing of the lumen of penile and pelvic vessels, (b) an impairment of endothelium-dependent NO-dependent corporal smooth muscle relaxation, and (c) corporal smooth muscle tissue alteration (fibrosis and degeneration of smooth muscle cells) resulting in ED *(25,26)*. Nevertheless, aging is a process that, in itself, induces functional and morphological modifications, which have to be taken into account when appraising ED *(1,15,23)*.

Findings from animal and human studies clearly indicate that the global erectile response is altered both as a result of atherosclerotic vascular disease development and during the aging process. Atherosclerotic disease, diabetes, and aging are commonly associated and induce structural and functional modifications that can take place at the level of the endothelium, vascular smooth muscle and extracellular matrix of blood vessels and/or cavernosal tissues *(24,25,27–29)*.

VASCULAR FACTORS OF ED

Vascular disease is the most common cause of organic ED and is most often the result of medical disorders that affect the arterial system *(1)*. The most common etiologic factors, which can also be combined, are atherosclerosis, hyperlipidemia with vascular stenosis of the penile arteries, smoking, diabetes, hypertension, and vascular surgery *(30)*. Other vascular factors include venous leaks and degenerative changes, like Peyronie's disease *(31)*. In addition, traumatic pelvic and perineal injury can result in ED *(32)*. Recently, perineal arterial compression during cycling has been proposed to be associated with ED *(33,34)*.

Erectile failure caused by venous insufficiency in the presence of adequate arterial inflow can be termed veno-occlusive ED. The importance of direct injury to the sinusoidal endothelium and smooth musculature at the cellular level has become apparent in the pathogenesis of veno-occlusive ED *(35)*. Such damage limits the ability of the smooth muscle to relax within the corpora, resulting in reduced sinusoidal dilation. Any factor leading to an alteration of the fibroelastic component of the trabeculae can result in incomplete venous occlusion with subsequent venous leakage and erectile failure *(35)*. Ischemic injury resulting from priapism with subsequent fibrosis of the erectile tissue will also subsequently result in ED.

NEUROGENIC FACTORS OF ED

Neurogenic ED can be defined broadly as an inability to sustain or maintain a penile erection because of neurologic impairment or dysfunction *(36)*. Underlying etiologies can include diabetic neuropathy and vasculopathy, multiple sclerosis, Parkinson's disease, hereditary peripheral neuropathies, chemically induced neuropathies, spina bifida, radical retropubic prostatectomy, spinal cord injury, cerebrovascular accidents, Alzheimer's disease, and lumbar disk herniation *(36)*.

Diabetes has been associated with corpus cavernosum smooth muscle changes, such as increased connective tissue synthesis and atrophy of smooth muscle within the corpus cavernosum in humans and animal models *(37)*. These structural changes can be correlated with an increased incidence of veno-occlusive dysfunction and erectile failure, consistent with systemic peripheral vascular disease observed in diabetes *(36)*. Transforming growth factor (TGF)-β_1 has been implicated in the connective tissue changes in ED *(38)*. In addition to the earlier-mentioned changes, advanced glycation end products have been documented in human corpus cavernosum biopsies from diabetic patients *(39)*.

ED is a frequent complication of prostate cancer therapy, particularly radical prostatectomy *(40)*. ED is reported to occur in 66% of men after a non-nerve-sparing procedure, in 59% after a unilateral nerve-sparing procedure, and 56% after a bilateral nerve-sparing procedure *(41)*. External beam radiation is associated with a nearly 50% reduction in erectile function *(40)*.

HORMONAL FACTORS OF ED

Testosterone is thought to primarily stimulate libido at the levels of the central nervous system *(42)*. Bagatelle et al. reported on normal men who had a significant decrease in sexual desire, fantasy, spontaneous erections, and masturbation after a few weeks of androgen suppression by a GnRH antagonist. These changes were not found when the subjects received androgen therapy simultaneously with the GnRH antagonist *(43)*.

ED is a common condition in the elderly population. Results of the Massachusetts Male Aging Study (MMAS) indicate that the most strongly associated variable to ED is age *(15)*. The prevalence of complete ED in this study tripled in men between ages 40 and 70 yr.

There is a considerable controversy regarding the role of androgens in erectile function. Animal studies using the rat model showed that penile cavernosal and spongiosal cells undergo apoptosis (programmed cell death) in response to castration. In a follow-up study, testosterone activated *de novo* DNA synthesis in the penis of castrated adult rats, including cavernosal cells *(44)*.

Korenman et al. found no difference in serum bioavailable testosterone levels between older men with and without ED. Therefore, they have proposed that ED and secondary hypogonadism are two common independent disorders of the aging male *(45)*. Similarly, the MMAS showed no significant correlation between ED and serum testosterone levels (either free, albumin-bound, or total). The only hormonal decline that correlated with ED in this study was that of dehydroepiandrosterone *(15)*. Data from animal and human studies indicate that low-normal range concentrations of testosterone are sufficient to maintain sexual activity, and that there is a threshold level of testosterone, above which there is no further improvement in response to therapy *(46)*. Administration of testosterone to normal eugonadal men enhances penile rigidity but does not change circumference or frequency of erections during nocturnal penile testing *(47)*. In hypogonadal men, it improves libido and sexual performance *(48)*.

It should be kept in mind that androgen deficiency, especially in elderly men, is not the most common cause of ED. There are other common vascular, neurological, and psychological, iatrogenic factors that are likely to coexist with androgen deficiency and prevent beneficial effects of androgen replacement therapy.

MEDICATIONS AS CAUSES OF ED

Although many prescription medications have been implicated in disorders of sexual desire, arousal, and orgasm, medications to treat hypertension and psychiatric disorders are most frequently cited as contributing to these dysfunctions *(49)*.

Antihypertensive Medications. The majority of antihypertensive medications have been implicated in sexual disorders. However, some substances are more likely than others to cause ED. For example, diuretics (e.g., chlorthalidone, hydrochlorothiazide, and spironolactone), central antiadrenergic agents (e.g., clonidine, methyldopa, reserpine), and guanethidine are commonly cited as causes of ED *(49)*. However, β-blockers, with the exception of propranolol, are less likely to cause ED, but can cause desire disorders *(49)*. Angiotensin-converting enzyme inhibitors may be least likely to cause ED. In addition, minoxidil, hydralazine, prazosin, and furosemide rarely cause sexual side effects, although hydralazine and prazosin have been associated with priapism in case reports *(49)*.

Psychiatric Medications. Psychiatric medications also commonly affect sexual function. Antidepressants (e.g., amitriptyline, amoxapine, clomipramine, desipramine, nortriptyline, protriptyline) have frequently been associated with ED and can cause a delayed or absent orgasmic response *(49)*. Similar side effects have been reported with selective serotonin reuptake inhibitors, such as fluoxetine and sertraline. Antipsychotic medications (e.g., thioridazine, chlorpromazine), without exception, have the potential for disrupting sexual response. Lithium and monoaminooxidase inhibitors may impair sexual desire and erectile function.

Many other prescription medications in diverse therapeutic classes are frequently cited as causing sexual dysfunctions. These include carbamazepine, digoxin, disulfiram, and ketoconazole *(49)*. In addition, antihyperlipidemic agents like clofibrate and gemfibrozil have been associated with ED. The statins appear to have a lower risk *(50)*. Hormonal agents, including antiandrogens, LH-RH analogs, and estrogens, also increase the risk of ED *(50)*. Other drugs associated with ED include protease inhibitors, cytotoxic agents, and H2-receptor antagonists *(50,51)*.

Psychogenic Causes of ED

Psychogenic ED frequently coexists with other sexual dysfunctions, notably hypoactive sexual desire, and with major psychiatric disorders, particularly depression and anxiety disorders *(52)*. In the latter cases, a primary diagnosis may be difficult to establish, and concomitant treatment of the patient's psychiatric disorder may be indicated as the initial step in management.

Many men with ED also have comorbid depression, and the relation between them appears to be bidirectional; the occurrence of either disorder may cause, result from, or exacerbate the other *(15,18,53)*. There are five models, not mutually exclusive, that describe a possible relation between ED and depression. First, ED may lead to "secondary" depression in vulnerable individuals. Studies have shown that men with ED are more likely to report depressive symptoms than are men without ED *(15,54)*. Second, ED can be symptomatic of a "primary" depressive episode. That is, men who are depressed frequently manifest symptoms of ED. Furthermore, some men with major depressive disorder develop a reversible loss of nocturnal penile tumescence, suggesting that depression can influence erectile neurophysiology *(55)*. Third, a common factor may be related to the development of both conditions. ED and depression frequently co-occur with other conditions, including diabetes, hypertension, cardiovascular disease, neurologic disorders (e.g., parkinsonism, multiple sclerosis), and endocrine disorders (e.g., adrenal, thyroid, gonadal). Numerous epidemiologic studies have indicated that the concurrence of depressive symptoms, particularly major depressive disorder, increased the risk of ischemic heart disease and mortality *(53)*. Other data showed that depression was a significant, independent risk factor for the development of symptomatic ischemic heart disease in otherwise healthy individuals *(56)*. Conversely, medical illness can precipitate depression in a predisposed individual. Significantly, ED, depression, and vascular disease share a number of risk factors, including smoking, obesity, dyslipidemia, and a sedentary lifestyle *(15)*. Fourth, ED can be an adverse effect of medication treatments for these conditions, including antidepressants, antihypertensives, cardiac drugs, and numerous other agents *(57)*. Between 5 and 80% of patients taking antidepressants experience side effects related to sexual function *(53)*. Similarly, between 10 and 50% of men taking antihypertensives experience ED while on therapy *(57)*. Finally, as relatively prevalent conditions, ED and depression can be coincidentally comorbid and, thus, etiologically unrelated *(53)*.

The significance of psychosocial factors in the etiology of ED has been highlighted in epidemiological studies. In the MMAS, ED was significantly associated with depressive symptoms, pessimistic attitudes, or a negative outlook on life *(15)*. Similarly, in the National Health and Social Life Survey, ED was significantly associated with emotional stress and a history of social coercion *(20)*. These studies underline the significant effects of psychosocial factors in the etiology of ED.

Generally, psychosocial determinants of ED are divided into immediate and remote causes *(20)*. Immediate causes include performance anxiety (or fear of failure), lack of adequate stimulation, and relationship conflicts. Among the remote or early developmental causes, various researchers have emphasized the role of sexual trauma in childhood, sexual identity or orientation issues, unresolved partner or parental attachments, and religious or cultural taboos *(20)*.

Frequently, interpersonal and relationship factors have been associated with ED. Communication difficulties, lack of intimacy or trust, and power conflicts have been emphasized as frequent concomitants of arousal difficulties in both sexes *(52)*. Loss of sexual attraction has also been implicated.

An expanded classification system for psychogenic ED has been proposed by the nomenclature committee of the International Society of Impotence Research. This new classification is intended to broaden the previously limited focus of psychogenic ED and incorporates clinical features (general vs situational ED) and hypothesized etiologic mechanisms (central excitation vs inhibition) of psychogenic ED. Recent studies have strongly implicated the role of central excitatory and inhibitory mechanisms in the control of male sexual arousal *(58)*. These concepts are incorporated into the proposed classification system.

In addition to the clinical subtypes of generalized vs situational, psychogenic ED can be characterized as lifelong (primary) or acquired (secondary). Primary psychogenic ED refers to the lifelong inability to achieve successful sexual performance, whereas secondary psychogenic ED occurs after a period of satisfactory sexual performance *(52)*.

Primary psychogenic ED is relatively rare and usually associated with a chronic pattern of sexual or interpersonal inhibition. Psychogenic ED may also be classified as secondary to substance abuse or a major psychiatric disorder.

CONCLUSION

The dramatic progress in the field of basic research of erectile physiology and pathophysiology during the last few years has led to exciting new insights and has resulted in revolutionary changes of treatment modalities in the individual with ED. In addition, clinical studies could successfully demonstrate the association of ED with other medical conditions. Hopefully, both basic and clinical research in this field will help in optimizing therapeutic approaches for the individual patient in the future. In this regard, a multidisciplinary approach using evidence-based guidelines is key for the thorough evaluation and effective treatment of the ED patient and his partner.

REFERENCES

1. NIH Consensus Development Panel on Impotence. NIH Consensus Conference: Impotence. JAMA 1992;270:83–90.
2. Benet AE, Melman A. The epidemiology of erectile dysfunction. Urol Clin North Am 1995;22:699–709.
3. Aytac IA, McKinlay JB, Krane RJ. The likely worldwide increase in erectile dysfunction between 1995 and 2025 and some possible policy consequences. BJU Int 1999;84:50–56.
4. Lue TF. Physiology of penile erection and pathophysiology of erectile dysfunction and priapism. In: Walsh PC, Retik AB, Vaughan ED, Wein AJ, eds. Campbell's Urology, 8th ed., vol. 2, Saunders, Philadelphia, 2002, pp. 1591–1618.
5. Saenz de Tejada I. Anatomy, physiology, and pathophysiology of ED. In: Jardin A, Wagner G, Khoury S, eds. Erectile Dysfunction. 5th ed., Plymbridge Distributors, Plymouth, UK, 2000, pp. 65–102.
6. Goldstein I, and the Working Group for the Study of Central Mechanisms in Erectile Dysfunction. Male sexual circuitry. Sci Am 2000;283:70–75.
7. Breza J, Aboseif SR, Orvis BR, et al. Detailed anatomy of penile neurovascular structures: surgical significance. J Urol 1989;141:437–443.
8. Lue TF. Erectile dysfunction. N Engl J Med 2000;342:1802–1813.
9. Rajfer J, Aronson WJ, Bush PA, et al. Nitric oxide as a mediator of relaxation of the corpus cavernosum in response to nonadrenergic, noncholinergic neurotransmission. N Engl J Med 1992;326:90–94.
10. Cox JD, Kim NN, Traish AM, et al. Arginase-boronic acid complex highlights a physiological role in erectile function. Nat Struct Biol 1999;6:1043–1047.
11. Bivalacqua TJ, Hellstrom WJ, Kadowitz PJ, et al. Increased expression of arginase II in human diabetic corpus cavernosum: in diabetic-associated erectile dysfunction. Biochem Biophys Res Commun 2001;283:923–927.
12. Chitaley K, Wingard CJ, Clinton Webb R, et al. Antagonism of Rho-kinase stimulates rat penile erection via a nitric oxide-independent pathway. Nat Med 2001; 7:119–122.

13. Mills TM, Chitaley K, Wingard CJ, et al. Effect of Rho-kinase inhibition on vasoconstriction in the penile circulation. J Appl Physiol 2001;91:1269–1273.
14. Araujo AB, Durante R, Feldman HA, et al. The relationship between depressive symptoms and male erectile dysfunction: cross-sectional results from the Massachusetts Male Aging Study. Psychosom Med 1998;60:458–465.
15. Feldman HA, Goldstein I, Hatzichristou DG, et al. Impotence and its medical and psychosocial correlates: results of the Massachusetts Male Aging Study. J Urol 1994;151:54–61.
16. Chun J, Carson CC. Physician-patient dialogue and clinical evaluation of erectile dysfunction. Urol Clin North Am 2001;28:249–258.
17. Burchardt M, Burchardt T, Anastasiadis AG, et al. Erectile dysfunction is a marker for cardiovascular complications and psychological functioning in men with hypertension. Int J Impot Res 2001;13:276–281.
18. Seidman SN, Roose SP, Menza MA, et al. Treatment of erectile dysfunction in men with depressive symptoms: results of a placebo-controlled trial with sildenafil citrate. Am J Psychiatry 2001;158:1623–1630.
19. Tiefer L, Schuetz-Mueller D. Psychological issues in diagnosis and treatment of erectile disorders. Urol Clin North Am 1995;22:767–773.
20. Laumann EO, Paik A, Rosen RC. Sexual dysfunction in the United States: prevalence and predictors. JAMA 1999;281:537–544.
21. Usta MF, Erdogru T, Tefekli A, et al. Honeymoon impotence: psychogenic or organic in origin? Urology 2001;57:758–762.
22. Araujo AB, Johannes CB, Feldman HA, et al. Relation between psychosocial risk factors and incident erectile dysfunction: prospective results from the Massachusetts Male Aging Study. Am J Epidemiol 2000;152:533–541.
23. Lewis RW, Hatzichristou DG, Laumann E, et al. Epidemiology and natural history of erectile dysfunction; risk factors including iatrogenic and aging. In: Jardin A, Wagner AH, Khoury S, Giuliano F, Padma-Nathan H, Rosen M, eds. Erectile Dysfunction, Health Publication Ltd, Plymouth, 2000, pp. 21–51.
24. Verbeuren TJ, Jordaens FH, Zonnekeyn LL, et al. Effect of hypercholesterolemia on vascular reactivity in the rabbit. I. Endothelium-dependent and endothelium-independent contractions and relaxations in isolated arteries of control and hypercholesterolemic rabbits. Circ Res 1986;58:552–564.
25. Kim JH, Klyachkin ML, Svendsen E, et al. Experimental hypercholesterolemia in rabbit induces cavernosal atherosclerosis with endothelial and smooth muscle cell dysfunction. J Urol 1994;151:198–205.
26. Behr-Roussel D, Bernabe J, Compagnie S, et al. Distinct mechanisms implicated in atherosclerosis-induced erectile dysfunction in rabbits. Atherosclerosis 2002;162:355–362.
27. De Angelis L, Marfella MA, Siniscalchi M, et al. Erectile and endothelial dysfunction in Type II diabetes: a possible link. Diabetologia 2001;44:1155–1160.
28. Azadzoi KM, Saenz de Tejada I. Hypercholesterolemia impairs endothelium-dependent relaxation of rabbit corpus cavernosum smooth muscle. J Urol 1991;146:238–240.
29. Taddei S, Virdis A, Mattei P, et al. Aging and endothelial function in normotensive subjects and patients with essential hypertension. Circulation 1995;91:1981–1987.
30. McVary K, Carrier S, Wessells H, and the Subcommittee on Smoking and Erectile Dysfunction Socioeconomic Committee, Sexual Medicine Society of North America. Smoking and erectile dysfunction: evidence-based analysis. J Urol 2001;166:1624–1632.

31. DePalma RG, Schwab F, Druy EM, et al. Experience in diagnosis and treatment of impotence caused by cavernosal leak syndrome. J Vasc Surg 1989;10: 117–121.
32. Munarriz RM, Yan QR, Nehra A, et al. Blunt trauma: the pathophysiology of hemodynamic injury leading to erectile dysfunction. J Urol 1995;153:1831–1840.
33. Marceau L, Kleinman K, Goldstein I, et al. Does bicycling contribute to the risk of erectile dysfunction? Results from the Massachusetts Male Aging Study (MMAS). Int J Impot Res 2001;13:298–302.
34. Sommer F, Schwarzer U, Klotz T, et al. Erectile dysfunction in cyclists. Is there any difference in penile blood flow during cycling in an upright versus a reclining position? Eur Urol 2001;39:720–723.
35. Rao DS, Donatucci CF. Vasculogenic impotence. Arterial and venous surgery. Urol Clin North Am 2001;28:309–319.
36. Nehra A, Moreland RB. Neurologic erectile dysfunction. Urol Clin North Am 2001;28:289–308.
37. Burchardt T, Burchardt M, Karden J, et al. Reduction of endothelial and smooth muscle density in the corpora cavernosa of the streptozotocin induced diabetic rat. J Urol 2000;164:1807–1811.
38. Moreland RB. Is there a role of hypoxemia in penile fibrosis: a viewpoint presented to the Society for the Study of Impotence. Int J Impot Res 1998;10: 113–120.
39. Jiaan DB, Seftel AD, Fogarty J, et al. Age-related increase in an advanced glycation end product in penile tissue. World J Urol 1995;13:369–375.
40. Siegel T, Moul JW, Spevak M, et al. The development of erectile dysfunction in men treated for prostate cancer. J Urol 2001;165:430–435.
41. Stanford JL, Feng Z, Hamilton AS, et al. Urinary and sexual function after radical prostatectomy for clinically localized prostate cancer: the Prostate Cancer Outcomes Study. JAMA 2000;283:354–360.
42. Wallen K. Sex and context: hormones and primate sexual motivation. Horm Behav 2001;40:339–357.
43. Bagatell CJ, Heiman JR, Rivier JE, et al. Effects of endogenous testosterone and estradiol on sexual behavior in normal young men. J Clin Endocrinol Metab 1994;78:711–716.
44. Shabsigh R, Raymond JF, Olsson CA, et al. Androgen induction of DNA synthesis in the rat penis. Urology 1998;52:723–728.
45. Korenman SG, Morley JE, Mooradian AD, et al. Secondary hypogonadism in older men: its relation to impotence. J Clin Endocrinol Metab 1990;71: 963–969.
46. Bhasin S. The dose-dependent effects of testosterone on sexual function and on muscle mass and function. Mayo Clin Proc 2000;75(Suppl):S70–S76.
47. Carani C, Scuteri A, Marrama P, et al. The effects of testosterone administration and visual erotic stimuli on nocturnal penile tumescence in normal men. Horm Behav 1990;24:435–441.
48. Wang C, Swedloff RS, Iranmanesh A, et al. Transdermal testosterone gel improves sexual function, mood, muscle strength, and body composition parameters in hypogonadal men. Testosterone Gel Study Group. J Clin Endocrinol Metab 2000; 85:2839–2853.
49. Finger WW, Lund M, Slagle MA. Medications that may contribute to sexual disorders. A guide to assessment and treatment in family practice. J Fam Pract 1997; 44:33–43.

50. Ralph D, McNicholas T. UK management guidelines for erectile dysfunction. BMJ 2000;321:499–503.
51. Chatterjee R, Andrews HO, McGarrigle HH, et al. Cavernosal arterial insufficiency is a major component of erectile dysfunction in some recipients of high-dose chemotherapy/chemo-radiotherapy for haematological malignancies. Bone Marrow Transplant 2000;25:1185–1189.
52. Rosen RC. Psychogenic erectile dysfunction. Urol Clin N Am 2001;28: 269–278.
53. Nurnberg HG, Seidman SN, Gelenberg AJ, et al. Depression, antidepressant therapies, and erectile dysfunction: clinical trials of sildenafil citrate (Viagra) in treated and untreated patients with depression. Urology 2002;60:58–66.
54. Shabsigh R, Klein LT, Seidman S, et al. Increased incidence of depressive symptoms in men with erectile dysfunction. Urology 1998;52:848–852.
55. Nofzinger EA, Thase ME, Reynolds CF 3rd, et al. Sexual function in depressed men. Assessment by self-report, behavioral, and nocturnal penile tumescence measures before and after treatment with cognitive behavior therapy. Arch Gen Psychiatry 1993;50:24–30.
56. Ford DE, Mead LA, Chang PP, et al. Depression is a risk factor for coronary artery disease in men: the precursors study. Arch Intern Med 1998;158:1422–1426.
57. Keene LC, Davies PH. Drug-related erectile dysfunction. Adverse Drug React Toxicol Rev 1999;181:5–24.
58. Bancroft J. Central inhibition of sexual response in the male: a theoretical perspective. Neurosci Biobehav Rev 1999;23:764–784.
59. Shabsigh R, Anastasiades A. Erectile dysfunction. Ann Rev Med 2003;54: 153–168.

2 Erectile Dysfunction
The Scope of the Problem

Culley C. Carson, MD

CONTENTS
>   INTRODUCTION
>   PREVALENCE OF ED
>   ETIOLOGY OF ED
>   RISK FACTORS FOR ED
>   RESULTS OF ED
>   CLINICAL EVALUATION
>   CONCLUSION
>   REFERENCES

INTRODUCTION

Throughout history, men have been dealing with the problems termed sexual dysfunction, impotence, and erectile dysfunction (ED). ED is a difficult and challenging condition affecting millions of men in the United States and throughout the world. In the 1990s and in the 21st century, ED has been defined as the consistent inability to obtain and maintain a penile erection sufficient to permit satisfactory sexual intercourse *(1)*. In the latter half of the 20th century, the issue of ED changed from a subject little discussed and poorly understood to an active area of medical, psychological, and pharmacological research and development. Indeed, the pejorative term "impotence" has been replaced with ED and erectile difficulties. During these

From: *Contemporary Cardiology: Heart Disease and Erectile Dysfunction*
Edited by: R. A. Kloner © Humana Press Inc., Totowa, NJ

years, the physiology and molecular biology of erection and ED has been carefully studied, and translational research has led to not only an elucidation of the physiology of erection but also to significant progress in the diagnosis and treatment of men with ED. Basic scientific investigation has clarified the anatomy, physiology, and pharmacology of the corpus cavernosum as well as the neurophysiology and vascular physiology of erectile function. Similarly, the mechanism of erection and its dependence upon the neurogenic, arterial, and venous systems to produce erectile rigidity continues to be studied. Further, the importance of androgen support of erectile function, both in the corpus cavernosum level and in the central nervous system, is being examined both clinically and in the basic science laboratories. Investigations into smooth muscle physiology, endothelial cell function, and central nervous system control with the identification of neurotransmitters, such as nitric oxide (NO) and vasoactive intestinal polypeptide, in the corpus cavernosum have led to the design, development, and use of specific pharmacological agents to recreate the normal physiology of the corpus cavernosum and restore erectile function in men previously termed "impotent."

PREVALENCE OF ED

In the United States as well as the rest of the world, ED is highly prevalent. The Massachusetts Male Aging Study (MMAS) particularly has documented the high prevalence, which reaches 52% in men over age 40 yr. MMAS was the first large population-based study of ED in the United States (2). The initial data were collected during 1987–1989 and established a cohort of 1709 men, of whom 1156 were re-interviewed during 1995–1997 (2). The baseline study included questions related to erectile function, such as frequency and quality of erections. The follow-up questionnaire included items related to erectile function plus a single question subjective global self-assessment that classified ED as ranging from none to complete.

The MMAS found that the combined prevalence of mild, moderate, and severe ED was 52% among this cohort of men aged 40 to 70 yr.

This prevalence increases with age and exceeds 70% in men over age 65 yr. The MMAS recorded depression, unhappiness with life, and pessimistic attitudes as significant risk factor predictors for ED (2). With increasing age, there was an increase in ED but, surprisingly, also a significant decrease in libido or desire for sexual activity. Nonmarried men appear to be at higher risk. A subsequent follow-up study of these same men 8 yr later showed that the incidence and prevalence of ED

Table 1
Worldwide Prevalence of Erectile Dysfunction

Population	Age (yr)	%
Cologne, Germany	30–80	19.2
Spain	25–70	18.9
Perth, Australia	40–69	33.9
Krimpen, Netherlands	50–78	11.0
London, UK	16–78	19.0

Data from ref. 6.

increases with age and that not smoking and regular exercise are factors that predict maintenance of erections as men age. With extrapolation of these data, it is estimated that more than 30 million men in the United States suffer from some degree of ED. The results of a large scale epidemiological study of sexual dysfunction in men throughout the United States demonstrated a high prevalence of ED in men of all ages, with as many as 31% of men complaining of some degree of ED.

Laumann et al. studied 1410 men and 1749 women ages 18–59 yr through analysis of the data from the National Health and Social Life Survey *(3)*. Overall, ED occurred in 5% of men, low sexual desire in 5% of men, and 21% of men, most often in the younger age group, suffered from premature ejaculation. The study demonstrated that sexual dysfunction is a significant public health concern and is widespread in Western society, influenced by health-related and psychological factors. Stress-inducing events influence and increase sexual dysfunction *(3)*. There is a strong association between sexual dysfunction and impaired quality of life on quality-of-life questionnaires. The Men's All Race Sexual Health Study investigated the differences among racial groups and the prevalence of ED *(4)*. Early data from this study confirm that white, black, and Hispanic Americans are equally at risk for ED and that risk factors for the three groups are similar.

Worldwide, epidemiological studies have confirmed the high prevalence rates in men of all ages (Table 1). Aytac et al. *(5)* calculated that the worldwide prevalence of ED will probably increase from 152 million men in 1995 to 322 million in 2025. Much of this increase of 170 million will occur in the developing world, that is, Asia, Africa, and South America, and is associated with the aging world population. Other related changes may be contributing to the increase of ED because it is associated with other diseases that are reaching epidemic proportions, such as obesity and diabetes.

Aytac et al. concluded that this likely increase in the prevalence of moderate to severe ED combined with newly available drug treatments will pose a major challenge for healthcare policy makers to develop and implement policies to alleviate ED. This will be a major problem, particularly in countries in which national health systems are already under stress from existing government funding priorities. Despite this high prevalence, fewer than 10% of men have received therapy for ED.

Despite these revolutions in the understanding and treatment of ED, there are many men who have not sought help for ED and many physicians who are uneasy and resistant to investigation and treatment of ED. Part of the problem includes the issues of men's health. It is estimated that in the United States, men have more than 150 million fewer doctor visits then women, even excluding prenatal visits. This partially accounts for not only the reluctance for ED treatment but also the lower life expectancy for men compared with women. Marwick surveyed patient's expectations and experiences in discussion of sexual issues with their physicians and found that 71% of patients stated that they believed that physicians would not recognize ED as a medical problem, whereas 68% of patients feared that discussing sexuality with their physicians would embarrass their physicians *(7)*.

Since the introduction of sildenafil in 1998, there has been a revolution in the treatment of ED throughout the world. The scientific and marketing efforts of physicians and the pharmaceutical industry have increased the presentation rates of ED by 250, 55, 103, 279, and 90% in the United States, Germany, UK, Mexico, and Spain, respectively, compared with the pre-sildenafil launch period *(7)*. Similarly, prescriptions for the treatment of ED before the introduction of sildenafil were slightly greater than 4 million with the majority of men with ED being treated with intracavernous alprostadil. Shortly after the introduction of sildenafil in the United States, the prescriptions for ED increased 438% to more than 19 million between April 1998 and December 1999 *(7)*. This increase was led by physicians and media who educated the public on the importance of ED and the ability to treat ED effectively. Numerous studies have demonstrated the improvement in quality of life for patients with ED treatment. In 1999, Parkerson et al. studied 1073 men in the United States and Europe with ED who were treated with intracavernous alprostadil *(8)*. These patients were followed for 19 month, and there was a demonstrated improvement in mental status in all groups despite a decrease in physical status associated with increasing age. Interestingly, social status also increased in Europe whereas it did not in the United States. In 1999, Litwin et al. reviewed the quality of life of 438 men undergoing treatment for carcinoma of the prostate with X-ray therapy or radical prostatectomy *(9)*. These patients included not only nerve-sparing but also non-nerve-sparing radical prostatectomy patients. An evaluation was conducted using the UCLA prostate cancer index. Sexual function during follow-up increased in the first year for all groups whereas function decreased slightly for radiation therapy patients in the second year. However, sexual function improved in all patients, but response was related to age, prediagnosis ED, and non-nerve-sparing radical prostatectomy. It has been estimated that 1 in 10 men worldwide have ED and that it is the most common chronic medical disorder in men over the age of 40 yr.

Patients and their partners must be educated in lifestyle issues that preserve erectile function and, indeed, optimize the response to agents for the treatment of ED. Smoking is one of the most important lifestyle issues that can impact on erectile function. In its follow-up publication, the MMAS reported an increase in ED with smoking in addition to other risk factors such as diabetes, heart disease, and hypertension *(2)*. Indeed, the incidence of ED increased among smokers with some stability in onset if men stopped smoking. The Health Professions Follow-Up Study reported by Bacon et al. examined 32,287 men and demonstrated a relative risk of ED of 2.2 (95% CI, 1.9–2.5) in men who smoked. Indeed, the effects of smoking in the laboratory, and in clinical research, have been widely published *(9)*. Smoking appears to enhance prostacyclin production, increase platelet vessel wall interaction, and reduce endothelium-mediated forearm vessel dilation in chronic human smokers *(10,11)*. Smoking has also been demonstrated to decrease endothelial nitric oxide synthase (NOS) activity and impair the release of NO. Finally, there has been a demonstrated increase in superoxide ion-mediated endothelium-derived relaxing factor degradation in smokers *(10)*.

Therefore, it is important to educate patients that ED can be treated in greater than 80% of men and that lifestyle changes may improve erections or at least stabilize ED. Expectations of excellent outcomes and success with low morbidity and risks are the norm *(12)*. Patients should also be educated and instructed that lifestyle counseling may assist their longevity and healthiness and may also improve not only erectile function but response to ED treatment. These counseling points should include smoking cessation, moderate alcohol intake, reduction in fat and cholesterol, exercise, improvement and compliance with cardiovascular and diabetic medications, stress reduction, depression treatment, and an optimism of ED treatment outcomes and resolution with appropriate management.

ETIOLOGY OF ED

ED has both organic and psychogenic etiologies. When Masters and Johnson published their sentinel work on sexual dysfunction, they felt that organic causes accounted for approximately 10% of the incidence of ED in American men, and psychogenic causes accounted for 90% *(12)*. Now we know that about 60% of patients have organic ED, which we define as vasculogenic, neurologic, hormonal, or smooth muscle abnormalities, including stress and depression. Less than 40% of men truly have psychogenic ED. In fact, we may be labeling some causes as psychogenic simply because we cannot yet identify a specific organic cause. We do know that patients with psychogenic causes, specifically stress disorders and depression, have an overactivity of α-agonists in their corpora cavernosal smooth muscle tissue, resulting in a chemical imbalance inhibiting corpus cavernosum smooth muscle relaxation.

RISK FACTORS FOR ED

When completing a history of a patient with ED, one should inquire about the patient's libido. Physicians used to think that if a patient had decreased desire that this automatically resulted from low levels of androgen hormones, such as testosterone. Indeed, this is not the case because libido level is a far better marker for depression and stress than it is for hypogonadism. Less than 50% of patients who truly are hypogonadal, with testosterone levels less than 100 ng/dL, have low libido, whereas greater than 80% who are depressed have low libido *(14)*. Therefore, although the physician should ask about libido, the patient's response cannot eliminate the need for a testosterone determination. It is also important to determine what medications patients are taking. Medications most often associated with ED are antihypertensives, although antidepressants, particularly the selective serotonin reuptake inhibitor (SSRI) medications, are also culprits. Smoking is also one of the most common risk factors for ED *(12)*.

The Treatment of Mild Hypertension Study examined a group of people with mild-to-moderate hypertension that had not been treated previously and compared various families of antihypertensives with placebo *(15)*. Patients were followed for 2 yr, and among the questions examined was that of erectile function. The incidence of ED was lowest with α-blockers represented by doxazosin, which was the only antihypertensive class to have less ED than placebo.

Studies in our laboratory confirmed this finding. When we reviewed the effect of antihypertensive agents on relaxation of the corpus cavernosum smooth muscle in vitro, we found that classes of agents most likely to preserve or be hospitable to erectile function included the α-blockers, angiotensin-converting enzyme inhibitors, and calcium channel blockers, in that order. This is important because modification of antihypertensives and careful selection of agents may preserve erectile function in some patients with significant hypertension.

Diabetes is another major cause for ED. Although it is clear that ED increases as patients age, diabetes is associated with ED at a younger age. A patient who has been diabetic, especially those who have been insulin dependent, for more than 10 yr has greater than a 50% chance of having significant ED. Further, ED is more common with diabetic complications, and, indeed, sildenafil is less effective in men with poorly controlled diabetes or those with multiple diabetes-related complications.

Depression also affects erectile function significantly. The MMAS examined classes of depression, with 1 being minimally depressed and 5 maximally depressed. In class 5 depressions, 60% of men age 61–70 yr had ED. In contrast, ED incidence is less than 10% if a patient is not depressed and is in the 40–50-yr age group *(2)*.Thus, depression is an additive risk factor to age for ED.

Atherosclerosis is perhaps one of the most common causes of ED in the aging male. It has been clearly demonstrated that high levels of cholesterol are destructive to the endothelial cells of the corpus cavernosum that produce the NO *(15)*. Reducing cholesterol levels in laboratory animals demonstrates significant improvement in corpus cavernosum smooth muscle relaxation *(16)*. Similarly, statin drugs have been demonstrated to be helpful in-patients with early ED from hypercholesterolemia.

Testosterone levels are also important in libido as well as corpus cavernosum smooth muscle activity. Testosterone levels change substantially with age *(14)*. Beginning at about age 50 yr, testosterone begins to decline with a subsequent increase in sex hormone-binding globulin that results in a marked diminution of free and bioavailable testosterone. Because NOS activity decreases substantially with a decrease in testosterone level, androgen levels are critical for erectile function. Indeed, animal studies suggest that NOS decreased almost 50% in castrated rats. Such a decrease was prevented or reversed by testosterone replacement. Similarly, there are changes in smooth muscle relaxation in the hypogonadal laboratory animal. Clearly, NO production requires adequate levels of testosterone.

Neurogenic causes of ED are also significant and common. Most often, peripheral neuropathy from diabetes is a cause of ED. Other neurogenic causes of ED include radical prostatectomy where the nerves that supply the penis with signals for corpus cavernosum smooth muscle dilation are damaged during the pelvic surgical procedure *(17)*. Other pelvic surgical procedures, such as radical colectomy and cystectomy, may also produce this nerve damage, as does pelvic radiation therapy. Neurologic conditions such as multiple sclerosis, stroke, and spinal cord injury have high prevalence of ED.

Other causes of ED, which are significant but less frequently encountered, include venogenic or venous leak *(18)*. Venous leak, or venous incompetence, occurs when the emissary veins draining the corpora cavernosa do not restrict the venous outflow artery from the corpora and allow excessive venous drainage overcoming the arterial inflow. This may be seen as a cause of primary ED or because of conditions, such as aging, priapism, perineal trauma, or Peyronie's disease.

Chronic illnesses are also associated with ED, but many of these patients have concerns regarding their chronic illnesses that override erectile function. Diseases such as multiple sclerosis, Alzheimer's disease, and renal and hepatic failure produce a significant incidence of ED. Indeed, the endocrine abnormalities of renal failure that include hyperprolactinemia and hypogonadism respond best to renal transplantation but can be treated medically in some patients *(19)*.

RESULTS OF ED

What are the results and impact of ED on patients and their partners? Litwin et al. looked at the quality of life measures for patients with ED and their partners *(9)*. Not only were erections deficient, but there was also significant psychological impact on the patient, including decreases in self-confidence, self-esteem, and emotional well-being and an increase in depression. Problems with marital interaction stress within the couple were significantly increased as was the bother score for sexual dysfunction. A subsequent measurement of decreased libido in both patient and partner were identified. Fifty-seven percent of patients reported having difficulty with erections and subsequently developing a loss of interest or loss of sexual desire. Also interesting was the socioeconomic impact of ED on these men. Men in the higher socioeconomic ranges had fewer problems and less bother scores than men in the lower socioeconomic levels. In measuring the impact of ED on the sexual partner, the changes are similar, with a decrease in libido, sexual drive, and marital harmony and an increase in depression and inability to discuss sexual issues. This may result in a loss of communication between the partners and can be disastrous to any marital relationship.

Partners are also affected by the chronic diseases that result in ED. Many wives fear they will harm their spouses. This is especially true after cerebrovascular accident or myocardial infarction, where the female partner feels that the stress of sexual activity may, in fact, be detrimental to her husband's health.

The pattern of ED begins with decreased penile rigidity and frequency of erectile function and coitus. Patients rarely see their physicians for the first 2 yr after sexual dysfunction begins *(20)*. Although the average frequency of normal patients in the adult range is between one and two encounters every 4–8 wk, patients with ED may have sexual activity less than once yearly. As this frequency decreases, the emotional distance between the partners begins to increase. Their emotional dissatisfaction with their relationship decreases and both of their libidos begin to decline. The frequency of other intimate acts consequently diminishes with a decrease in hugging, kissing, touching, and even talking. Thus, the impact on the couple and their relationship is substantial *(20)*.

ED is a chronic common problem that has a major impact on patients and their partners. It is something that physicians and health care workers must identify because there are excellent ways of effectively treating these patients and resolving their ED before marital discord and couple disharmony ensue. The most important method for caring for these patients is identifying the problem, and identifying the problem can only begin by asking the patient and/or his partner, "Do you have erectile problems; are there problems with your sexual function?" By beginning a dialog with your patients, something can be done to help both patients and partners.

Despite the stress on organic ED, pure psychogenic ED occurs, and, in those patients with organic ED, an emotional aspect of sexual function is virtually always present. The problems of sexuality overlap into relationship issues; self-esteem; moral and cultural values; and patient fears about their bodies, aging, and psychological health. Clearly, the appropriate management and understanding of psychological issues are essential for appropriate evaluation and treatment of patients, gaining their trust, and providing state-of-the-art therapy for patients with sexual concerns and dysfunction.

As a first step, a physician–patient dialogue must be initiated to fully evaluate the clinical abnormalities associated with ED. This begins with a face-to-face interview, a sympathetic history-taking with privacy and physician concern to maintain patient trust, comfort, and openness. A knowledgeable professional medical staff must be available to answer questions that patients initially may be embarrassed to ask physicians. Facilitating this interaction using a standardized questionnaire may open discussions, provide comfort for the patient in initiating conversation, and allow physicians to evaluate the severity of ED. Available standardized questionnaires include the Brief Male Sexual Function Inventory for Urology, the more frequently used International Index of Erectile Function (IIEF), and its short form, the five-question Sexual Health Inventory for Men (SHIM; refs. *21* and *22*). After initiating treatment, such outcomes questionnaires as the Erectile Dysfunction Inventory of Treatment Satisfaction may be useful *(23)*. The Brief Male Sexual Function Inventory for Urology is composed of 11 questions developed to measure sexual drive, erectile function, problem assessment, and overall sexual satisfaction *(22)*. It is a brief, clinically validated and standardized self-administered questionnaire that works well in the office setting. The IIEF, a cross-culturally and psychometrically validated questionnaire, is widely used in clinical trials for medications and other interventions for ED. This 15-item questionnaire is evaluated for multiple domains, including erectile function, ejaculatory function, and desire. Erectile function is graded by severity, based on a scale from 6 to 30. The shorter five-question SHIM is, perhaps, the easiest for patients to take and for physicians to evaluate as a screening instrument (Fig. 1). The Erectile Dysfunction Inventory of Treatment Satisfaction questionnaire, not designed for initial evaluation, is useful for identifying the patient and partner satisfaction from treatment modalities initiated for ED.

In addition to a comfortable, safe environment for the patient to discuss the issue with a physician, an interview with the partner may be helpful in evaluating ED. The partner may provide insight into sexual difficulties, relationship problems, and underlying health concerns that the patient may be uneasy about discussing. This may also identify the partner's approach to and value of intimacy and sexual function in the relationship *(24)*.

The physician–patient interaction, relationship, and interview have been discussed widely, and Marwick has documented that patients are clearly uneasy in bringing up the subject of ED or sexual problems with their physicians *(7)*. Marwick demonstrated that greater than 70% of patients felt that it would be embarrassing to discuss sexual problems and that physicians themselves would be embarrassed and find the problems of ED trivial or insignificant. Therefore, the emphasis is for the physician to initiate questioning and begin the discussion of erectile function in patients seen both for routine visits and treatment of diagnoses associated with risk factors for ED. The use of the SHIM in the office before the visit may facilitate this interaction and initiate a conversation regarding ED.

1. How do you rate your confidence that you could get and keep an erection?

Very low	Low	Moderate	High	Very high
1	2	3	4	5

2. When you had erections with sexual stimulation, how often were your erections hard enough for penetration (entering your partner)?

No sexual activity	Almost never or never	A few times (much less than half the time)	Sometimes (about half the time)	Most times (much more than half the time)	Almost always or always
0	1	2	3	4	5

3. During sexual intercourse, how often were you able to maintain your erection after you had penetrated (entered) your partner?

Did not attempt intercourse	Almost never or never	A few times (much less than half the time)	Sometimes (about half the time)	Most times (much more than half the time)	Almost always or always
0	1	2	3	4	5

4. During sexual intercourse, how difficult was it to maintain your erection to completion of intercourse?

Did not attempt intercourse	Extremely difficult	Very difficult	Difficult	Slightly difficult	Not difficult
0	1	2	3	4	5

5. When you attempted sexual intercourse, how often was it satisfactory for you?

Did not attempt intercourse	Almost never or never	A few times (much less than half the time)	Somtimes (about half the time)	Most times (much more than half the time)	Almost always or always
0	1	2	3	4	5

SCORE: Add the numbers corresponding to questions 1–5. If your score is 21 or less, you may want to give this form to your healthcare professional to determine if you have ED. If so, you may want to discuss safe and effective treatment options with your doctor

Fig. 1. Sexual health inventory for men over the past 6 mo. (Adapted from ref. *21, 22,* and Kloner et al. J Urol 2003;170:S46–S50.)

CLINICAL EVALUATION

The adequate evaluation for ED continues to evolve. Before the introduction of sildenafil, there was an emphasis on a goal-directed approach to male sexual dysfunction that included careful identification of the etiology of the ED *(25)*. The goal of this approach was to identify a specific etiology such that more invasive, costly, uncomfortable treatment modalities could be applied based on the patient's treatment goals. In the era of managed care, cost consciousness, and with minimally invasive safe and effective oral medications, extensive evaluation of patients is no longer the first line for patients presenting with ED. However, it is critically important to review the patient's history carefully to identify underlying risk factors, medications, and lifestyle factors that may contribute to ED with hopes that modifying these risk factors will facilitate further treatment with oral agents.

A full sexual history is critical with special attention to risk factors and medications *(20)*. This should be followed by a thorough physical examination, laboratory studies, and appropriate clinical diagnostic studies. ED may be caused by various etiologies or combinations of factors. A history should include a careful sexual history to elicit these possible causes *(25)*. Patients should be queried regarding morning erections, nocturnal erections, erectile quality, and erections during masturbation, and ejaculatory function. Open-ended questions are best for this purpose because they provide the most spontaneous, accurate, and detailed information regarding the current status of erectile function, onset of ED, and surrounding precipitating factors.

Patients who complain of loss of libido or sexual desire may be considered as at risk for hypogonadism. Low libido, however, may be caused by medications, hypochondriasis, stress, anxiety, or depression *(14)*. Low libido clearly requires evaluation to identify those patients with androgen deficiency of the aging male or other causes of hypogonadism. Those patients with chronic renal failure, especially on chronic dialysis, may have low libido caused by low testosterone and high prolactin levels *(19)*. These abnormalities can be treated medically to decrease prolactin and increase testosterone levels.

A history of ejaculatory dysfunction must also be elicited to identify those patients with premature ejaculation or delayed ejaculation. Younger men more often complain of premature ejaculation whereas those in the older age group more often have difficulties with retarded ejaculation or even absent ejaculation. This may be caused by natural aging, lack of androgen, neurologic abnormalities, medications, or pelvic surgery. Patients with retrograde ejaculation must be suspected

Table 2
Modifiable Risk Factors for Erectile Dysfunction

Diabetes mellitus
Cardiovascular disease
Spinal cord injury
Cigarette smoking
Depression
Atherosclerosis
Hypertension
Pelvic surgery/trauma
Medications
Arthritis
Peripheral vascular disease
Renal failure
Substance abuse
Endocrine abnormalities
Peptic ulcer disease

of having diabetes mellitus, may be using α-blocking medication, or may have had previous urologic or neurologic surgery *(20)*.

Medical problems associated with ED may include those listed in Table 2. Each of these should be discussed with the patient during history taking. Any condition associated with cardiac disease, hypertension, diabetes, or lipid abnormalities can be associated with ED. Indeed, atherosclerosis is a risk factor in 70% of men greater than age 60 yr, and ED occurs in diabetic men at 10–15 yr after onset and affects 50% of diabetic men *(16)*. ED in Type 1 diabetes is often of neurogenic etiology, whereas Type 2 diabetics more often have vascular problems or combinations of etiologies.

Medications are also frequently causes of ED. Some of the medications associated with ED are listed in Table 3. Most often, antihypertensives and antidepressant (SSRIs) medications are the culprits. Recreational drugs, such as cocaine, marijuana, alcohol, and tobacco, also have the potential for causing ED.

Additional history should include history of penile trauma, priapism, curvature of the penis from Peyronie's disease, or congenital corporal disproportion. Depression and anxiety can often be identified in this initial phase of the examination.

Physical examination of patients with ED should be focused on the genitalia. A general inspection of body habitus to identify hair distribution, obesity or overweight, and secondary sex characteristics should

Table 3
Medications Associated With Erectile Dysfunction

β-adrenergic antagonists
Thiazide diuretics
Verapamil
Naproxen
Amitriptyline
Digoxin
Phenytoin
Hydralazine
Clofibrate
Indomethacin
Cimetidine
Omeprazole
Metoclopramide
Famotidine
Lithium
Antidepressants (SSRIs)[a]
Antiandrogen hormones
Recreational drugs (marijuana, cocaine, and heroin)

[a]Selective serotonine reuptake inhibitors

be identified. Patients with severe obesity should be suspected of having sleep apnea or high estrogen levels, which may be associated with ED. Testicular size and consistency, as well as penile anatomy, should be examined carefully. Patients with small or soft testes should be suspected of hypogonadism, and lesions of the shaft of the penis can be identified in those patients with Peyronie's disease. A brief neurologic examination should be performed with an evaluation of sensation of lower extremities, deep tendon reflexes, and perineal sensation. A bulbocavernosus or cremasteric reflex as well as sphincter tone on rectal examination can be quantified. Digital rectal examination to identify prostate size, consistency, nodularity, pain, or prostatitis should be conducted. If questions arise regarding penile sensation, biothesiometry of the glans penis and penile shaft can be performed in the office with this vibratory sensation device *(26)*. Results should be compared with an age-adjusted normogram to identify those patients with decreased glans penis sensation.

Once a careful physical examination is completed, laboratory investigation should be tailored to the individual patient and goals of therapy. In patients who have not had recent health evaluation, fasting blood glucose should be measured to identify patients at risk for diabetes mellitus. This is especially important in those patients with a family history of diabetes or those patients with personal histories of polyuria or polydipsia. In known diabetics, an Hb A1c can evaluate control and medical compliance with diabetic therapy. Similarly, laboratory studies can include a lipid profile to identify those patients with hypercholesterolemia. In those patients with suggestive history, a thyroid profile can be obtained as well. Most importantly, however, is an evaluation of hormone status. Hypogonadism, though only found in a small number of patients, should be evaluated in all patients with ED *(27)*. An initial screening of morning total testosterone should be performed to identify testosterone level. It is important to perform this as a morning evaluation because testosterone concentration peak occurs between 8 and 10 a.m. Repeat testosterone levels with a free testosterone, luteinizing hormone, and prolactin level should be performed if testosterone is suspicious. Buvat and Lemaire reviewed endocrine screening results in 1022 patients with ED and found that limiting testosterone evaluation to those patients with abnormal physical examinations or decreased libido would miss 40% of patients with low testosterone *(27)*. They recommend testosterone determinations for all men over age 50 yr. Other hormonal studies associated with decreased libido and decreased sexual function include dehydroepiandrosterone (DHEA) and DHEA sulfate, which can be evaluated. Reiter et al. demonstrated that replacement of DHEA in patients with low DHEA and normal testosterone may improve sexual desire and libido substantially in addition to improving sexual performance and erectile function *(28)*.

With this basic group of studies, including history, physical examination, questionnaires, and laboratory studies, the majority of patients can be identified as having ED and started on appropriate oral medications for treatment. However, if oral medications are unsuccessful, patients are interested in their underlying ED etiology, or surgical intervention is contemplated, further evaluation may be required (Table 4). This evaluation may include the standard studies of nocturnal penile tumescence monitoring (NPT), arterial and venous studies, including color Doppler arterial studies, and ultimately cavernosography, and selective pudendal arteriography.

NPT monitoring was first described in the 1970s by Fisher for separation of organic and psychogenic ED patients. It is well known that normal men have significant erectile function during rapid eye movement sleep. A total of four to six erections occur during the usual night's sleep with base and tip rigidity greater than 55% and sustained for at

Table 4
Diagnostic Tests for Erectile Dysfunction

Body system	Test
Neurologic testing	
Somatic nerves	Biothesiometry
	Nerve conduction velocities
	Evoked potentials
Autonomic nerves	Cardiovascular reflex tests
	Sympathetic skin response
	Corpus cavernosum electromyography
	Thermal threshold testing
	Urethroanal reflex latency
	Nocturnal penile tumescence
Vascular testing	
Arteriogenic	Penile brachial index
	Pharmacopenile duplex ultrasonography
	Selective pudendal arteriography
Veno-occlusive	Intracavernous injections
	Pharmacopenile duplex ultrasonography
	Dynamic infusion cavernosometry and cavernosography
Psychogenic ED	Nocturnal penile tumescence

Abbreviations: ED, erectile dysfunction.

least 10 min. The RigiScan recording device (Timm Medical, Augusta, GA) provides an economical, safe, noninvasive home-monitoring device for screening patients with NPT monitoring studies (29). Although controversy remains regarding the diagnostic accuracy of NPT evaluation, it may be useful in separating patients with organic and psychogenic ED and for use in medical legal situations. False/negative studies may be found in those patients with depression, sleep disorders, sleep apnea, sleep-altering medications, smoking, and caffeine use. The overall accuracy of nocturnal penile tumescence monitoring is approximately 80% (29). An abnormal NPT test should be confirmed with at least two nights of study and subsequent independent validation studies.

Although specific widely available clinical studies for neurogenic testing except for tactile testing have limited availability, such studies as dorsal nerve conduction velocities and sacral nerve-evoked potentials may be useful in some patients and are available at research institutes and ED centers. Vascular studies to identify functional abnormalities of the arterial and venous systems can be used with accurate determination of vascular function and anatomy. Older studies using hand-held Doppler with penile brachial index identification appear to be inaccurate and poorly reproducible. However, the use of duplex ultrasound color Doppler flow studies with intracavernous injection of vasoactive agents can carefully evaluate both the arterial and venous systems that produce erections in a functional fashion. In 1985, Lue and Broderick reported the combination of intracavernous injections of vasoactive agents with duplex ultrasonography providing high-resolution sonography and pulsed Doppler blood flow analysis to evaluate the penile arteries and provide information regarding venous outflow incompetence. This non-invasive technique measures cavernous arterial diameter, detects abnormalities in cavernous bodies, such as fibrosis and calcifications, and evaluates venous outflow. In 1990, Mueller et al. compared selective internal iliac arteriography with duplex Doppler ultrasound sonography for arteriogenic ED *(30)*. In the 43 men evaluated, selective arteriography and duplex sonography correlated in 91% of cases, with duplex ultrasound providing higher accuracy than selective arteriography for the diagnosis of arteriogenic ED. Duplex ultrasonography can also identify venous leak ED/veno-occlusive dysfunction in an indirect fashion. If veno-occlusive dysfunction is suspected from initial studies, dynamic infusion cavernosography and cavernosometry can be performed to identify areas of veno-occlusive dysfunction and suggests surgical or nonsurgical intervention.

In those patients with suspected traumatic injuries to the arterial supply of the penis, selective pudendal arteriography in combination with intracavernous injection can provide an accurate review of the penile arterial anatomy and identify those patients who are candidates for arterial revascularization. Duplex Doppler studies can identify those patients in whom arteriography may be helpful. Ideal candidates for this procedure include those with a single solitary obstructive lesion of the pudendal arterial system who are less than age 40 yr and nonsmokers who have no other significant vascular disease risk factors such as diabetes or hypercholesterolemia.

CONCLUSION

ED is currently treatable with safe effective oral medication that can restore not only erectile function but also quality of life for men with sexual problems. The most important part of evaluation of patients with ED is asking the patients about their erectile status. Although there are many clinical diagnostic studies, laboratory studies, and possible findings on physical examination, the most important part of evaluation and treatment is taking an adequate history and eliciting an erectile problem from patients. An adequate physician–patient rapport is an important starting point for successful treatment of ED.

REFERENCES

1. Padma-Nathan H. Diagnostic and treatment strategies for erectile dysfunction: the 'Process of Care' model. Int J Impot Res 2000;(Suppl 12)4:S119–S121.
2. Feldman H, Goldstein I, Hatzichristou D. Impotence and its medical and psychological correlance: results of the Massachusetts Male Aging Study. J Urol 1994; 151:54–61.
3. Laumann EO, Paik AM, Rosen RC. Sexual dysfunction in the United States: prevalence and predictors. JAMA 1999;281:537–546.
4. Carson CC, West S, Glasser DB, et al. Prevalence and correlates of erectile dysfunction in a United States nation-wide population-based sample. J. Urol 2002; 167 (Suppl):29.
5. Aytac IA, Araujo AB, Johannes CB, et al. Socioeconomic factors and incidence of erectile dysfunction: findings of the longitudinal Massachusetts Male Aging Study. Social Sci Med 2000;51:771–778.
6. Carson CC. New developments on the diagnosis and treatment of erectile dysfunction. In: Kirby RS and O'Leary MO, eds. Hot Topics in Urology ISIS Medical Publishers, Oxford, 2003.
7. Marwick C. Survey says patients expect little help on sex. JAMA 1999;281: 2173–2174.
8. Parkerson GR Jr., Willke RJ, Hays RD. An international comparison of the reliability and responsiveness of the Duke Health Profile for measuring health-related quality of life of patients treated with alprostadil for erectile dysfunction. Med Care 1999;37:56–67.
9. Litwin MS, Nied RJ, Dhanani N. Health-related quality of life in men with erectile dysfunction. J Gen Intern Med 1998;13:159–166.
10. McVary KT, Carrier S, Wessells H. Subcommittee on Smoking and Erectile Dysfunction Socioeconomic Committee, Sexual Medicine Society of North America. Smoking and erectile dysfunction: evidence-based analysis. J Urol 2001;166:1624–1632.
11. Sharlip I. Is smoking an independent risk factor for erectile dysfunction? Int J Impot Res 2001;13(Suppl 5):S51.
12. Derby CA, Mohr BA, Goldstein I, et al. Modifiable risk factors and erectile dysfunction: can lifestyle changes modify risk? Urology 2000;56:302–306.
13. Masters WH, Johnson VE. Human Sexual Inadequacy. Little Brown, Boston, 1970.
14. Morales A, Heaton JWP, Carson CC. Andropause: a misnomer for a true clinical entity. J Urol 2000;163:705–712.
15. Sullivan ME, Keoghane SR, Miller MA. Vascular risk factors and erectile dysfunction. BJU Int 2000;87:838–845.
16. Kim JH, Klyachkin ML, Svendsen E, et al. Experimental hypercholesterolemia in rabbits induces cavernosal atherosclerosis with endothelial and smooth muscle cell dysfunction. J Urol 1994;151:198–205.

17. Begg CB, Riedel ER, Bach PB, et al. Variations in morbidity after radical prostatectomy. N Engl JMed 2002;346:1138–1144.
18. Kerfoot WW, Carson CC, Donaldson JT, et al. Investigation of vascular changes following penile vein ligation. J Urol 1994;152:884–887.
19. Carson CC, Patel MP. The epidemiology, anatomy, physiology, and treatment of erectile dysfunction in chronic renal failure patients. Adv Renal Replace Ther 1999;6:296–309.
20. Chun J, Carson CC. Physician/patient dialogue and clinical evaluation of erectile dysfunction. Urol Clin N Am 2001;28:249–258.
21. Rosen RC, Riley A, Wagner G, et al. The International Index of Erectile Function (IIEF): a multidimensional scale for assessment of erectile dysfunction. Urology 1997;49:822–828.
22. O'Leary M, Fowler FJ, Lenderking WR, et al. Brief male sexual function inventory for urology. Urology 1995;46:697–703.
23. Althof SE, Corty EW, Levine SB, et al. EDITS: development of questionnaires for evaluating satisfaction with treatments for erectile dysfunction. Urology 1999;53: 793–799.
24. Finkle AL, Thompson R. Urologic counseling. In: male sexual impotence. Geriatrics1972;27:67–72.
25. Carson CC. Erectile dysfunction in the 21st century: whom we can treat, whom we cannot treat and patient education [review]. Int J Impot Res 2002;14(Suppl 1): S29–S34.
26. Kirby RS. Basic assessment of the patient with erectile dysfunction. In: Kirby CC, Goldstein I, eds. Textbook of Erectile Dysfunction ISIS Medical Publishers, Oxford, 1999, pp. 195–205, 2002.
27. Buvat J, Lemaire A. Endocrine screening in 1022 men with erectile dysfunction: clinical significance and cost effective strategy. J Urol 1997;158:1764–1769.
28. Reiter WJ, Pycha A, Schatzl G. Serum dehydroepiandrosterone concentrations in men with erectile dysfunction. Urology 2000;55:755–758.
29. Allen RP, Smolev JK, Engel RM, et al. Comparison of RigiScan and formal nocturnal penile tumescence testing in the evaluation of erectile rigidity. J Urol 1993;149:1265–1268.
30. Mueller SC, Wallenberg HV, Voges GE, et al. Comparison of selective internal ileac pharmacoangiography, penile brachial index, and duplex sonography with pulsed doppler analysis for the evaluation of vasculogenic impotence. J Urol 1990;143:928–939.

3   Erectile Dysfunction and Cardiovascular Risk Factors

Robert A. Kloner, MD, PhD

CONTENTS

INTRODUCTION
HYPERTENSION
LIPID ABNORMALITIES
SMOKING
DIABETES
HOW COMMON IS ED AMONG MEN WITH CORONARY HEART DISEASE?
REFERENCES

INTRODUCTION

Erectile dysfunction (ED), the consistent inability of a man to achieve an erection satisfactory for sexual activity, has been estimated to afflict, to some degree, 52% of male adults between the ages of 40 and 70 yr in the United States *(1)*. Millions of men in the United States suffer with ED. Although there are numerous causes of ED (vascular, psychogenic, neurologic, endocrine, structural, traumatic, and drug-related) in men over age 50 yr, the most common cause is thought to be vascular *(2–4)*. This chapter reviews the connection between ED and vascular disease and the connection between ED and risk factors for atherosclerosis.

For a normal erection to occur, there must be an increase in blood supply to the corpora cavernosa, the erectile bodies of the penis. This process requires vasodilation of the arteries, arterioles, and sinusoids

From: *Contemporary Cardiology: Heart Disease and Erectile Dysfunction*
Edited by: R. A. Kloner © Humana Press Inc., Totowa, NJ

Table 1
Cardiovascular Risk Factors Associated With ED

Smoking
Low HDL; High total cholesterol
Hypertension
Diabetes
Obesity
Lack of physical activity

that supply the penis *(5)*. For normal vasodilation to occur, the endothelium of the blood vessels must be intact. The endothelial cells and nerve cells within the corpus cavernosum release nitric oxide (NO) that allows relaxation of the smooth muscle cells within the vasculature of the penis *(6)*. Furthermore, damage to the endothelium eventually may lead to atherosclerotic plaques, which result in stenoses that physically block blood flow into the corpus cavernosum.

The term endothelial dysfunction (another ED) implies that the endothelium does not function normally in its ability to respond to stimuli or release NO properly for normal vasodilatation. It is one of the earliest processes in the spectrum of atherosclerosis. Endothelial dysfunction also involves abnormalities of the endothelial lining that can cause increased cell adhesion to the surface of the blood vessel, attracting neutrophils and macrophages, and increasing permeability to lipids. In the United States, endothelial dysfunction often occurs at a young age, at least in part because of the high fat and salt content of the US diet.

The risk factors for the development of endothelial dysfunction, and eventually frank atherosclerotic plaques, include smoking, lipid abnormalities, diabetes, hypertension, obesity, and lack of physical activity. Because the development of endothelial dysfunction and atherosclerosis is a systemic disease, when one vascular bed is affected, it is likely that other vascular beds are affected as well. Therefore, the same cardiovascular risk factors that are associated with coronary artery disease (CAD) are associated with endothelial dysfunction and atherosclerosis of blood vessels that supply the penis (Table 1; Figs. 1 and 2). An erection is basically a vascular event, and factors that inhibit vasodilation of the blood vessels to the penis inhibit that event.

Studies by Virag et al. *(7)* and the Massachusetts Male Aging Study (MMAS) by Feldman et al. *(1)* were some of the first modern studies to link ED with risk factors for atherosclerosis. Virag et al. showed that

ED = ENDOTHELIAL = ERECTILE
       DYSFUNCTON   DYSFUNCTION

Fig. 1. ED may represent both endothelial dysfunction as well as erectile dysfunction.

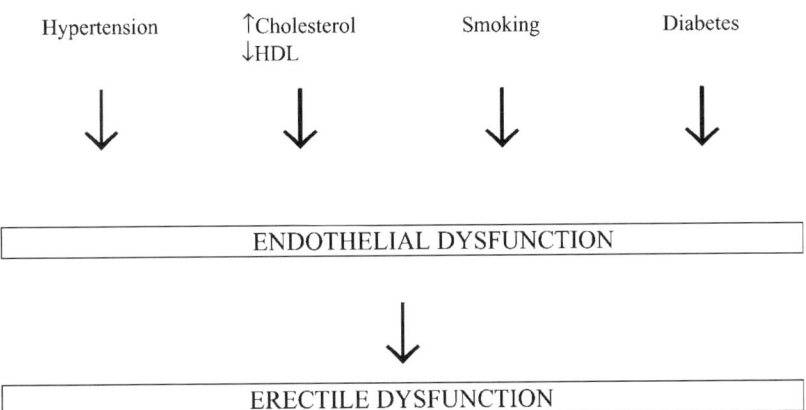

Fig. 2. Vascular risk factors, such as hypertension, lipid abnormalities, smoking, and diabetes, cause endothelial dysfunction. This results in the inability of the arteries to dilate normally with certain stimuli, and results in increased endothelial permeability to lipids and increased adhesion for macrophages, white blood cells, and platelets. Endothelial dysfunction is perhaps the earliest phase of atherosclerosis and persists throughout the spectrum of atherosclerotic lesion development.

smoking, lipid abnormalities, and diabetes were more common in men with ED than in the general population (7). In addition, when these investigators measured the penile blood pressure index (the ratio between blood pressure in the penis vs blood pressure in the brachial artery), they observed an additive decline in this ratio as risk factors were added. The MMAS (1,8) showed that patients with heart disease and risk factors for heart disease (lipid abnormalities, hypertension, diabetes, and smoking) were more likely to have ED.

HYPERTENSION

Most (1,8–11), but not all, studies (7) have shown an association between hypertension and ED. In the original MMAS (1), which was performed in men ages 40–70 yr, the age-adjusted probability of complete ED was greater in men with treated hypertension (15%) vs the entire cohort (9.6%). Bulpitt et al. (9) described a study of 302 patients in which ED was observed in 6.9% of normotensive men, 17.1% of men with untreated hypertension, and 24.6% of men with treated hypertension. Buchardt et al. *(10)* recently showed that 68.3% of men with hypertension demonstrated some degree of ED. Also, the severity of ED was worse in patients with hypertension than in the general population. Jensen et al. *(12)* studied the prevalence and etiology of ED in 101 male hypertensive patients over 4 months and observed that 27% of men with hypertension had ED vs 4% of men in the same general population. Studies of Doppler ultrasonography of the penile arteries, with or without papaverine injections, suggested that in 89% of these hypertensive patients the cause of ED was arterial dysfunction.

One interesting and perhaps paradoxical observation among these studies is that treated hypertensive patients often were no better or perhaps even demonstrated worse ED *(9)*. This paradox is explained, in part, by the concept that some of the antihypertensive medicines that are used may actually worsen ED.

The thiazide diuretics, such as chlorthalidone and hydrochlorothiazide, β-blockers, and centrally acting antihypertensive agents, are the most likely agents to be associated with ED *(11–14)*. Calcium channel blockers and angiotensin-converting enzyme inhibitors are less likely to induce ED. There have been a few recent reports suggesting that the angiotensin receptor blockers actually may improve ED in hypertension patients *(15)*.

Patients with hypertension and ED should not be denied their antihypertension medicines because of concern for developing ED. The treatment of hypertension has been shown to unequivocally reduce coronary heart disease, stroke, and hypertensive heart disease. The good news is that oral phosphodiesterase-5 inhibitors work quite effectively in hypertensive men on most of the antihypertensive agents.

LIPID ABNORMALITIES

In the MMAS, a low high-density lipoprotein (HDL) level correlated with development of age-adjusted ED; a high HDL level appeared to be protective *(1)*. In a study by Wei et al. *(16)*, 3250 men ages 25–83 yr were followed for a mean of 22 months after the first presentation of dyslipidemia, at which time they initially did not have ED. An increase in total cholesterol >240 mg/dL was associated with a 1.83 times greater risk of ED compared with men who had a total cholesterol of <180 mg/dL. Men with an HDL of >60 mg/dL had a lower (0.3 times) risk of ED vs men with an HDL of <30 mg/dL. Every 1 mmol/L increase in total cholesterol was associated with a 1.32 times increase in the risk of ED; every 1 mmol/L increase in HDL was associated with a 0.38 decrease in risk of ED. A follow-up study to the MMAS *(8)* demonstrated that ED developed prospectively in those men with a high Framingham risk score—one component of which is a high total cholesterol.

Evidence showing that lipid lowering will reduce or reverse ED is sparse. One study *(17)* observed that pravastatin and lovastatin (both powerful lipid-lowering agents) improved nocturnal penile tumescence in middle-aged men. In contrast, Rizvi et al. *(18)* showed that statins and fibrates themselves can actually cause ED. Both obesity and lack of physical exertion have been associated with ED as well as hypertension and lipid abnormalities *(8)* Derby et al. *(19)* prospectively examined the effect of lifestyle changes on ED. Two of the factors he studied were sedentary lifestyle and obesity. Men ages 40–70 yr (n = 593) who did not have ED at baseline were given questionnaires at baseline (1987–1989) and then at follow-up (1995–1997). If patients had obesity at baseline, they were more likely to have it at follow-up independent of subsequent weight loss. Continuation of physical activity or the initiation of physical activity did improve erectile function. The authors suggest that certain midlife changes in lifestyle (other than physical activity) may have been too late to have a beneficial effect on ED. In other words, after years of damage to the endothelium from noxious factors, it may be too late to reverse ED by lifestyle modification alone. Although there is still some controversy in this regard; this controversy will be seen when discussing the issue of smoking.

SMOKING

In the original MMAS *(1)* smoking markedly increased the age-adjusted probability of developing complete ED in men with treated heart disease. In the follow-up study *(8)* from this group, which studied men without ED at baseline and then about 8 yr later, smoking nearly doubled the chance of developing ED. Surprisingly, even passive cigarette smoke exposure and cigar smoking increased the probability of developing ED. McVary et al. *(20)* reported a comprehensive review of the literature in which smoking doubled the likelihood of a man developing moderate-to-complete ED.

Smoking has well-known adverse effects on the endothelium and vascular function *(20–28)*. Aromatic compounds and free radicals from cigarette smoke decrease endothelial nitric oxide synthase (eNOS), which adds to any existing NO deficiency, and elicit superoxide-mediated NO degradation. This reduction in NO increases penile vascular smooth muscle tone and promotes flaccidity. Besides this mechanism, nicotine can promote hypercoagulability, increase platelet aggregation, and release of free fatty acids and catecholamines. Cigarette smoke remains a major risk factor for the development of atherosclerosis *(22,23)*, including that of the hypogastric–cavernous arterial bed. Both nicotine and carbon monoxide also have direct toxic effects on the vascular endothelium. Most studies support the concept that cigarette smoking is deleterious to normal erectile function *(23–29)*.

In Derby's study *(19)*, reductions in smoking did not lower the incidence of ED. However, in a study of over 4000 United States Army Vietnam-era veterans, Mannino et al. *(24)* found that the prevalence of ED among men ages 31–49 yr was similar in former smokers and men who had never smoked, whereas it was significantly higher in current smokers. Guay et al. *(30)* reported improved penile tumescence and rigidity within 1 month of smoking cessation in younger patients who were heavy smokers. Thus, the best advice is that young people should not smoke in the first place, and if they do, they should quit. Quitting in midlife may simply be too late for some patients, in which the endothelial damage already has occurred.

DIABETES

Diabetes is a well-known risk factor for ED *(1)*. In one study, the prevalence rates of ED were 83% by the time diabetic men were in their late 60s *(31)*. Diabetes contributes to ED by accelerating vascular disease as well as by inducing neuropathy *(31–33)*. The onset of ED occurs earlier in diabetic patients than the general population. In one study, by age 43 yr, 47% of diabetic men had ED *(31)*. ED increases dramatically with duration of diabetes. There is a general lack of data regarding whether tight control of diabetes can improve erectile function.

In general, there is a lack of data examining the effect of control of cardiovascular risk factors on ED. With the advent of very effective oral therapy, it is unlikely that large trials will be able to examine this issue. There was one interesting study recently that did suggest that risk factor modification would enhance the ability of sildenafil to improve erections. Guay et al. *(33)* optimized treatment of comorbid medical conditions in men with ED over a course of >6 month. Patients received lifestyle advice regarding smoking and alcohol. Also, they optimized treatment of hypertension, hyperlipidemia, hypogonadism, and diabetes. Efficacy with sildenafil appeared to be improved in certain subgroups. The percent of patients with hypertension that responded was 83%, which is higher than previously reported (>70%). Patients who had hypogonadism treated with testosterone had a greater success rate with sildenafil at 85% vs those without testosterone (75%).

Theoretically, treatment with oral therapy for ED might have an interesting effect regarding therapy for certain cardiovascular risk factors. For example, hypertensive patients who avoid antihypertensive medicines because of the potential side effect of ED might be more inclined to take their medicine if they know the oral agent, like sildenafil, will work even if they are on antihypertensive medicines. Thus, one advantage of effective oral therapy for ED is the possibility of better compliance with antihypertensive medicines.

HOW COMMON IS ED AMONG MEN WITH CORONARY HEART DISEASE?

It has been suggested that ED is very common among men with established CAD or even those with underlying but not clinically established disease *(34–37)*. The frequency of ED among men who have had a myocardial infarction or coronary artery bypass surgery is often placed at greater than 60%. One angiographic trial of men with CAD observed that the severity of ED correlated with the number of diseased coronary arteries *(34)*. Patients with single vessel CAD had fewer problems with ED than men with multivessel CAD.

Recently, we studied the prevalence of ED in a population of men with chronic, stable, CAD *(38)*. Patients were asked to fill out the five-question questionnaire, the Sexual Health Inventory for Men (SHIM), which is based on the International Index of Erectile Function questionnaire. The five questions focus on the ability to attain and maintain an erection. Usually, completing the questionnaire took approximately 5 min or less. Seventy-six men participated, with a mean age of 64 yr. Of these participants, 24 men had undergone previous coronary artery bypass surgery; 29 had previous percutaneous coronary angioplasty with or without stenting or other intervention. Hypertension was present in 17 men and diabetes in 11. About half of the men were taking β-blockers; greater than 90% were on statins for lipid lowering, and 28% were taking diuretics. Seventy percent (53 of 76) had a SHIM score of ≤21, which is a score indicative of ED. Severe ED (a score of ≤7) was present in 19 of 76, or 25% of the men. Because the questionnaire reflected successful sildenafil therapy in four patients who had a previous history of ED, if these four were included as having had ED, then 57 of 76 (75%) of these men with chronic CAD had ED or recent histories of ED. These results suggested that ED is a very common problem in the population of men with stable CAD (Figs. 3 and 4). Despite this observation, it has been my general impression

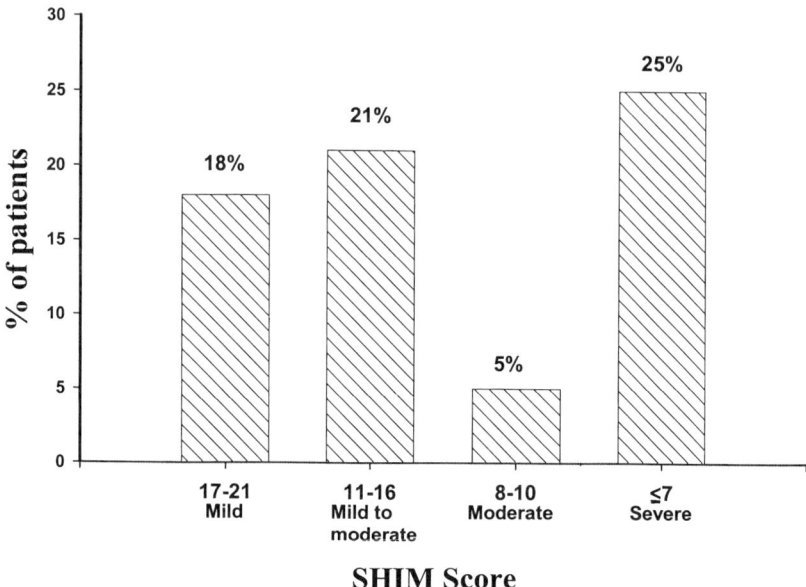

Fig. 3. The degree of ED among men with chronic artery disease who had a SHIM score of ≤21. Note that the most common category was severe ED at 25% of the men (reproduced from ref. *38*).

that most cardiologists do not ask their patients about ED. Many of the patients in our cohort had never discussed ED with their health care provider. The SHIM is a useful and inexpensive technique for "breaking the ice" with not only the cardiac patient, but any patient.

ED may be a marker for occult CAD or for risk factors for CAD. Pritzker *(35)* recently described the results of an intriguing preliminary report called "The Penile Stress Test: A Window to the Hearts of Man?" These investigators reviewed results of stress tests, risk factor analysis, and coronary angiography in 50 cardiac asymptomatic men with ED of presumed vascular origin between the ages of 40 and 60 yr. Multiple cardiovascular risk factors were identified in 80%. Exercise testing was positive (electrocardiogram) in 28 of 50 patients. Coronary angiography performed in 20 patients showed left main coronary obstruction or three-vessel disease in six patients, two-vessel disease in seven patients, and single-vessel CAD in seven patients. Only 15 of the 50 patients had seen a physician in the previous 2 yr. The results suggest that there is a high prevalence of coronary risk factors and significant CAD in coronary asymptomatic men with ED. Hence, ED may be a marker for occult coronary artery disease and/or risk factors for it.

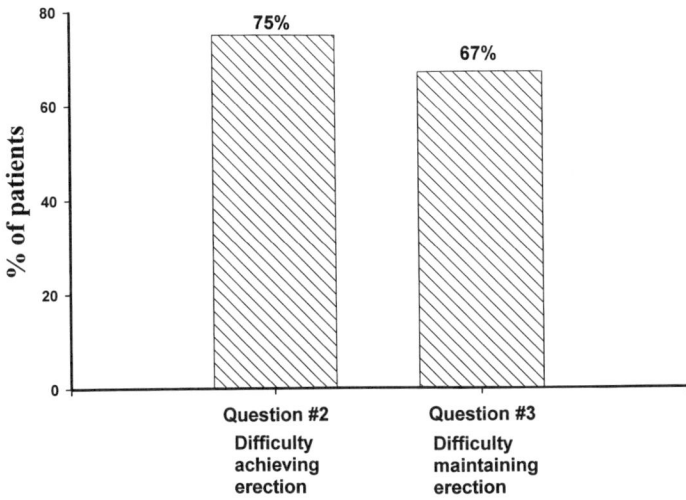

Fig. 4. Percent of coronary patients who reported difficulty achieving or maintaining an erection based on the SHIM questionnaire (reproduced from ref. *38*).

These findings suggest that ED is common in the coronary patient, and this is likely related to the concept that endothelial dysfunction and atherosclerosis are systemic disorders *(36)*. Damage to the endothelium by smoking, hypertension, lipid abnormalities, and diabetes affects blood vessels throughout the body, including those supplying the heart and the genitals. It is important that health care workers ask patients with CAD or risk factors for CAD about their sexual health and ED. Conversely, health care workers should ask their patients with ED about their cardiovascular health and about risk factors for CAD and ED. Because some men are seeking help from their health care provider for the first time, to obtain oral therapy for ED, the physician has an opportunity here to explore the issue of cardiovascular risk factors. The physician may diagnose for the first time hypertension, lipid abnormalities, or diabetes in such patients. Or the physician may discover that the patient smokes. Identifying these risk factors and then treating them in the man presenting with ED may actually save the patient's life and at least slow down the progression of vascular disease.

REFERENCES

1. Feldman HA, Goldstein I, Hatzichristou DG, et al. Impotence and its medical and psychosocial correlates: results of the Massachusetts Male Aging Study. J Urol 1994;151:54–61.

2. Morley JE, Kaiser FE. Impotence in elderly men. Drugs Aging 1992;2:330–344.
3. Sullivan ME, Keoghane SR, Miller MAW. Vascular risk factors and erectile dysfunction. BJU Int 2001;87:838–845.
4. Bortolotti A, Parazzini F, Colli E, et al. The epidemiology of erectile dysfunction and its risk factors. Int J Androl 1997;20:323–334.
5. Jarow J, Kloner RA, Holmes AM. Viagra M. Evans and Company, Inc. New York, 1998, pp. 1–150.
6. Burnett AL. Nitric oxide in the penis: physiology and pathology. J Urol 1997;157: 320–324.
7. Virag R, Bouilly P, Frydman D. Is impotence an arterial disorder? A study of arterial risk factors in 440 impotent men. Lancet 1985;8422:181–184.
8. Feldman HA, Johannes CB, Derby CA, et al. Erectile dysfunction and coronary risk factors: prospective results from the Massachusetts Male Aging Study. Prev Med 2000;30:328–338.
9. Bulpitt CJ, Dollery CT, Carne S. Change in symptom of hypertensive patients after referral to hospital clinic. Br Heart J 1976;38:121–128.
10. Burchardt M, Burchardt T, Baer L, et al. Hypertension is associated with severe erectile dysfunction. J Urol 2000;164:1188–1191.
11. Williams GH, Croog SH, Levine S, et al. Impact of antihypertensive therapy on quality of life: effect of hydrochlorothiazide. J Hypertens 1987;5(Suppl 1): S29–S35.
12. Jensen J, Lendorf A, Stimpel H, et al. The prevalence and etiology of impotence in 101 male hypertensive outpatients. Am J Hypertens 1999;12:271–275.
13. Grimm RH, Grandits GA, Priueas RJ, et al. Long-term effects on sexual function of five antihypertensive drugs and nutritional hygienic treatment in hypertensive men and women in the Treatment of Mild Hypertension Study. (THOMS) Hypertension 1997;29:8–14.
14. Wassertheil-Smoller S, Blaufox MD, Oberman A, et al., for the TAIM Research Group. Effects of antihypertensives on sexual function and quality of life: the TAIM Study. Ann Intern Med 1991;114:613–620.
15. Fogari R, Zoppi A, Poletti L, et al. Sexual activity in hypertensive men treated with valsartan or carvedilol: a crossover study. Am J Hypertens 2001;14:27–31.
16. Wei M, Macera CA, Davis DR, et al. Total cholesterol and high density lipoprotein cholesterol as important predictors of erectile dysfunction. Am J Epidemiol 1994;140:930–937.
17. Rosen RC, Weiner DN. Cardiovascular disease and sleep-related erections. J Psychosom Res 1997;42:515–516.
18. Rizvi K, Hampson JP, Harvey JN. Do lipid-lowering drugs cause erectile dysfunction? A systematic review. Fam Pract 2002;19:95–98.
19. Derby CA, Mohr BA, Goldstein I, et al. Modifiable risk factors and erectile dysfunction: can lifestyle changes modify risk? Urology 2000;56:302–306.
20. McVary KT, Carrier S, Wessells H, the Subcommittee on smoking and erectile dysfunction, Socioeconomic Committee, Sexual Medicine Society of North America. Smoking and erectile dysfunction: evidence-based analysis. J Urol 2001; 166:1624–1632.
21. Jeremy JY, Mikhallidis DP, Thompson CS, et al. The effect of cigarette smoke and diabetes mellitus on muscarinic stimulation of prostacyclin synthesis by the rat penis. Diabetes Res 1986;3:467–469.
22. Shabsigh R, Fishman IJ, Schum C, et al. Cigarette smoking and other vascular risk factors in vasculogenic impotence. Urology 1991;38:227–231.

23. Rosen MP, Greenfield AJ, Walker TG, et al. Cigarette smoking: an independent risk factor for atherosclerosis in the hypogastric-cavernous arterial bed of men with arteriogenic impotence. J Urol 1991;145:759–763.
24. Mannino DM, Klevens RM, Flanders WD. Cigarette smoking: an independent risk factor for impotence? Am J Epidemiol 1994;140:1003–1008.
25. Ledda A. Cigarette smoking, hypertension and erectile dysfunction. Curr Med Res Opin 2000;16(Suppl 1):S13–S16.
26. Juenemann K-P, Lue TF, Luo J-A, et al. The effect of cigarette smoking on penile erection. J Urol 1987;138:438–441.
27. Jacobs MC, Lenders JW, Kapma JA, et al. Effect of chronic smoking on endothelium-dependent vascular relaxation in humans. Clin Sci 1993;85:51–55.
28. Levine LA, Gerber GS. Acute vasospasm of penile arteries in response to cigarette smoking. Urology 1990;36:99–100.
29. Mersdorf A, Goldsmith PC, Diederichs W, et al. Ultrastructural changes in impotent penile tissue: a comparison of 65 patients. J Urol 1991;145:749–758.
30. Guay AT, Perez JB, Heatly GJ. Cessation of smoking rapidly decreases erectile dysfunction. Endocrine Pract 1998;4:23.
31. Klein R, Klein BEK, Lee KE, et al. Prevalence of self-reported erectile dysfunction in people with long-term IDDM. Diabetes Care 1996;19:135–141.
32. De-Tejada IS, Goldstein I, Azadzoi K, et al. Impaired neurogenic and endothelium-mediated relaxation of penile smooth muscle from diabetic men with impotence. N Engl J Med 1989;320:1025–1030.
33. Guay AT. Sexual dysfunction in the diabetic patients. Int J Impot Res 2001;13(Suppl 5):S47–S50.
34. Greenstein A, Chen J, Miller H, et al. Does severity of ischemic coronary disease correlate with erectile function? Int J Impot Res 1997;9:123–126.
35. Pritzker MR. The penile stress test: a window to the hearts of man? 72nd Scientific Sessions of the American Heart Association, November 7–10, 1999; Atlanta, Georgia. Abstract 104561.
36. O'Kane PD, Jackson G. Erectile dysfunction: is there silent obstructive coronary artery disease? Int J Clin Pract 2001;55:219–220.
37. Kirby M, Jackson G, Betteridge J, et al. Is erectile dysfunction a marker for cardiovascular disease? Int J Clin Pract 2001;155:614–618.
38. Kloner RA, Mullin SH, Shook T, et al. Erectile dysfunction in the cardiac patient: how common and should we treat? J Urol 2003;170:S46–S50.

4 Psychologic Aspects of Erectile Dysfunction in Heart Patients

Raymond C. Rosen, PhD

CONTENTS

INTRODUCTION
DEPRESSION AND ED IN PATIENTS WITH HEART DISEASE
THE ROLE OF STRESS AND ANXIETY
OTHER PSYCHOLOGICAL OR INTERPERSONAL FACTORS
OTHER SEXUAL DYSFUNCTIONS
COMBINING MEDICAL AND PSYCHOLOGICAL APPROACHES
POTENTIAL BENEFITS OF ADDRESSING PSYCHOLOGICAL ASPECTS OF ED
CONCLUSION
REFERENCES

INTRODUCTION

Erectile dysfunction (ED) is strongly related to both physical and psychological risk factors. Epidemiologic studies have highlighted the prevalence of psychosocial factors in the etiology of ED. In the Massachusetts Male Aging Study (MMAS) *(1)*, ED was significantly associated with self-reported depressive symptoms (OR = 2.88), pessimistic attitudes (OR = 3.89), or a negative outlook on life (OR = 2.30; Table 1). Depressed mood was found to be a significant predictor of ED, even after potential confounding factors had been controlled for (OR = 3). Similar findings were reported for the National

From: *Contemporary Cardiology: Heart Disease and Erectile Dysfunction*
Edited by: R. A. Kloner © Humana Press Inc., Totowa, NJ

Table 1
Psychosocial Predictors of ED

National Health and Social Life Survey (n = 1202)		Massachusetts Male Aging Study (n = 1265)	
Variable	OR	Variable	OR
Perceived health	2.82*	Marital change	1.41
Emotional stress	3.56*	Employment change	1.42
Household income	2.11*	Depressive symptoms	2.88*
Sexual coercion	3.52*	Unhappiness with life	2.30*
Prepubertal coercion	3.13*	Pessimistic attitude	3.89*

*$p < 0.05$.

Health and Social Life Survey (2), in which ED was significantly associated with self-reported emotional stress (OR = 3.56) and a history of sexual coercion (OR = 3.52). Socioeconomic factors, including a decrease in household income over the past 5 yr, also were significantly associated with the incidence of ED in this study. Overall, these studies underscore the independent and interactive effects of psychosocial factors in the etiology of ED.

Men with heart disease are at special risk for ED for several reasons: (a) there may be a direct causal association between cardiovascular risk factors (e.g., hypertension, hypercholesterolemia) and ED; (b) cardiovascular drugs (e.g., β-blockers, diuretics) can interfere with erection or other aspects of sexual function; (c) patients with heart disease are at increased risk for depression, which may, in turn, lead to ED—depression and ED have been strongly linked in a number of studies, as have cardiovascular disease and depression; (d) other psychological factors or reactions to illness (e.g., anxiety, relationship distress) may interfere with sexual function; and (e) cardiovascular disease and ED may not be directly related but are both commonly associated with aging.

In evaluating the link between cardiovascular disease and ED, it should also be noted that psychological reactions, such as depression or anxiety, might be observed as either causes or consequences of sexual dysfunction or both. Furthermore, these psychological reactions to ED can affect the patient's cardiac function either directly or indirectly via their adherence to medication or other lifestyle factors. In a recent large-scale study of men with Type 2 diabetes and ED (3), it was found that erectile difficulties correlated strongly with depression, increased emotional distress, and lack of adherence to their diabetes care. Patients with diabetes and ED in this study were less motivated and involved in their diabetes care compared with patients without ED. We have previously observed that patients with hypertension are frequently noncompliant with antihypertensive medication because of concerns about sexual side effects. As noted above, patients with ED are also likely to experience depression as a result of their condition, and this psychological reaction may adversely affect the course of their cardiac disease. For these reasons, male patients with cardiovascular disease should be routinely evaluated for ED, and treatment should be provided whenever indicated.

Case Vignette 1

Dan B. is a 58-yr-old married accountant with a 4-yr history of ED. He reports increasing difficulty in achieving or maintaining erections and has not had sexual intercourse for the past 18 month. The patient's medical history is significant for hypertension and hypercholesterolemia for the past 10 yr. He has been treated with several medications, including statins, diuretics, and β-blockers, and has been attempting to lose weight (current weight = 215 lbs). The patient's occupation is moderately stressful, particularly because of the accounting investigations of recent months. He is mildly depressed and has experienced sleep difficulties and loss of energy for the past year. His wife has experienced menopausal symptoms for the past several years and has little interest in sex.

This chapter reviews the major psychological factors associated with ED in patients with cardiovascular disease. In particular, we will consider, in detail, the role of depression as either cause or consequence of ED in patients with heart disease. Stress, anxiety, and relationship difficulties are other psychosocial factors frequently associated with ED in these patients. Partner relationship issues are also important to consider, as illustrated by case vignette 1. Although ED typically is associated with a combination of organic (i.e., vascular) and psychologic factors in patients with heart disease, it may occasionally result from psychogenic factors alone. Accordingly, we consider briefly mechanisms and management approaches for psychogenic ED. Many patients may benefit from combined medical and psychological approaches for ED and these are briefly reviewed. Finally, potential psychological and interpersonal benefits of treating ED in patients with heart disease are considered.

DEPRESSION AND ED IN PATIENTS WITH HEART DISEASE

Depression and heart disease have been linked in many studies, most of which have shown increased morbidity and mortality in patients with cardiovascular disease and depression *(4–6)*. Depression is not only common in patients with heart disease but it significantly impacts on the prognosis and course of the patient's illness *(7,8)*. The association may be mediated directly via the neuroendocrine effects of depression on cardiovascular function or indirectly via changes in lifestyle or lack of medical adherence. Although a detailed discussion of the mechanisms involved is beyond the scope of the present chapter, it is evident that patients with heart disease are at increased risk for depression and that the presence of depression adversely affects the course and outcome of their cardiovascular disease.

Given the increased rate of depression in patients with heart disease, it is not surprising that ED is also common in these patients. The relationship between ED and depression in patients with heart disease has been specifically addressed in two recent reviews *(9,10)*. Roose and Seidman *(9)* have proposed four potential mechanisms to account for the association between ED and depression in patients with heart disease: (a) depression can lead directly to a loss of erectile function via the neuroendocrine effects of the disease; (b) ED may be caused by underlying organic (e.g., vascular) causes, and depression may result from the loss of sexual function and associated psychological consequences; (c) both ED and depression may be consequences of another underlying condition (e.g., hypothyroidism); and (d) ED and depression may be coincidentally comorbid because of the association with aging in both disorders.

Based on findings from the MMAS *(1,11)*, Goldstein *(10)* has proposed an interactive model to account for the relationship between ED, cardiovascular disease and depression. This model posits a mutually reinforcing relationship between these three factors, with additional influences from demographic, lifestyle, and other factors (e.g., medication use). As shown, this model posits a mutually reinforcing relationship between these three factors, with additional influences from demographic, lifestyle, and other health factors (e.g., medication use). Based on this model, the author proposes that patients with cardiovascular disease should be routinely screened for both depression and ED. Because depression and ED are likely to be associated with the outcome of treatment for cardiovascular disease, he argues further that patients with cardiovascular disease and ED should be treated directly for their sexual difficulties. Although there is strong evidence for improved mood after treatment of patients with ED *(12)*, to date this has not been specifically shown to improve cardiac outcomes in patients with ED and heart disease.

From a clinical perspective, a number of factors need to be taken into account. First, the nature and severity of the patient's depression should be clinically evaluated. Potential suicide risk, vegetative symptoms, and other aspects of the patient's depression should be carefully assessed. A psychiatric consultation should be obtained whenever indicated. Because ED may be a presenting symptom of major depression, the first priority should be a careful mental status assessment and appropriate referral as needed. After this, specific aspects of the patient's erectile and/or other sexual difficulties should be evaluated and their relationship to the patient's depression explored. Did the sexual problems appear before or after onset of the mood disorder? Is there a loss of libido in addition to ED, and, if so, did these problems develop in any particular order? Older depressed men commonly experience loss of libido as a component of their depression, and this may lead to a secondary loss of erectile function over time. Did the sexual problems develop or increase in response to antidepressant medication use? Selective serotonin reuptake inhibitors (SSRIs) and other antidepressant drugs have a high rate of adverse sexual side effects *(13)*, including loss of orgasm, decreased desire, and erection difficulties. Unfortunately, antidepressant therapy for the patient's depression may lead to worsening of the sexual difficulties in many instances.

Case Vignette 2

Max P. is a 64-yr-old construction engineer who suffered a myocardial infarction (MI) 1 yr ago. The patient has a 15-yr history of hypertension and coronary artery disease (CAD). The patient has had difficulty in returning to work since the MI and is reluctant to engage in vigorous activity despite a satisfactory recovery. The patient and his wife have had difficulty in resuming sexual activity, and he experiences intermittent erectile failure. Viagra (50 mg) is moderately effective, although the patient is reluctant to use the drug because of fear of triggering another heart attack. He is moderately depressed and has recently begun taking Zoloft 50 mg/d (Pfizer Inc., New York, NY).

Relationship conflicts can be a contributing factor to the patient's depression or ED or may be a result in some cases. Depression or dysphoric mood impacts negatively on social and interpersonal relationships. Depressed men typically avoid making new relationships or may withdraw emotionally or physically from their ongoing relationships. They are less likely to initiate positive social activities and often become sexually or socially unassertive. Men with both ED and depression are especially likely to withdraw from all forms of sexual expression or physical intimacy, as illustrated by case vignette 2. Partner reactions may be more or less accepting of these changes, which may, in turn, elicit a range of emotional responses in the patient ranging from rejection to anger and hostility. These and other couple's issues may exacerbate the effects of depression and associated ED in patients with heart disease.

Despite the complex dynamics involved, recent studies strongly support the value of direct treatment of erectile difficulties in men with both depression and ED. In one study involving middle-aged men with ED and subsyndromal depression *(12)*, we found that direct treatment of ED with sildenafil led to marked improvements in both erectile function and mood. Partner relationships were also improved and a high rate of positive response to sildenafil (>70%) was observed overall in the study. Other recent studies have shown that depressed men being treated with SSRIs who develop sexual problems in association with their antidepressant medication also respond well to treatment with sildenafil *(14)*. Overall, these studies suggest that direct treatment of ED in men with both depression and ED is likely to be effective and may have significant positive effects on both mood and sexual function in these patients. However, the presence of ED in patients with heart disease should always be regarded as a potential marker or symptom of depression, which should lead to further clinical investigation of the patient's depression. Physicians should also bear in mind that antidepressant medications might cause or exacerbate sexual difficulties in depressed patients *(13)*.

THE ROLE OF STRESS AND ANXIETY

In addition to depression, patients with heart disease frequently show increased levels of anxiety or psychological distress *(15)*. Stress or anxiety may be present as part of an overall "type A" personality profile, or the patient may have a specific anxiety reaction to the diagnosis or treatment of heart disease. This is especially apparent in patients who suffer a stroke or MI or who have frequent episodes of angina pectoris or dyspnea. As illustrated by case vignette 2, "heart" patients are often concerned that sexual activity could lead to another stroke or heart attack and may develop a pattern of sexual avoidance and secondary ED as a result. Patients also typically lack information or education

Table 2
Common Clinical Concerns of the Cardiac Patient
(adapted from ref. 16)

Increased "life stress" because of coronary event
Increased anxiety and overprotectiveness in the partner
Avoidance of previously unsatisfactory sexual activity
Fear of harming partner
Fear of coital coronary
Fear of "harmful effects of sexual activity"
Anxiety about safety of ED therapy (e.g., sildenafil)

---

about the potential risks associated with sexual activity, and this may contribute significantly to their anxiety.

Friedman *(16)* has reviewed the role of anxiety and psychological distress in mediating sexual problems in patients with heart disease. This author notes that patients with cardiovascular disease are at increased risk for anxiety disorders generally and that panic disorder in particular is common in patients with more severe forms of heart disease. As with depression, fear or anxiety has been linked to an increased incidence of ED either directly via increased sympathetic tone or indirectly via the related effects on sexual avoidance or other interpersonal or psychological mechanisms. Patients with a history of MI (and their partners) are often anxious about the potential harmful effects of sexual activity or other forms of physical activity. These patients often avoid all forms of sexual activity following their recovery. Table 2 summarizes common anxieties or clinical concerns encountered in the cardiac patient.

Friedman *(16)* has emphasized the need to address these issues directly in the context of cardiac rehabilitation. He notes that normal signs of sexual arousal, such as increased heart rate or respiration, may easily be misinterpreted by male patients or their partners as cardiac symptoms. Anxious patients are also more likely to experience sexual performance anxiety, which can lead to a loss of erection or premature ejaculation. Loss of libido and associated relationship conflict may further exacerbate sexual performance difficulties in these patients. Heart patients with sexual dysfunction may be reluctant to use sildenafil or other ED therapies because of concerns about the cardiac safety of the medications. For these reasons, it is strongly recommended that partners be included in the rehabilitation process from the outset and that sexual issues be addressed whenever necessary. Patients with more severe anxiety or sexual performance difficulties may benefit from specialized referral to address these issues.

OTHER PSYCHOLOGICAL OR INTERPERSONAL FACTORS

Psychosocial determinants of sexual dysfunction are traditionally divided into immediate and remote causes. Immediate causes include performance anxiety or fear of failure, lack of adequate stimulation, and relationship conflicts. Performance anxiety has been especially emphasized as a major cause of psychogenic ED in patients with or without medical illness *(17)*. As first described by Masters and Johnson *(18)*, performance anxiety includes the adoption of a "spectator role" in which the individual's attention is focused predominantly on sexual performance and away from erotic stimulation. This cognitive distraction from sexually arousing cues was viewed by Masters and Johnson as central to arousal difficulties in both sexes and formed the basis of their "sensate focus" approach to treatment. Among the remote or early developmental causes of arousal disorders, various authors have emphasized the role of childhood sexual trauma, sexual identity or orientation issues, unresolved partner or parental attachments, and religious or cultural taboos.

Interpersonal and relationship factors have also been associated frequently with ED *(19)*. Communication difficulties, lack of intimacy, or trust and power conflicts have been emphasized as frequent concomitants of arousal difficulties in both sexes. Loss of sexual attraction has also been implicated in some studies. Relationship conflicts may be a consequence as well as a cause of ED for many couples. It has frequently been observed that ED is most sexually debilitating for couples with limited sexual repertoires and few alternatives to intercourse. In particular, performance demands and fear of failure are increased markedly for individuals or couples who lack alternative means of sexual satisfaction to penile–vaginal intercourse. For these individuals, the male's inability to achieve a firm and lasting erection typically results in a complete cessation of all sexual activity. This, in turn, may lead to diminished sexual desire in one or both partners and increased distance or conflict in the relationship. A "vicious cycle" phenomenon frequently ensues, as the loss of sexual or affectionate interaction is associated with increased performance demands and interpersonal distress.

Increased genital stimulation may be necessary for some men to achieve an adequate erection and may augment the effects of pharmacological therapy. Among older men, in particular, there is an increasing need for direct, tactile stimulation of the penis, along with a decreasing responsiveness to psychogenic forms of stimulation. Thus, the older male may require extended manual or oral stimulation of the penis to achieve adequate erection for intercourse. The female partner is frequently unaware of this important physiological change in her partner and may misattribute his lack of arousal to sexual disinterest or her loss of sexual attractiveness to her partner. When informed of the need for change in this area, older couples frequently have difficulty in modifying or adapting their traditional sexual script. Many of these couples have minimal experience of foreplay or nonintercourse forms of sexual stimulation.

In considering the role of psychological or psychosocial factors in ED in older men with heart disease, traditional male attitudes to sexuality need to be considered. Men with erectile difficulties (and their partners) are often resistant to psychological explanations or interventions. As noted by Zilbergeld (20), men with ED typically experience both shame and guilt in association with their sexual dysfunction, and organic explanations of the disorder are obviously more appealing. These patients frequently present with the request: "Tell me it's not all in my head, doc!" For this reason, most men (and their partners) are more likely to accept a referral for psychological or couple's counseling when combined with medical treatment for the disorder.

OTHER SEXUAL DYSFUNCTIONS

Male patients with heart disease (or their partners) may have other sexual dysfunctions in addition to ED. These include anorgasmia or delayed ejaculation in the male and arousal or penetration difficulties in the female. Although precise data are lacking on the relative prevalence of these problems in patients with heart disease and ED, many cases present with concomitant sexual problems in one or both partners. Again, a thorough assessment is important in determining the history of these problems and their temporal relationship to the patient's ED. In some instances, ED may develop secondary to anorgasmia in the male or in response to chronic penetration difficulties (i.e., dyspareunia) in the female partner. Treatment of the male's erectile difficulties with sildenafil (or other medical therapy) may serve only to reinitiate or exacerbate these underlying problems. Whenever possible, these problems should be identified and addressed before the initiation of medical treatment with sildenafil.

It is particularly important to address penetration or lubrication difficulties in the female partner before initiation of treatment for the male's ED. In cases of dyspareunia (painful intercourse) or vaginismus (involuntary spasm or contractions of the vagina), a complete gynecological evaluation for the woman is recommended at the outset. Depending upon the severity of the problem and results of the physical and psychosexual evaluation, medical or sex therapy interventions should be initiated, and the couple should be counseled to avoid attempting intercourse initially. The male may wish to try sildenafil in conjunction with manual (either self- or partner stimulation) or oral stimulation but should be strongly discouraged from attempting intercourse until sufficient progress has been made in treating the sexual dysfunction in the partner. Some women report a recurrence of the penetration problem when the male begins to use sildenafil (or other medical therapy) and intercourse is resumed. Although generally less debilitating than dyspareunia or vaginismus, arousal or lubrication difficulties might also make resumption of intercourse difficult or painful for the partner. This is particularly common in postmenopausal women not taking hormonal replacement. Again, these problems should be addressed directly before the introduction of sildenafil or other ED therapies.

Sexual desire problems in either partner can be particularly difficult to address *(21)*. In some instances, the lack of interest or desire for sex becomes apparent as a form of "resistance" or noncompliance with the prescribed medical therapy. If either partner is found to have low desire that predates or is a major causal factor for the male's ED, couple's or sex therapy should be specifically addressed to this problem. Medical treatments (e.g., sildenafil) can be prescribed in such cases, although the primary focus of treatment should be on the underlying sexual desire disorder. Desire problems can also be caused by undiagnosed endocrine factors (e.g., hypogonadism), medication use, relationship conflicts, or depression, as noted above. In each instance, the desire disorder should be separately addressed either prior to, or in conjunction with, the patient's ED.

COMBINING MEDICAL AND PSYCHOLOGICAL APPROACHES

Case Vignette 3

Bill K. is a 49-yr-old married stockbroker with a history of CAD and recent coronary bypass surgery. The patient complains of increasing erection difficulties and loss of libido since undergoing his bypass surgery 2 yr ago. He is currently maintained on statin and β-blocker therapy, in addition to intermittent use of benzodiazepines for anxiety.

He reports increasing marital distress and is concerned that his wife may be having an affair with a colleague at work. The patient has experienced moderate success in achieving erection with sildenafil (50 mg) but has not attempted sexual intercourse with his wife for several months. His libido is markedly reduced and he notes that his wife is avoiding him sexually and emotionally. The patient feels anxious and helpless about his situation.

Despite the availability and effectiveness of medical treatments for ED, there is growing recognition of the limits of pharmacological therapy in many instances and the need for combining medical and psychological approaches. At times, treatment of ED with sildenafil or other medical therapy serves only to reveal or highlight other sexual problems, such as lack of sexual desire or anorgasmia. Sexual problems in the partner or other couple's issues may come to light after successful (or unsuccessful) use of sildenafil, as demonstrated in case vignette 3. Leiblum *(22)* has proposed that success rates with sildenafil may be significantly lower in couples for whom there has been chronic sexual or marital conflict, lack of desire in one or both partners, or significant psychiatric illness in either partner. Several authors have recommended combined use of sildenafil and counseling approaches in such cases, particular in cases of low desire, sexual initiation difficulties, or the presence of other sexual dysfunctions in either partner *(22)*. Controlled trials of combination drug and nondrug therapy for sexual dysfunction unfortunately have not been performed to date.

A careful clinical assessment should be performed in advising a couple whether or not to begin using sildenafil (or other medical treatment) before, or in conjunction with, counseling for one or more of the above problems. There are presently no clearcut guidelines or criteria to be followed in making this decision. In some instances, a resumption of sexual activity may lead to reduced tension in the relationship, thereby facilitating more effective communication and problem solving around couples' issues. However, in other instances attempts at sexual intercourse are likely to increase or exacerbate underlying conflicts or tensions, and should be postponed until significant progress has been made in other areas. Particularly in cases involving extramarital affairs or sexual activity outside of the primary relationship, the introduction of medical treatments for ED should be handled with special care.

For couples with less serious sexual or relationship problems, physicians or health care clinicians may provide simple guidelines for enhancing relationship satisfaction and for improving communication around sexual issues. For example, couples should be encouraged to communicate more directly with one another about their sexual preferences and priorities. Simple suggestions for increasing emotional and physical intimacy can be offered, such as taking more time to talk about personal issues and sharing personal feelings more frequently. Many couples experience romance loss along with sexual intimacy, and suggestions can be made for developing a more romantic approach to lovemaking. Some of these recommendations can be provided by a physician, cardiac nurse, or physician assistant *(23)*. Referral for more specialized couples or sex therapy is advised when physicians or health care providers are uncomfortable in addressing couples' or sexual issues, or if more serious sexual or relationship problems are encountered.

POTENTIAL BENEFITS OF ADDRESSING PSYCHOLOGICAL ASPECTS OF ED

There are several potential benefits of addressing psychological aspects of ED in patients with heart disease. First, compliance is likely to be better and treatment outcomes improved if these issues are directly addressed. As noted above, sildenafil is less likely to be effective in patients with significant performance anxiety, partner conflicts, lack of libido or other sexual problems. Sexual problems in the partner should be separately assessed in all cases and appropriate referral made, when indicated. The presence of ED in patients with heart disease may be symptomatic of depression or anxiety, and these underlying problems should be separately addressed in all cases. At times, direct treatment of the patient's ED with sildenafil or other medical therapy will result in significant improvements in mood or interpersonal functioning *(12)*. In other cases, it will be necessary for patient's to be referred for psychiatric evaluation and/or consultation. Additionally, addressing psychological aspects of ED in patients with heart disease can play an important role in maintaining or enhancing the patient/physician relationship.

CONCLUSION

Loss of erection is one of the most salient losses or impairments experienced by many men in response to illness or aging. Men vary greatly in their ability to compensate or adjust to such losses and in the psychological coping style they display. The significance of the loss is also highly variable, as some men experience ED as equivalent to a loss of masculinity or male identity. ED can also be associated with significant performance anxiety or concerns about cardiac safety. It can be caused by, or impact significantly on, stresses in the partner relationship. These issues should be carefully assessed in all cases.

There is a complex and clinically important relationship between depression and ED in heart patients. In general, patients with cardiovascular disease are susceptible to various depressive disorders, including major depressive disorder, minor depression, and dysphoric mood disorder. Depression may play a role in the genesis or outcome of the patient's cardiovascular disease and may be a contributing factor to the occurrence of ED. This chapter has reviewed the complex interaction between cardiovascular disease, ED, and depression, as well as the need to address all three aspects in all cases. Similarly, we have considered the role of stress and anxiety in both cardiovascular disease and ED. Cardiac rehabilitation programs need to include greater emphasis on risks and benefits of sexual activity, and educational intervention should be provided for both patients and partners.

Finally, we have emphasized the potential value of combining medical and psychological approaches for ED in these patients. By addressing psychological or interpersonal issues, treatment compliance is likely to be enhanced and better outcomes achieved. Even in cases with a predominant organic (e.g., vascular) ED etiology, attention to psychological factors may lead to more effective use of sildenafil or other medical therapies.

REFERENCES

1. Feldman HA, Goldstein I, Hatzichristou DG, et al. . Impotence and its medical and psychosocial correlates: results of the Massachusetts Male Aging Study. J Urol 1994;151:54–61.
2. Lauman EO, Paik A, Rosen RC. Sexual dysfunction in the United States: prevalence and predictors. JAMA 1999;281:6:537–544.
3. DeBarardis G, Franciosi M, Belfiglio M, et al. Erectile dysfunction and quality of life in type 2 diabetic patients. Diabetes Care 2002;25:284–291.
4. Aromaa A, Raitasalo R, Reunanen A, et al. Depression and cardiovascular diseases. Acta Psychiatry Scand Suppl 1994;377:77–82.
5. Ariyo AA, Haan M, Tangen CM, et al. for the Cardiovascular Health Study Collaborative Research Group. Depressive symptoms and risks of coronary heart disease and mortality in elderly Americans. Circulation 2000;102:1773–1779.
6. Schultz R, Beach SR, Ives DG, et al. Association between depression and mortality in older adults: the Cardiovascular Health Study. Arch Intern Med 2000; 160:1761–1768.
7. Frasure-Smith N, Lesperance F, Talajic M. Depression and 18-month prognosis after myocardial infarction. Circulation 1995;91:999–1005.
8. Bush DE, Ziegelstein RC, Tayback M, et al. Even minimal symptoms of depression increase mortality risk after acute myocardial infarction. Am J Cardiol 2001; 88:337–341.

9. Roose SP, Seidman SN. Sexual activity and cardiac risk: Is depression a contributing factor? Am J Cardiol 2000;86(Suppl)38F–40F.
10. Goldstein I. The mutually reinforcing triad of depressive symptoms, cardiovascular disease, and erectile dysfunction. Am J Cardiol 2000;86(Suppl): 41F–45F.
11. Araujo AB, Durante R, Feldman HA, et al. The relationship between depressive symptoms and male erectile dysfunction: cross-sectional results from the Massachusetts Male Aging Study. Psychosom Med 1998;60:458–465.
12. Seidman SN, Roose SP, Menza MA, et al. Treatment of erectile dysfunction in men with depressive symptoms: results of a placebo-controlled trial with sildenafil citrate. Am J Psychiatry 2001;158:1623–1630.
13. Rosen R, Lane R, Menza M. Effects of SSRIs on sexual function: a critical review. J Clin Psychopharmacol 1999;19:67–85.
14. Nurnberg G, Seidman S, Gelenberg A, et al. Toward clarifying the relationship between treatments for depression and erectile dysfunction: a review of 4 studies using sildenafil citrate in depressed men. J Urol 2002.
15. Weissman MM, Markowitz JS, Ouellette R, et al. Panic disorder and cardiovascular/ cerebrovascular problems: results from a community survey. Am J Psychiatry 1990; 147:1504–1508.
16. Friedman S. Cardiac disease, anxiety and sexual functioning. Am J Cardiol 2000;86(Suppl):46F–50F.
17. Rosen RC, Leiblum SR, Spector I. Psychologically-based treatment for male erectile disorder: A cognitive-interpersonal model. J Sex Marital Ther 1994;20:67–85.
18. Masters WH, Johnson VE. Human Sexual Inadequacy. Little Brown, Boston, 1970.
19. Rosen RC, Leiblum SR. Erectile disorders: historical trends and clinical perspectives. In: Rosen RC, Leiblum SR, eds. Erectile Disorders: Assessment and Treatment. Guilford Press, New York, 1992, pp. 3–26.
20. Zilbergeld B. The New Male Sexuality. Bantam Books, New York, 1992.
21. Rosen RC, Leiblum SR. Treatment of sexual dysfunction: an integrated approach. J Consulting Clin Psychol 1995;63:877–890.
22. Leiblum SR. After sildenafil: bridging the gap between pharmacologic treatment and satisfying sexual relationships. J Clin Psychiatry 2002;63(Suppl 5):17–22.
23. Albaugh J, Amargo I, Capelson R, et al. Health care clinicians in sexual medicine: focus on erectile dysfunction [review]. Urol Nurs 2002;22:217–231.

5 Management of Erectile Dysfunction
An Overview

Harin Padma-Nathan, MD

CONTENTS
INTRODUCTION
SILDENAFIL CITRATE
NEW PDE5 INHIBITORS: EFFICACY, SAFETY,
 AND COMPARATIVE PERSPECTIVES
COMPARATIVE PERSPECTIVES ON THE THREE
 PDE5 INHIBITORS
CONCLUSION
REFERENCES

INTRODUCTION

The evolution of the management of erectile dysfunction (ED) over the past quarter century is a reflection of the convergence of dramatic medical discoveries that encompass both basic and clinical sciences. Underlying the elegance of simplicity of the current ED management is the impact of such discoveries as the role of the nitric oxide cyclic guanosine monophosphate pathway in regulating vascular and penile trabecular smooth muscle, the role of phosphodiesterase type-5 (PDE5) in regulating this cyclic guanosine monophosphate, and, ultimately, the serendipitous discovery of sildenafil citrate, a highly potent and highly selective inhibitor of this enzyme *(1)*. What was once a field made complex by highly invasive and somewhat artificial diagnostic testing (nocturnal erections studies, duplex ultrasonography, and cavernosometry) is

From: *Contemporary Cardiology: Heart Disease and Erectile Dysfunction*
Edited by: R. A. Kloner © Humana Press Inc., Totowa, NJ

now more effectively and readily managed by generalists and specialists in much the same way. In fact, the approach to ED management is surprisingly similar around the world. Assessment today is focused on the history and physical examination in all patients followed by simple laboratory studies (serum testosterone, lipid profile, and glycated hemoglobin) in a select few. The First International Consultation on Erectile Dysfunction, in part sponsored by the World Health Organization, has recommended a step-wise approach to the management of ED, particularly nonhormonal ED, with initial therapy being oral medications, followed by local therapies, such as penile injection therapy, intraurethral applications, and vacuum constriction devices *(2)*. The therapy of last resort in most, but not all, men is the implantation of a penile prosthesis. This chapter focuses on medical therapies, particularly first-line oral medication therapy.

Medical therapy with oral medications today is primarily PDE5 inhibitor therapy with sildenafil citrate. In addition, in Europe, the centrally acting dopamine agonist sublingual apomorphine (Uprima, Abbott Laboratories, Abbott Park, IL) is available. It is effective in approximately 30–40% of men with mild or psychogenic ED as well as select men with organic erectile dysfunction *(3,4)*. It has about 2–6% of the oral therapy market in Europe. It is not approved in the United States. The cardiovascular effects of this and other non-PDE5 inhibitor therapies are discussed in another chapter. In the near future, two new PDE5 inhibitors, vardenafil and tadalafil, will be available in Europe and most likely the United States. This chapter focuses on sildenafil but also examines other PDE5 inhibitors in advanced development.

Local therapies may be considered in patients who fail oral medication, who have specific contraindications to oral therapy, or who experience adverse events from oral therapy. Intracavernosal injection therapy is clearly the most effective local pharmacological therapy. The direct injection into the corpora cavernosa of vasoactive agents, primarily alprostadil (the synthetic version of prostaglandin E1) is associated with broad efficacy (60–70%) and relative safety *(5)*. The side effects associated with injection therapy are primarily local and include pain, priapism (a prolonged and eventually ischemic erection), and scar tissue formation over time. The intraurethral application of alprostadil is an alternative to injection therapy but is associated with much lower efficacy (30–40%) and systemic (hypotension) as well as the afore-mentioned local side effects *(6)*. Both of these local therapies are considerably more expensive than oral therapy. More recently, a topical therapy of a proprietary combination of alprostadil and a percutaneous absorption enhancer has been in development *(7)*.

Clearly, the most pervasive and effective therapy for erectile dysfunction is sildenafil citrate. Recently, the 4-yr clinical experience with sildenafil in the management of erectile dysfunction was reviewed extensively and is detailed in the following sections *(8)*.

SILDENAFIL CITRATE

Sildenafil citrate (Viagra, Pfizer Inc., New York, NY) was approved for the management of ED by the United States Food and Drug Administration in April 1998. It has had a dramatic impact on the breath and scope of ED management globally. In fact, as of March 31, 2002, more than 16 million patients with ED have been treated with sildenafil, with over 100 million prescriptions issued by more than 500,000 physicians (on file, Pfizer). The following is a summary of the 4-yr efficacy and safety experience with sildenafil *(9)*.

Overall Efficacy of Sildenafil in the Treatment of ED
POOLED, DOUBLE-BLIND CLINICAL TRIAL RESULTS

The following is an 11-study clinical trial analysis that encompasses a total of 1329 patients who received placebo and 1338 patients who received sildenafil *(9)*. Patient characteristics (age, ethnic group, body mass index [BMI], smoking status, and ED duration and etiology) were similar for the two treatment groups. Sildenafil treatment was associated with significantly higher mean scores for individual International Index of Erectile Function (IIEF) questions assessing ability to achieve (Q3, Fig. 1) and maintain (Q4, Fig. 2) an erection satisfactory for sexual performance and for the six questions comprising the Erectile Function (EF) domain of the IIEF (EF domain, Fig. 3; p values < 0.02 vs placebo). A significant treatment effect was demonstrated across all patient subgroups characterized by demographic factors (Figs. 1A, 2A, 3A) such as race/ethnic group (white, black, Hispanic, Asian), age (<65 yr and ≥65 yr), and BMI (<30 and ≥30 kg/m^2); ED characteristics (Figs. 1B, 2B, 3B), including etiology (organic, mixed, psychogenic), severity at baseline (mild-to-moderate, severe), and ED duration (≤2 yr, >2 yr to ≤5 yr, >5 yr); and concomitant occurrence (Figs. 1C, 2C, 3C) of other medical conditions (diabetes, ischemic heart disease, peripheral vascular disease, postradical prostatectomy, hypertension, or depression) or concomitant use of medications known to be associated with ED (antihypertensives or antidepressants).

After 12 wk of treatment, 46.5 to 87% of patients in the subgroups receiving sildenafil indicated that treatment had improved their erec-

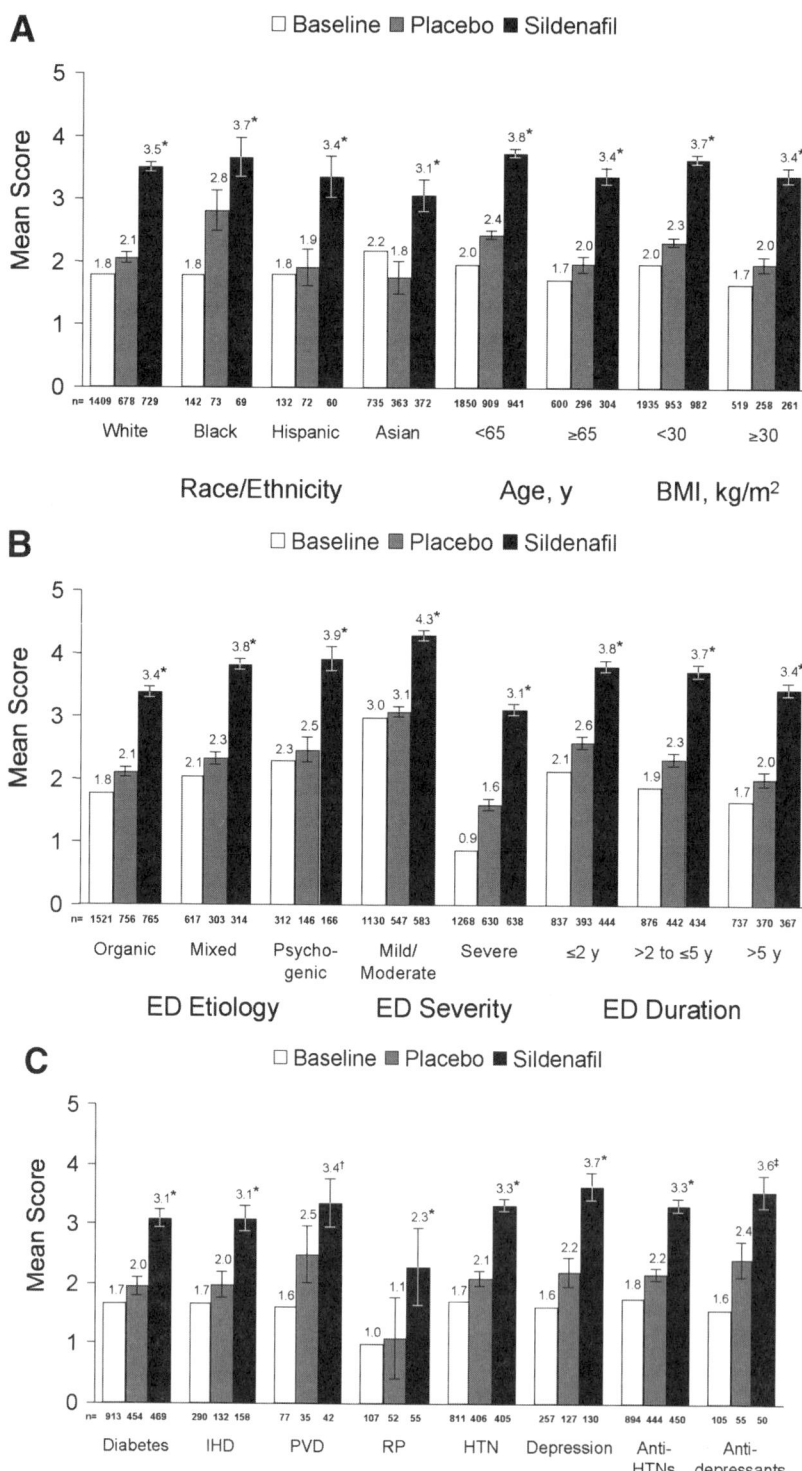

tions compared with 11.3 to 41.3% of patients in subgroups receiving placebo ($p < 0.001$). Likewise, in the six trials in which sexual event log data were collected, significantly greater percentages of attempts at intercourse that were successful were reported by patient subgroups receiving sildenafil (52.6–80.1%) compared with patient subgroups receiving placebo (14.0–34.5%, $p < 0.0001$).

LONG-TERM EFFECTIVENESS

Effectiveness was maintained in patients electing to continue open-label treatment with sildenafil for their ED in three long-term extension studies. In these three studies, a total of 89% of patients who had previously completed double-blind and open-label extension studies completed an additional 1 yr of open-label treatment and chose to continue taking sildenafil. Greater than 95% of these patients reported satisfaction with treatment effect on erections and improvement in ability to engage in sexual activity at the end of 1 yr (Fig. 4). Of the 11% of patients who discontinued treatment, 2% discontinued for treatment-related reasons (1.6% for insufficient response; 0.4% for adverse events).

In one of the three extension studies ($n = 979$), treatment was extended for an additional 2 yr. Satisfaction with treatment effect on erections and improvement in ability to engage in sexual activity was reported by greater than or equal to 95% of patients at the end of 1, 2, and 3 yr of open-label treatment with sildenafil (Fig. 5). Most patients were receiving 100 mg sildenafil (84% at study start, 87% at 1 yr, 87% at 2 yr, and 88% at 3 yr). Over the 3-yr period, 32% of patients discontinued treatment. However, only 6.7% of discontinuations were treatment-related (5.7% from insufficient response and 1% from treatment-related adverse events), suggesting that both tolerability and

---

Fig. 1. (*opposite*) Overall baseline mean score and least squares mean ± SE scores at end of treatment for question 3 (ability to achieve erections) of the International Index of Erectile Function. Scores ranged from 1 (never/almost never) to 5 (always/almost always) with a response of 0 indicating "did not attempt sexual intercourse." **A** shows scores for subgroups characterized by patient characteristics, **B** shows scores for subgroups characterized by ED characteristics, **C** shows scores for subgroups characterized by concomitant medical conditions/ medications.

BMI, body mass index; IHD, ischemic heart disease; PVD, peripheral vascular disease; RP, radical prostatectomy; HTN, hypertension; anti-HTNS, antihypertensives. *$p < 0.0001$, †$p < 0.02$, ‡$p < 0.0002$. ED severity categories of mild to moderate (IIEF erectile domain score, 11–25) and severe ED (IIEF erectile domain score, ≤10) (from ref. 9).

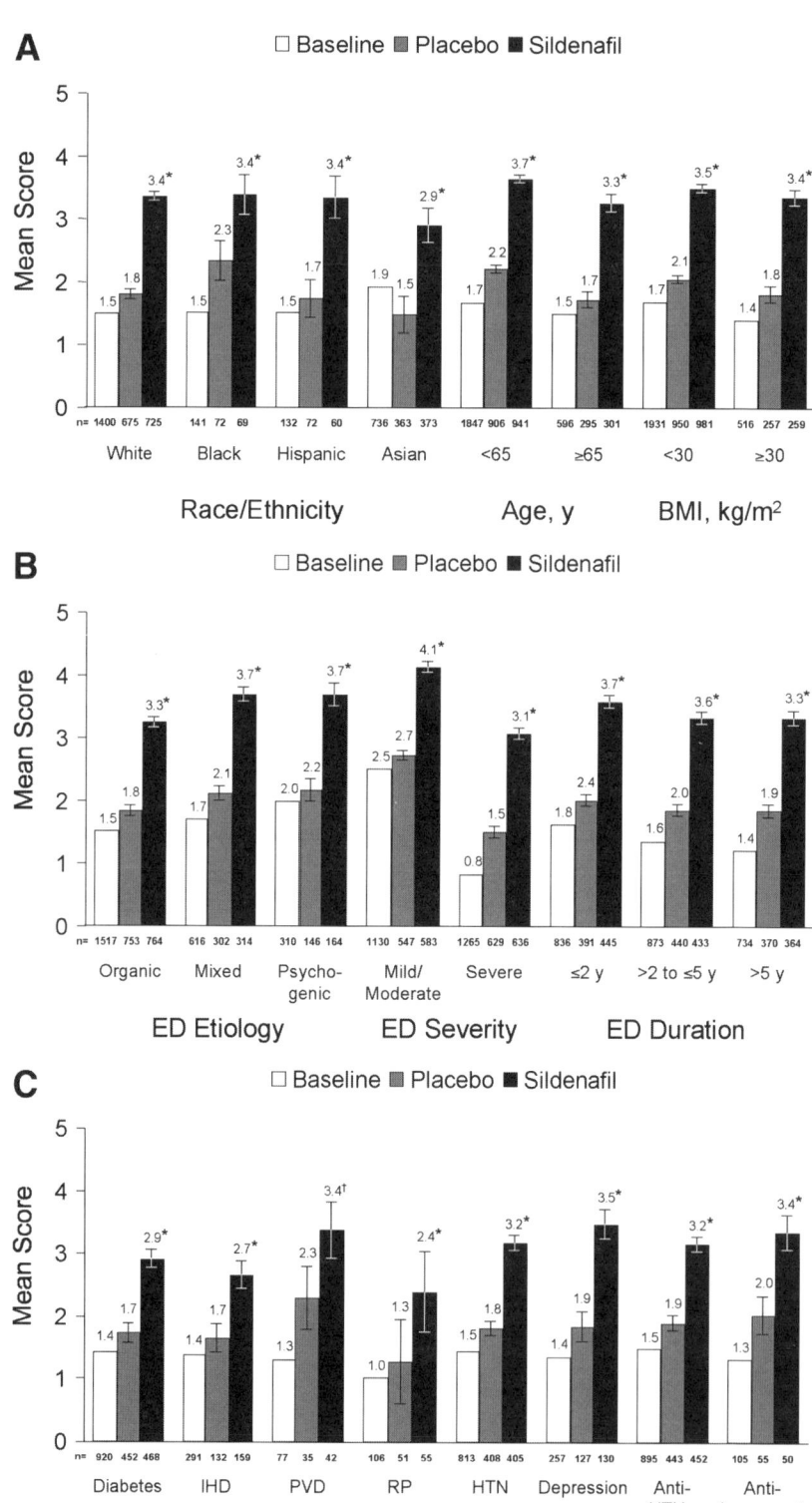

effectiveness were maintained with long-term sildenafil treatment. The remaining 25.3% of patients discontinued for reasons not related to treatment (e.g., nontreatment-related adverse events, lost to follow-up, withdrawn consent, and protocol violations).

The high level of effectiveness of sildenafil in the broad spectrum of patient populations with ED reported in these 11 pooled randomized trials has been mirrored in accounts of sildenafil use in the clinical practice setting *(10–12)*.

Numerous studies have assessed the effectiveness of sildenafil in specific patient populations, particularly populations that have been shown to be at increased risk for ED. The following summaries examine the populations of interest to the readership of this book *(9)*.

ISCHEMIC HEART DISEASE

Like ED, the rate of ischemic heart disease increases with age, escalating from 0.4% for men aged less than 45 yr to 8% for men ages 45–64 yr to 19% for men 65 yr or older *(13)*. Additional shared risk factors for ED and cardiovascular disease include hypertension, diabetes, dyslipidemia, and smoking. A significant correlation between the number of occluded coronary vessels and erectile function in patients with ischemic heart disease has also been demonstrated *(14)*. As in the pooled analysis reported earlier, a favorable response to sildenafil in patients with ischemic heart disease and ED has been observed in other published reports in this patient population. Sildenafil produced a significant improvement in erectile function (GEQ and IIEF Q3 and Q4, $p = 0.0001$) in a double-blind, placebo-controlled trial of sildenafil in men with ED and cardiovascular disease who were receiv-

---

Fig. 2. (*opposite*) Overall baseline mean score and least squares mean ± SE scores at end of treatment for question 4 (ability to maintain erections) of the International Index of Erectile Function. Scores ranged from 1 (never/almost never) to 5 (always/almost always) with a response of 0 indicating "did not attempt sexual intercourse." **A** shows scores for subgroups characterized by patient characteristics, **B** shows scores for subgroups characterized by ED characteristics, and **C** shows scores for subgroups characterized by concomitant medical conditions/medications.

BMI, body mass index; IHD, ischemic heart disease; PVD, peripheral vascular disease; RP, radical prostatectomy; HTN, hypertension; anti-HTNs. antihypertensives. *$p < 0.0001$,† $p < 0.005$.

ED severity categories of mild to moderate (IIEF erectile domain score, 11–25) and severe ED (IIEF erectile domain score, ≤10) (from ref. 9).

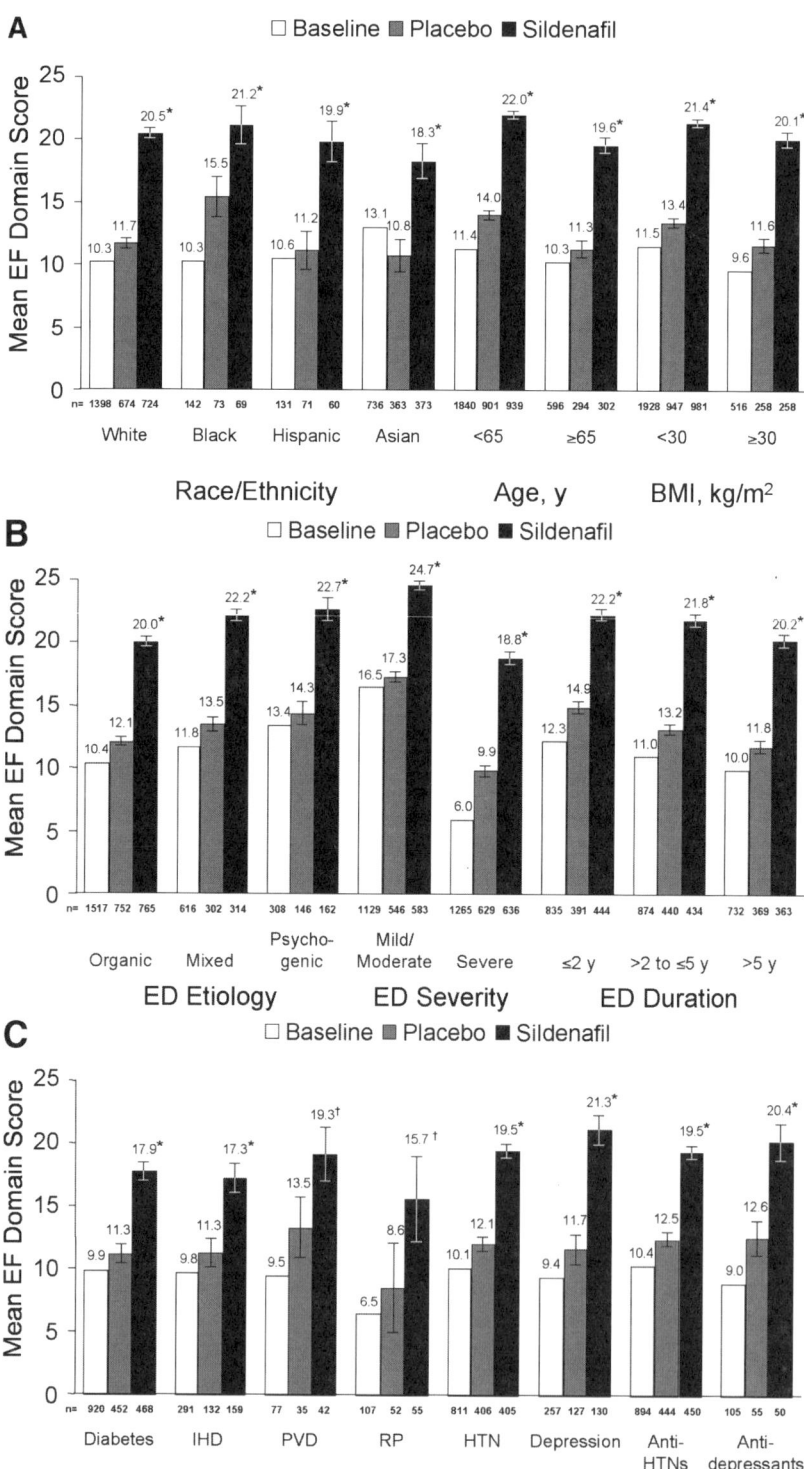

ing β-blockers and/or angiotensin-converting enzyme inhibitors and/or calcium channel blockers, but not nitrates *(15)*. In an earlier subanalysis of patients with ischemic heart disease and ED who received sildenafil (5–200 mg) or placebo for 4 wk to 6 month in nine randomized trials, sildenafil use was associated with significant improvements in all efficacy parameters analyzed (GEQ and IIEF Q3, Q4, and EF domain, $p < 0.0001$; ref. *13*).

Recent guidelines for managing ED in patients with cardiovascular disease emphasize the need to assess the risk of triggering further cardiovascular events with the return to sexual activity *(16)*. Patients considered at low cardiac risk include those who are asymptomatic with fewer than three risk factors for coronary artery disease (CAD) (excluding age and gender), postsuccessful coronary revascularization, or postmyocardial infarction (>6–8 wk) or who have controlled hypertension, mild valvular disease, mild stable angina, or New York Heart Association (NYHA) class I congestive heart failure. The guidelines suggest that all first-line ED therapies, with the exception of sildenafil for patients taking nitrates, may be considered for these patients *(16)*.

A recent study using these guidelines reported a favorable treatment outcome with sildenafil in 70 patients with cardiovascular disease and ED who were assessed and prescribed sildenafil in a cardiac outpatient clinic *(17)*. Patients included 18 men with mild stable angina on medical therapy, 6 with controlled hypertension, 41 who had undergone successful coronary angioplasty or bypass surgery, and 5 with congestive heart failure (NYHA class I/II [$n = 4$]; NYHA class III/IV [$n = 1$]); 10 patients also had diabetes. Sildenafil (50-mg dose in 60; 100-mg

---

Fig. 3. (*opposite*) Overall baseline mean score and least squares mean ± SE scores at end of treatment for the EF domain (questions 1–5 and 15) of the International Index of Erectile Function. Total domain score ranged from 1 to 30; scores for individual questions ranged from 1 (never/almost never) to 5 (always/almost always) with a response of 0 indicating "did not attempt sexual intercourse." **A** shows scores for subgroups characterized by patient characteristics, **B** shows scores for subgroups characterized by ED characteristics, and **C** shows scores for subgroups characterized by concomitant medical conditions/medications.

BMI, body mass index; IHD, ischemic heart disease; PVD, peripheral vascular disease; RP, radical prostatectomy; HTN, hypertension; anti-HTNs, antihypertensives. $*p < 0.0001, †p < 0.001$. [from Carson et al., Urology, 2002] ED severity categories of mild to moderate (IIEF erectile domain score, 11–25) and severe ED (IIEF erectile domain score, ≤10) (from ref. *9*).

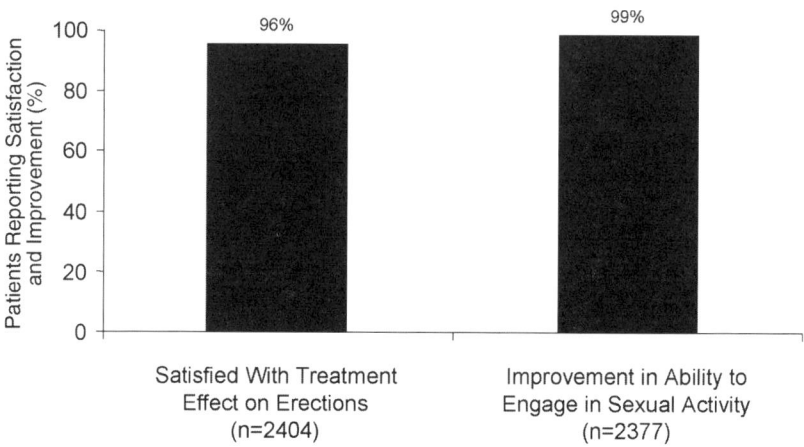

Fig. 4. Patients reporting satisfaction with treatment effect on erections and improvement in ability to engage in sexual activity at end of 1-yr open-label treatment with sildenafil (from ref. 9).

dose in 10) was effective in 67 of these 70 patients. Sildenafil was also generally well tolerated, with only one patient reporting abnormal vision and three patients reporting headache or flushing. No patients reported angina during sexual intercourse.

PERIPHERAL VASCULAR DISEASE

Peripheral vascular disease, also called peripheral arterial disease, an atherosclerotic syndrome resulting in arterial occlusions in vessels other than the coronary or intracranial vascular beds, affects an estimated 8–12 million people in the United States *(18,19)*. Overall, 86% of the men with peripheral vascular disease had some degree of ED, which was quite similar to the high rate of ED reported in 26 of 31 (84%) patients with aorta-iliac occlusive disease *(20)*. Erectile function improved significantly with sildenafil in men with ED and peripheral vascular disease. We noted a twofold increase in mean scores for IIEF Q3, Q4, and EF domain in men with ED and peripheral vascular disease over pretreatment scores with sildenafil.

HYPERTENSION

Both systemic vascular disease and antihypertensive drug therapy are thought to contribute to the increased occurrence of ED in men with hypertension. ED has been reported in an estimated 8–17% of men with untreated hypertension and up to 61% of men receiving antihypertensive therapy. Although most classes of antihypertensive agents

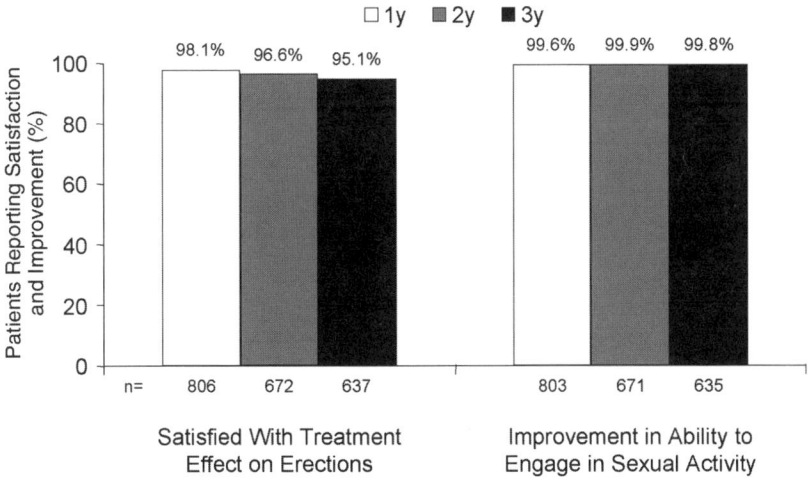

Fig. 5. Patients reporting satisfaction with treatment effect on erections and improvement in ability to engage in sexual activity at end of 1, 2, and 3 yr of open-label treatment with sildenafil (from ref. 9).

have been reported to cause ED, nonselective β-blockers, potassium-sparing and thiazide diuretics, and centrally acting antihypertensives have been most commonly associated with ED *(21)*. Patient compliance with effective antihypertensive therapy may be compromised if sexual function is adversely affected by the medication.

Sildenafil has been found to be effective across all efficacy parameters analyzed in the subgroup of men with a history of hypertension as well as the subgroup of men with ED who were receiving concomitant antihypertensive therapy. An earlier subanalysis of 10 randomized sildenafil trials found sildenafil to be equally effective regardless of whether patients were receiving concomitant antihypertensive therapy or not *(22)*. Sildenafil treatment was also associated with significant increases in the ability to achieve and maintain erections compared with placebo ($p < 0.0001$) in a double-blind, placebo-controlled study in men with ED and stable cardiovascular disease; 83% of these men had hypertension *(15)*. A recently completed double-blind, placebo-controlled trial specifically assessed the efficacy of sildenafil in 562 men with ED who were taking two or more antihypertensive agents (two antihypertensives [$n = 324$], <3 antihypertensives [$n = 235$], and unspecified [$n = 3$]; ref. *23*). Mean scores on IIEF Q3, Q4, and EF domain improved significantly in sildenafil-treated patients compared with placebo-treated patients, significantly more sildenafil-treated patients reported improved erections (71% vs 18% of placebo-treated patients), and significantly more intercourse attempts were successful.

DIABETES

A reported 35–70% of men with diabetes also have ED *(23)*. Compared with men without diabetes, ED occurs at an earlier age *(24)*, and the age-adjusted probability of complete ED is nearly three times higher in men with treated diabetes. Vasculogenic and neurologic abnormalities are believed to be the primary causes for ED in diabetic men *(25)*. Four 12-wk, double-blind, placebo-controlled trials evaluating sildenafil in men with ED and underlying diabetes have been completed *(24–28)*. In the first two trials *(25,28)* 259 and 261 patients were randomized to placebo and sildenafil, respectively. Approximately 20% of patients had Type 1 diabetes, and 80% had Type 2 diabetes. In these studies, 51–56% of sildenafil-treated patients reported improved erections compared with 10–12% of patients randomized to placebo. The ability to achieve and maintain an erection sufficient for intercourse improved, although the mean scores, 2.8–3.2 (1.8–2.0 for placebo) for IIEF Q3 and 2.7–2.9 (1.6–1.7 for placebo) for IIEF Q4, were somewhat lower than that seen in the general clinical trial population of patients with ED *(1)*. The remaining two studies separately evaluated sildenafil in men with ED and Type 2 diabetes *(26)* or Type 1 diabetes *(27)*. The Type 2 diabetes study included 219 patients randomized to receive sildenafil ($n = 110$) or placebo ($n = 109$; ref. 26). After 12 wk of treatment, mean scores for GEQ; IIEF Q3, Q4, and EF domain; and the percentage of successful intercourse attempts had improved significantly for men receiving sildenafil compared with placebo ($p < 0.0001$). Moreover, sildenafil was effective in improving ED even in cases of poor glycemic control or multiple chronic complications. Efficacy was similar in the double-blind, placebo-controlled study of 188 men with Type 1 diabetes and ED *(27)*. The mean scores for IIEF Q3, Q4, GEQ, and the percentage of intercourse attempts that were successful improved significantly from baseline to end of treatment in patients receiving sildenafil compared with those receiving placebo ($p = 0.0001$).

A pooled analysis of these four trials allowed for evaluation of efficacy in subgroups defined by patient age (< 49 yr, 50–64 yr, and >65 yr), ED duration (<2 yr, 2–5 yr, and >5 yr), diabetes duration (Type 1 diabetes [< 20 and >20 yr] and Type 2 diabetes [<10 and >10 yr]), number of diabetic complications (cardiovascular, nephropathy, neuropathy, and retinopathy) and ED severity (mild–moderate or severe; refs. *29* and *30*). Although on-treatment scores for IIEF Q3,

Q4, and EF domain; GEQ; and percentage of intercourse attempts that were successful tended to be lower in patients who were older, who had ED that was severe or of longer duration, or who had diabetes of longer duration or with more complications, no significant differences in treatment effect across subcategories of age, ED duration, and diabetes duration, diabetic complications, and ED severity were found (interaction $p > 0.05$).

Overall Safety Profile of Sildenafil
DOUBLE-BLIND, PLACEBO-CONTROLLED TRIALS

Morales and colleagues *(31)* were the first to extensively evaluate the tolerability of sildenafil in phase II/III clinical trials. In these 18 double-blind, placebo-controlled trials, patients were randomized to receive sildenafil ($n = 2722$) or placebo ($n = 1552$) treatment for up to 6 month. Of the 11 trials where study drug was taken on an "as-needed" basis, five used a fixed-dosing schedule to provide insight on the safety of sildenafil by dose. Six trials used a flexible-dosing regimen whereby the starting dose of study drug (50 mg) could be adjusted to 25 mg or 100 mg based on efficacy and tolerability. Flexible-dosing schedules most closely resemble the dosing patterns used in clinical practice. In these flexible-dose trials, the incidences of the most commonly reported adverse effects (AEs; from all causes) were higher in sildenafil- vs placebo-treated patients. However, AEs were predominantly transient and mild or moderate in severity. In both the sildenafil- and placebo-treated groups, approximately two-thirds of AEs were classified as mild. Discontinuation rates from AEs of all causes were similar in the sildenafil (2.5%) and placebo (2.3%) treatment groups. Headache (1.1%), facial flushing (0.4%), and nausea (0.4%) were the most common AEs, leading to discontinuation in the sildenafil group, and headache (0.4%) was the most common AE, leading to discontinuation in the placebo group.

Overall, the results obtained from pooling data from 18 double-blind, placebo-controlled trials demonstrate that sildenafil is a well-tolerated oral therapy for ED (Table 2). AEs were mostly transient and mild to moderate in severity, and the rate of discontinuations from AEs were low and comparable between patients who received sildenafil and those who received placebo.

In a retrospective analysis of data pooled from 25 double-blind, placebo-controlled trials (18 of which were the phase II/III trials), Osterloh et al. examined the overall efficacy and safety of sildenafil in close to 6000 patients and in more detail among subgroups of patients stratified by existing comorbid conditions such as diabetes, hypertension, and ischemic heart disease (IHD; ref. *32*). The most commonly reported treatment-related AEs for all patients and for specific comorbidities are presented in Table 1. Markedly smaller percentages of sildenafil-treated patients with diabetes reported headaches (7.7%) and facial flushing (7.8%) compared with those for all patients combined (14.6% and 14.1%, respectively). By contrast, slightly larger proportions of sildenafil-treated patients with IHD reported headache (16.9%) and dyspepsia (8.3%) relative to those for the entire population of patients (14.6% and 6.2%, respectively). The proportions of patients reporting visual AEs were similar across sildenafil-treated patient subgroups (3.1–5.2%) and compared with all patients combined (5.2%; ref. *33*). Although these data suggest that patients may tolerate sildenafil differently based on existing comorbid conditions, the discontinuation rates from AEs were low across all subgroups: 1.9% for patients with diabetes, 2.3% in those with hypertension, and 3.6% in patients with IHD. The overall discontinuation rate from AEs was 2%.

OPEN-LABEL EXTENSION STUDIES

Patients who were compliant during the double-blind treatment period were eligible to continue with open-label sildenafil treatment for up to 2 yr. Morales et al. *(31)* reported on the tolerability of sildenafil in 10 open-label studies ($n = 2199$); Steers et al. *(34)* described the safety results from four of these open-label trials ($n = 1008$). In Morales et al. *(31)*, the most frequently reported AEs were mild or moderate and included headache (10%), facial flushing (9%), dyspepsia (6%), and respiratory tract infection (6%). AEs from all causes accounted for 2% of the discontinuations over a 1-yr period, and headache was the most common reason for discontinuation. In a subanalysis by Steers et al, 7% of patients reduced the dose of sildenafil or temporarily discontinued treatment because of AEs *(34)*. Serious adverse events (SAEs) occurred in 7% of patients and two patients died during the study. One patient died of an acute myocardial infarction (MI) (he had had a previous MI); the other died from a malignant melanoma. Neither death was considered treatment related by the investigators *(31)* (Table 3).

Ocular Safety of Sildenafil

Although sildenafil is a potent and selective inhibitor of PDE5, it also has an approximately 10-fold lower affinity for PDE6, which is present in high concentrations in the retina. Given that PDE6 is a key enzyme in the retinal phototransduction process, the overall safety of sildenafil

Table 1
Most Commonly Reported Treatment-Related Adverse Events for All Patients and by Comorbid Condition (8)

Adverse Event	Diabetes n (%)		Hypertension n (%)		IHD n (%)		All Patients n (%)	
	Placebo (n = 585)	Sildenafil (n = 743)	Placebo (n = 654)	Sildenafil (n = 928)	Placebo (n = 220)	Sildenafil (n = 362)	Placebo (n = 2373)	Sildenafil (n = 3545)
Headache	14 (2.4)	57 (7.7)	14 (2.1)	112 (12.1)	6 (2.7)	61 (16.9)	78 (3.3)	519 (14.6)
Facial flushing	9 (1.5)	58 (7.8)	21 (3.2)	119 (12.8)	1 (0.5)	49 (13.5)	44 (1.9)	499 (14.1)
Dyspepsia	7 (0.3)	38 (5.1)	3 (0.5)	50 (5.4)	1 (0.5)	30 (8.3)	17 (0.7)	221 (6.2)
Abnormal vision	1 (0.2)	23 (3.1)	2 (0.3)	47 (5.1)	3 (1.4)	19 (5.2)	8 (0.3)	185 (5.2)
Dizziness	4 (0.7)	9 (1.2)	10 (1.5)	23 (2.5)	0 (0.0)	5 (1.4)	25 (1.1)	79 (2.2)
Rhinitis	2 (0.3)	11 (1.5)	2 (0.3)	26 (2.8)	0 (0.0)	6 (1.7)	4 (0.2)	93 (2.6)

IHD, ischemic heart disease.
Adapted from Padma-Nathan et al., Urology, 2002.

Table 2
Most Commonly Reported Adverse Events After 3 Yr of Open-Label Sildenafil Treatment (8)

Adverse Event[a]	Treatment Related n (%)	Not Treatment Related n (%)	Total n (%)
Coronary artery disease	0 (0.0)	19 (2.0)	19 (2.0)
Prostate disorder	0 (0.0)	12 (1.3)	12 (1.3)
Dyspepsia	9 (0.9)	2 (0.2)	11 (1.2)
Carcinoma	0 (0.0)	9 (0.9)	9 (0.9)
Headache	9 (0.9)	0 (0.0)	9 (0.9)
Myocardial infarction	1 (0.1)	7 (0.8)	8 (0.8)
Abnormal vision	4 (0.4)	0 (0.0)	4 (0.4)
Facial flushing	4 (0.4)	0 (0.0)	4 (0.4)
Rhinitis	3 (0.3)	0 (0.0)	3 (0.3)
Congestive heart failure	0 (0.0)	2 (0.2)	2 (0.2)

[a]Serious adverse events and observed or volunteered adverse events that resulted in a change in sildenafil dose or a temporary/permanent discontinuation. Incidence rate was calculated using the total number of patients assessed for safety ($n = 955$).

in the visual system has been evaluated extensively in preclinical and clinical trials during the drug's development and in other well-designed studies conducted after sildenafil was approved for marketing.

CLINICAL STUDIES

Morales et al. (31) showed that, in the fixed-dose series of studies, the incidences of all causality and treatment-related abnormal vision were dose related, ranging from 1.0% at 25 mg to 11.1% at 100 mg of sildenafil for visual AEs from all causes, and from 0.3–10.7%, respectively, for treatment-related AEs. The majority of all visual AEs were mild or moderate in severity; only five patients reported SAEs. Only one patient discontinued treatment solely because of abnormal vision. In the flexible-dose series, 2.7% of sildenafil- and 0.4% of placebo-treated patients reported abnormal vision (e.g., blue "haze" around objects, decreased color discrimination, increased brightness of light) that were transient and dose related (data on file, Pfizer). Overall, results from Phase I/II/III acute treatment studies have demonstrated that there are mild, transient, and reversible changes in blue/green color discrimination. There were no clinically significant effects on visual

Table 3
Discontinuations by Year During 3 Yr of Open-Label Sildenafil Treatment

	Number of discontinuations (%)[a]			
	Yr 1	Yr 2	Yr 3	Total
Treatment related				
Insufficient response	23 (2.4)	17 (1.7)	16 (1.6)	56 (5.7)
Adverse event	5 (0.5)	3 (0.3)	2 (0.2)	10 (1.0)
Total	28 (2.9)	20 (2.0)	18 (1.8)	66 (6.7)
Not treatment related				
Adverse event	30 (3.1)	14 (1.4)	13 (1.3)	57 (5.8)
Lost to follow-up	21 (2.1)	17 (1.7)	18 (1.8)	56 (5.7)
Study violation	14 (1.4)	9 (0.9)	5 (0.5)	28 (2.9)
Withdrawn consent	17 (1.7)	16 (1.6)	16 (1.6)	49 (5.0)
Death	1 (0.1)	3 (0.3)	2 (0.2)	6 (0.6)
Other	29 (3.0)	11 (1.1)	12 (1.2)	52 (5.3)
Total	112 (11.5)	70 (7.2)	66 (6.7)	248 (25.3)
Grand Total	140 (14.3)	90 (9.2)	84 (8.6)	314 (32.1)

[a]Percentages were calculated using the total number of patients enrolled ($n = 97$).

function tests that included visual acuity, electroretinograms, intraocular pressure, and pupillometry *(35–37)*.

In long-term, open-label studies of up to 2 yr in duration, the overall incidence of abnormal vision remained low (2%), and there were no cumulative changes in visual function or structures in the eye *(38,39)*. Moreover, none of the patients discontinued because of visual AEs even after 2 yr of extended treatment. During the long-term, 3-yr, open-label treatment study, patients reported only four (<1%) occurrences (i.e., SAEs or AEs resulting in a dosage change) of visual disturbances and one (0.1%) patient reported conjunctivitis. Two events each were reported during the first and second years; there were no visual AEs during the third year. Thus, with up to 4 yr of sildenafil treatment, the occurrence of significant visual events has remained low.

POSTMARKETING CASE SERIES AND REPORTS

There have been rare reports (five cases) of patients who developed nonarteritic anterior ischemic optic neuropathy (NAION) after taking sildenafil *(40)*. Three of the patients developed NAION after using sildenafil for the first time; two others had been using sildenafil periodically for 1–2 yr. All five patients had optic discs with a small cup-to-disc ratio (e.g., 0.1). This anatomical configuration is more common in patients with NAION and has been implicated in the pathogenesis of the neuropathy. The investigators acknowledged that a definite causal relationship between sildenafil and NAION cannot be established given the large number of prescriptions that have been written for sildenafil and the overlap in the patient populations that are at risk for NAION and are also likely to be taking sildenafil.

In terms of special patient populations, there have been no reports of increased visual AEs in patients with diabetes, or preexisting eye disorders, including glaucoma and macular degeneration (41).

SUMMARY

Findings from the combined analysis of 11 double-blind trials of sildenafil in men with ED and a field experience in over 20 million men confirm the positive efficacy and safety profile of sildenafil. There are over 1500 published peer-reviewed articles and abstracts on sildenafil supporting the evidenced-based conclusion that it is the first-line therapy for men with ED until otherwise proven. Therefore, unless a patient has a specific contraindication (e.g., nitrate use), a trial with sildenafil is appropriate for virtually every patients presenting with ED.

NEW PDE5 INHIBITORS: EFFICACY, SAFETY, AND COMPARATIVE PERSPECTIVES

Similar to sildenafil, both vardenafil and tadalafil are both potent PDE5 inhibitors. They all have a contraindication in men receiving organic nitrates. The biochemical potency of a PDE5 inhibitor is described by its IC50—the concentration of the enzyme necessary to inhibit 50% of the enzyme activity. The IC50 of all three PDE5 inhibitors is within the same range of 1–10 nM. However, vardenafil appears to be more potent within this range (42,43). Regardless, the three appear to have equal clinical efficacy. In addition, sildenafil and vardenafil appear to demonstrate some mild PDE6 inhibitory properties at high doses. This is associated with mild transient visual disturbances and, at least in the case of sildenafil, is not associated with any significant acute or chronic effect in men with normal visual function or in men with macular degeneration, treated glaucoma, or non-proliferative diabetic retinopathy. Tadalafil is a PDE11 inhibitor. PDE11 is found in the anterior pituitary, testes, prostate and heart. It is unresolved as to whether PDE11 inhibition will cause alterations in sperm function or, more importantly, whether it will increase inotropism and myocardial oxygen consumption.

Vardenafil

Vardenafil is a potent selective PDE5 inhibitor. It is contraindicated in men taking organic nitrates *(44)*. A North American, phase 3, multicenter, randomized, double-blind, placebo-controlled, four-arm, parallel-group comparison of vardenafil 5, 10, and 20 mg vs placebo was recently published *(44)*. In this study, similar to sildenafil, patients were instructed to take study medication approx 1 h before intended sexual intercourse. Vardenafil is both chemically and pharmacologically nearly identical to sildenafil. It has a similar pharmacokinetic, efficacy and safety profile. This study consisted of 805 men at 54 study centers who completed baseline evaluations and were randomized to treatment with either placebo (n = 197) or vardenafil 5 mg (n = 205), 10 mg (n = 206), or 20 mg (n = 197). Over the course of 26 wk of therapy, 37% of all patients (297 of 805) discontinued. Of patients randomized to placebo, 54% discontinued, most commonly because of insufficient therapeutic effect (20%). Of patients randomized to vardenafil, 31% discontinued, most commonly because they were lost to follow-up (9%). Overall, patients were diagnosed with ED a mean of 3.6 yr before screening and experienced symptoms of ED an average of 2.3 yr before the clinical diagnosis was made. Sildenafil had been used previously by 71% (544 of 762), all of whom experienced improved erections during this treatment. Only 15 of 256 screening failures were caused by failure to respond to sildenafil. The following were observed medical conditions at screening: hypertension (37%), pure hypercholesterolemia (24%), and Type 2 diabetes.

Successful penetration increased from 40.9% at baseline to 80.5% at wk 12, and the ability to maintain an erection for successful intercourse increased from 14.7% at baseline to 64.5% at wk 12. All groups showed continued improvements vs baseline throughout the 26-wk treatment period, and differences between scores for placebo-treated patients and those randomized to vardenafil remained significant at all time points.

SIDE EFFECTS

In general, treatment with vardenafil was well tolerated *(44)* Most of the side effects were mild or moderate in intensity. The most commonly reported side effects associated with 20 mg vardenafil are headaches (18%), and flushing. Visual changes occurred in less than 2% of patients. There was a trend toward a greater decrease in blood pressure with vardenafil 10 mg and 20 mg than with placebo and vardenafil 5 mg. Nevertheless, mean blood pressure decreases in patients taking 5, 10, or 20 mg vardenafil were small, ranging from −3.6 to −6.6 mm Hg for supine SBP, −3.5 to −6.5 mm Hg for standing SBP, −3.5 to −4.8 mm Hg for supine DBP, and −2.1 to −4.5 mm Hg for standing DBP. It is expected, because of its chemical and pharmacological similarity to sildenafil, vardenafil will have similar cardiovascular effects, particularly with respect to central hemodynamics.

Tadalafil

Tadalafil (Cialis, Lilly ICOS LLC Bethel, WA) is a potent selective phosphodiesterase type 5 inhibitor with a mean terminal half-life of 17.5 h (20 h in men over age 65 yr). This is its distinguishing characteristic along with its PDE11 inhibitory properties. Recently, an integrated analysis of five randomized, double-blind, placebo-controlled, parallel group trials involving 1112 men conducted at 74 centers was published *(45)*. Patients were instructed to self-administer treatment as needed before sexual intercourse with no restrictions on food or timing of sexual intercourse. Men receiving organic nitrates were excluded. Mean patient age was 59 yr (range, 22–82). Hypertension was present in 30% of men, and 21% had diabetes.

EFFICACY AND SIDE EFFECTS

The proportion of successfully completed sexual attempts was 75% in men receiving 20 mg tadalafil compared with 32% on placebo. The most frequently reported side effects for the 20 mg tadalafil dose were headache (20%) and dyspepsia (17%), followed by back pain (9%), nasal congestion (5%), myalgia (7%), and flushing (5%). These events were mostly mild or moderate. One tadalafil-treated patient (0.1%) reported an episode of abnormal color vision *(45)*. Tadalafil is a mild vasodilator and may decrease systemic blood pressure accordingly. Publications regarding its effects on central hemodynamics, including coronary blood flow, left ventricular contractility, and myocardial oxygen consumption, are not yet available. This is a critical issue in light of its PDE11inhibitory properties.

EUROPEAN LABELING CONTRAINDICATIONS

Tadalafil has recently been approved in Europe. The current European labeling indications reflect this concern regarding the absence of data on its direct effect on the myocardium. It is not only contraindicated in men receiving organic nitrates but also in men with a unstable angina or angina occurring during intercourse, a recent MI (within 90 d) or stroke (within 5 month), uncontrolled hypertension, uncontrolled arrhythmias, uncontrolled hypotension, or the patients with Class II–IV (NYHA) congestive heart failure. In addition, because the inclusion criteria for the trials included men only in the low-risk profile of the Princeton Guidelines, it is suggested by the author that men with three or more risk factors (excluding gender and age) be evaluated by exercise treadmill testing before tadalafil use or that they receive sildenafil instead.

COMPARATIVE PERSPECTIVES ON THE THREE PDE5 INHIBITORS

It would appear that vardenafil is identical to sildenafil in clinically meaningful terms—it is identical with respect to efficacy, adverse event profile, and pharmacokinetics. Tadalafil is a longer-acting PDE5 inhibitor with PDE11 inhibitory properties. The effect of chronic PDE11 inhibition on subfertile men and on the heart remains to be determined in future studies. The duration of action of tadalafil appears to be at least 36 h *(46)* but, in fact, this one distinguishing property has not been examined further. It is probably true that it is effective for three half-lives (60 h) but also may have nitrate interaction for five half-lives or 100 h (men over 65 yr). Thus, tadalafil may also be inappropriate for men that are infrequently sexually active. It may be more suited for chronic dosing than for on-demand therapy where rapid action, such as associated with sildenafil, is needed. Only extensive field experience will tell if these new compounds will fare as well as sildenafil. Regardless, these new entrants in the class will offer more therapeutic options for our patients and should further expand the practice of sexual medicine.

CONCLUSION

The current management of ED has been revolutionized by the advent of oral medical therapy. The evidence-based support for first-line therapy is in favor of PDE5 inhibitors, and within this class the greatest efficacy, safety, and field experience would support sildenafil as the therapy of choice.

REFERENCES

1. Goldstein I, Lue TF, Padma-Nathan H, et al: Oral sildenafil in the treatment of erectile dysfunction. N Engl J Med 1998;338:1397–1404.
2. Jardin A, Wagner G, Khoury S, et al.,eds. Erectile Dysfunction, First International Consultation in Erectile Dysfunction. Health Publications Inc. Paris. 2000.

3. Giuliano F, Allard J. Apomorphine SL (Uprima1): preclinical and clinical experiences learned from the first central nervous system-acting ED drug. Int J Impot Res 2002;14(Suppl 1)S53–S56.
4. Abbott Laboratories. Uprima (apomorphine hydrochloride) Product Monograph. Abbott Urology International, 2001.
5. Linet OM, Ogrinc FG, Alprostadil Study Group. Efficacy and safety of intracavernosal alprostadil in men with erectile dysfunction. N Engl J Med 1996;334: 873–877.
6. Padma-Nathan H, Hellstrom WJ, Kaiser FE, et al. and the MUSE Study Group. Treatment of men with erectile dysfunction with transurethral alprostadil. N Engl J Med 1997;336:1–7.
7. Padma-Nathan H, Steidel C, Salem S, et al. The efficacy and safety of a topical alprostadil cream, Alprox-TD, for the treatment of erectile dysfunction: two Phase 2 studies in mild-to-moderate and severe ED. Int J Impot Res 2003;15:10–17.
8. Padma-Nathan H, guest ed. Sildenafil citrate (Viagra) and erectile dysfunction: a comprehensive four year update on efficacy, safety, and management options. Urology 2002;60:(Suppl):1–90.
9. Carson CC, Burnett AL, Levine LA, et al. The efficacy of sildenafil citrate (Viagra) in clinical populations: an update. Urology 2002;60:12–27.
10. Marks LS, Duda C, Dorey FJ. Treatment of erectile dysfunction with sildenafil. Urology 1999;53:19–24.
11. Guay AT, Perez JB, Jacobson J, et al: Efficacy and safety of sildenafil citrate for treatment of erectile dysfunction in a population with associated organic risk factors [published correction appears in J Androl 2002;23:113]. J Androl 2001;22: 793–797.
12. Jarow JP, Burnett AL, Geringer AM. Clinical efficacy of sildenafil citrate based on etiology and response to prior treatment. J Urol 1999;162:722–725.
13. Conti CR, Pepine CR, Sweeney M. Efficacy and safety of sildenafil citrate in the treatment of erectile dysfunction in patients with ischemic heart disease. Am J Cardiol 1999;83(Suppl 5A):29C–34C.
14. Greenstein A, Chen J, Matzkin H, et al. Does severity of ischemic coronary disease correlate with erectile function? Int J Impot Res 1997;9:123–126.
15. Olsson AM, Persson CA, and Swedish Sildenafil Investigators Group. Efficacy and safety of sildenafil citrate for the treatment of erectile dysfunction in men with cardiovascular disease. Int J Clin Pract 2001;55:171–176.
16. DeBusk R, Drory Y, Goldstein I, et al. Management of sexual dysfunction in patients with cardiovascular disease: recommendations of the Princeton Consensus Panel. Am J Cardiol 2000;86:175–181.
17. Jackson G. Sildenafil (Viagra) and cardiac patients: an open outpatient study. Heart 2001;85(Suppl I):P42.
18. Ouriel K. Detection of peripheral arterial disease in primary care. JAMA 2001; 286:1380–1381.
19. Hirsch AT, Criqui MH, Treat-Jacobson D, et al. Peripheral arterial disease detection, awareness, and treatment in primary care. JAMA 2001;286:1317–1324.
20. Cormio L, Edgren J, Lepantalo M, et al. Aortofemoral surgery and sexual function. Eur J Vasc Endovasc Surg 1996;11:453–457.
21. Keene LC, Davies PH. Drug-related erectile dysfunction. Adverse Drug React Toxicol Rev 1999;18:5–24.
22. Kloner RA, Brown M, Prisant LM, et al. Effect of sildenafil in patients with erectile dysfunction taking antihypertensive therapy. Sildenafil Study Group. Am J Hypertens 2001;14:70–73.

23. Mancia G, Pickering TG, Glasser DB, et al. Efficacy of VIAGRA® (sildenafil citrate) in men with erectile dysfunction and arterial hypertension who are taking multiple antihypertensive treatments. Presented at the17th Annual Scientific Meeting of the American Society of Hypertension; New York, NY; May 15–18, 2002.
24. Hirsch IB, Korenman SG, Stecher V, et al. Viagra (sildenafil citrate): efficacy and safety in the treatment of erectile dysfunction (ED) in men with diabetes. Diabetes 1999;48(Suppl):A–90.
25. De Berardis G, Franciosi M, Belfiglio M, et al. Erectile dysfunction and quality of life in type 2 diabetic patients: a serious problem too often overlooked. Diabetes Care 2002;25:284–291.
26. Boulton AJ, Selam JL, Sweeney M, et al. Sildenafil citrate for the treatment of erectile dysfunction in men with type II diabetes mellitus. Diabetologia 2001;44:1296–1301.
27. Murphy L, Stuckey B, Jadzinsky MN, et al. Efficacy of sildenafil citrate for erectile dysfunction in men with type I diabetes mellitus. Diabetes 2001;50 (Suppl 2):A99.
28. Rendell MS, Rajfer J, Wicker P, et al. Sildenafil for the treatment of erectile dysfunction in men with diabetes. JAMA 1999;281:421–426.
29. Korenman SG, Siegel RL, Stecher VJ, et al. Efficacy of sildenafil citrate in men with erectile dysfunction and diabetes mellitus: effect of patient age and disease duration. Presented at the 83rd Annual Meeting of the Endocrine Society; Denver, Colorado; June 20–23, 2001.
30. Korenman SG, Wohlhuter C, Sweeney M, et al. Sildenafil citrate for the treatment of erectile dysfunction in men with diabetes mellitus: stratification by diabetic complications. Presented at 83rd Annual Meeting of the Endocrine Society; Denver, Colorado; June 20–23, 2001.
31. Morales A, Gingell C, Collins M, et al. Clinical safety of oral sildenafil citrate (VIAGRA) in the treatment of erectile dysfunction. Int J Impot Res 1998;10:69–74.
32. Osterloh I, Gillies H, Siegel R, et al. Efficacy and safety of VIAGRA® (sildenafil citrate). Presented at: 4th Congress of the European Society for Sexual and Impotence Research, Rome, Italy, September 30-October 3, 2001.
33. Christiansen E, Guirguis WR, Cox D, et al. Long-term efficacy and safety of oral Viagra (sildenafil citrate) in men with erectile dysfunction and the effect of randomised treatment withdrawal. Int J Impot Res 2000;12:177–182.
34. Steers W, Guay AT, Leriche A, et al. Assessment of the efficacy and safety of Viagra (sildenafil citrate) in men with erectile dysfunction during long-term treatment. Int J Impot Res 2001;13:261–267.
35. Laties A, Ellis P, Mollon JD. The effects of sildenafil citrate (Viagra) on color discrimination in volunteers and patients with erectile dysfunction. Invest Ophthalmol Vis Sci 1999;40:S693.
36. Laties A, Ellis P, Koppiker N, et al. Visual function testing in patients and healthy volunteers receiving Viagra. Ophthalmic Res 1998;30(Suppl 1):177.
37. Yajima T, Yajima Y, Koppiker N, et al. No clinically important effects on intraocular pressure after short-term administration of sildenafil citrate (VIAGRA). Am J Ophthalmol 2000;129:675–676.
38. Laties A, Koppiker N, Smith M. Characterization of visual adverse events after dosing with sildenafil citrate. Invest Ophthalmol Vis Sci 2000;41:S592.
39. Zrenner E, Koppiker NP, Smith MD, et al. The effects of long-term sildenafil treatment on ocular safety in patients with erectile dysfunction. Invest Ophthalmol Vis Sci 2000;41:S592.

40. Pomeranz H, Smith K, Hart WJ, et al. Sildenafil-associated nonarteritic anterior ischemic optic neuropathy. Ophthalmology 2002;109:584–587.
41. Laties A, Fraunfelder FT. Ocular safety of Viagra (sildenafil citrate). Trans Am Optahal Soc 1999; 97 115–125.
42. Bishoff E, et al. The inhibitory selectivity of bovine and human recombinant phosphodiesterase isoenzymes. Int J Impot Res 2001;13(Suppl4):41.
43. Angulo J, et al. Characterization of vardenafil, a new PDE5 inhibitor for erectile dysfunction, and comparison of activity with sildenafil. Int J Impot Res 2001; 13(Suppl 4):24.
44. Hellstrom WJG, Gittleman M, Karlin G, et al. Vardenafil for treatment of men with erectile dysfunction: Efficacy and safety in a randomized, double-blind, placebo-controlled trial. J Androl 2002;23:763–771.
45. Brock GB, McMahon CG, Chen KK, et al. Efficacy and safety of tadalafil for the treatment of erectile dysfunction: results of an integrated analysis. J Urol 2002; 168:1332–1336.
46. Padma-Nathan H, Rosen RC, Shabsigh R, et al. Tadalafil (IC351) provides prompt response and extended period of responsiveness for the treatment of men with erectile dysfunction (ED). Annual meeting of the AUA, 2001, Anaheim, CA.

6 Sildenafil Citrate and the Nitric Oxide/Cyclic Guanosine Monophosphate Signaling Pathway

Ian H. Osterloh, MRCP, and Stephen C. Phillips, PhD

CONTENTS

INTRODUCTION
NO/cGMP SIGNALING PATHWAY
PDE5 INHIBITION BY SILDENAFIL
CONCLUSION
REFERENCES

INTRODUCTION

Cyclic nucleotides (cAMP and cGMP) play pivotal roles in a vast array of intracellular signaling pathways. Until the 1990s, cylic adenosine monophosphate (cAMP) was thought to be the most important cyclic nucleotide involved in regulation of smooth muscle activity in the cardiovascular and other organ systems. However, in the mid-to-late 1980s, scientists at Sandwich (the European Research Center of Pfizer Inc.) developed an interest in cyclic guanosine monophosphate (cGMP), which is now recognized as an important intracellular messenger that initiates complex signaling cascades, thereby regulating diverse physiological processes, such as vascular smooth muscle tone, homeostasis of

From: *Contemporary Cardiology: Heart Disease and Erectile Dysfunction*
Edited by: R. A. Kloner © Humana Press Inc., Totowa, NJ

intestinal fluid and electrolytes, and phototransduction in the retina *(1,2)*. Cellular levels of cGMP are controlled by the relative activities of guanylyl cyclases, which catalyze the synthesis of cGMP from guanosine triphosphate (GTP), and secondly by phosphodiesterases (PDEs), which hydrolyze cGMP to GMP. Nitric oxide (NO), a potent activator of soluble guanylyl cyclases (sGCs), is a central component of the cGMP-signaling pathway (Fig. 1). Other stimuli, such as atrial natriuretic peptide, can elevate cGMP by stimulating membrane bound guanylyl cyclase *(3,4)*.

Nitrates directly elevate cGMP levels. This underlies their vascular smooth muscle relaxation and antianginal effects *(5)*. However, agents that directly raise NO levels could cause unwanted problems as a result of increased free radical formation *(6)*. Furthermore, the clinical utility of nitrates is limited by numerous factors, including the development of tachyphylaxis *(7)*. Although the mechanism of induction of tachyphylaxis still is not resolved fully, scientists in Sandwich hypothesized that if they could develop an agent that worked further down the NO/cGMP pathway, that is, an agent that directly elevated cGMP levels without affecting NO levels, then it could have the beneficial properties associated with nitrates but, perhaps, without inducing tachyphylaxis.

In the mid-1980s, five families of PDEs were characterized, and a program was started to assess the feasibility of developing a potent and selective inhibitor of cGMP-specific phosphodiesterase type-5 (PDE5; *8*). PDE5 was chosen as the target because it was known to be present in vascular smooth muscle and in platelets. In theory, a selective inhibitor of PDE5 should elevate cGMP levels in both locations, resulting in vasodilatory effects and inhibition of platelet aggregation, properties that could be useful in treating various cardiovascular conditions, including angina.

In 1989, UK-92,480, now better known as sildenafil citrate (Viagra; Pfizer Inc., New York, NY), was synthesized in Sandwich; laboratory studies showed it to be a potent and selective inhibitor of PDE5 *(8)*. With the initial lead indication as angina, clinical development commenced in 1991 with single-dose healthy volunteer trials. These were fairly uneventful, although at doses of 150 mg and 200 mg, some minor and transient visual side effects were reported. Subsequent investigations (*see* "Vision") revealed these side effects to be the result of a weak inhibitory effect of sildenafil on PDE6, a cGMP-specific PDE exclusively located in photoreceptor cells. However, during the seventh clinical trial, in which healthy volunteers received placebo or various doses of sildenafil three times per day for 10 consecutive days, erections were reported as an adverse event *(8)*.

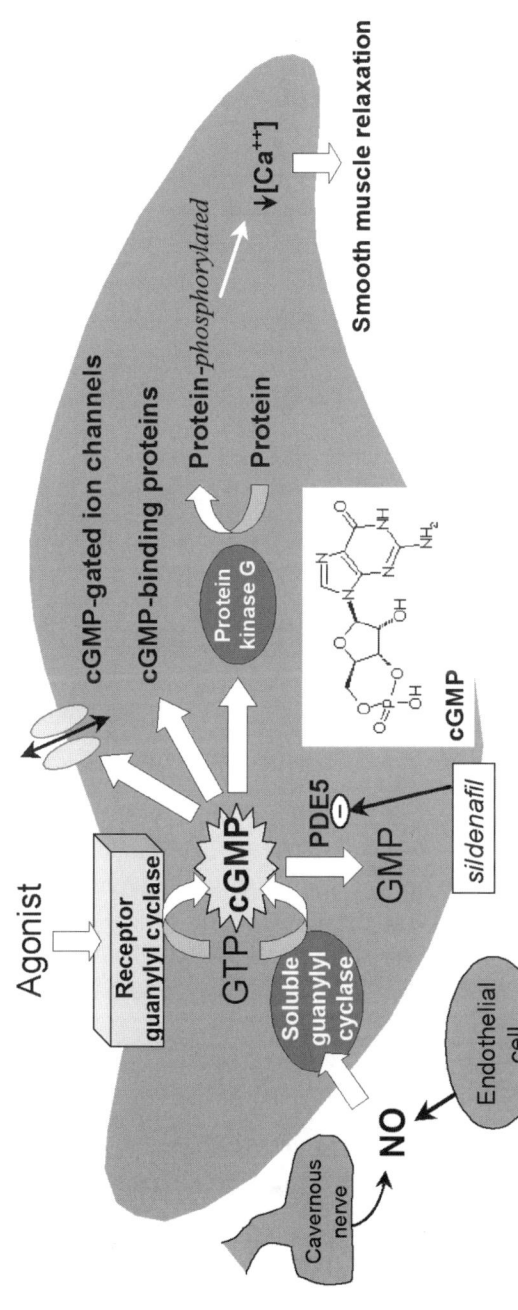

Fig. 1. The NO/cGMP signaling pathway showing stimuli promoting synthesis of cGMP, downstream intracellular signaling targets modulated by cGMP, and role of PDEs in cGMP breakdown. This pathway mediates relaxation of vascular smooth muscle and penile erection. PDE5 is the target for sildenafil and other PDE5 inhibitors in the treatment of ED. NO, nitric oxide; PDE, phosphodiesterase; cGMP, cyclic guanosine monophosphate; GMP, guanosine monophosphate; GTP, guanosine triphosphate.

It was not immediately obvious that such observations would have important clinical findings because the drug regimen producing this effect was quite intensive. Moreover, increased erectile activity in young healthy males would not necessarily translate into an ability to increase erectile response in older men with various medical illnesses affecting the health of blood vessels and the integrity of nerves.

However, simultaneously, Ignarro and others were reporting that NO is the neurotransmitter released from cavernous nerves during sexual stimulation *(9)*, and NO diffuses into smooth muscle cells of the penis, stimulating the production of cGMP and leading to corpus cavernosum smooth muscle relaxation, vasocongestion, and erection *(10,11)*. It remained to be shown that PDE5 was present in the smooth muscle of the corpus cavernosum, but the Pfizer team assumed this must be true if the erections reported in the volunteer study were drug-related. Moreover, the publication by Ignarro et al. was important because it indicated that if sildenafil was indeed facilitating the erectile response, then sexual stimulation was a prerequisite for this drug effect. The role of sexual stimulation probably explains the absence of reports of erections in earlier studies and had important implications for the design of clinical studies in men with ED.

In 1993, the first pilot study of sildenafil in men with ED was started, and, in late 1994, sildenafil entered phase IIB clinical trials. Sildenafil was first approved for the treatment of ED in 1998 and, interestingly, after a few years on the market and further preclinical and clinical studies, not only is PDE5 inhibition firmly established as a treatment of ED but there is renewed interest in the potential of PDE5 inhibition as a possible therapeutic approach to a number of cardiovascular conditions. The remainder of this chapter focuses on the mechanism of action of sildenafil in relation to the NO/cGMP signaling pathway and the relevance of this mechanism to erectile function.

NO/CGMP SIGNALING PATHWAY

Nitric Oxide

Organic nitrates have been a mainstay in the symptomatic management of coronary artery disease (CAD) since Brunton and Murrell used them to relieve angina in Britain in the mid-1800s *(12)*. The organic nitrates mediate hemodynamic and antianginal actions via vasodilation of capacitance veins and conductive arteries *(7)*. However, a century passed before it was determined that NO, liberated after denitration of the organic nitrate prodrug, was the active moiety in organic nitrates *(13)*.

ENDOGENOUS SYNTHESIS

From the 1980s onward, the endothelium began to be recognized not simply as a passive internal lining of blood vessels but for its active ability to modulate the tone of the adjacent smooth muscle by secreting a chemical signal. The chemical factor was known originally as endothelium-derived relaxing factor because of its source and vascular smooth muscle relaxation activity *(14)*, but in 1987 it was recognized that NO and endothelium-derived relaxing factor were one and the same entity *(15,16)*.

NO is produced by the catalytic actions of NO synthase (NOS) on the substrate L-arginine. There are three types of NOS: two calcium-dependent, low-output enzymes (type I or neurogenic [nNOS] and type III or endothelial, constitutive [eNOS]) and a calcium-independent, high-output enzyme (type II or inducible [iNOS]; *17*). All three isoforms have been found in vascular smooth muscle cells, depending on the blood vessel type *(18)*. In the corpus cavernosum of the human penis, the cavernous nerves express nNOS, and eNOS and iNOS are present in smooth muscle cells *(19,20)* and endothelial cells *(21)*.

PHYSIOLOGICAL EFFECTS

NO diffuses rapidly across cell membranes. Some of the many biochemically transformed species of NO are highly reactive and include transition metals such as hemoglobin (Fe^{2+})–NO and oxygen superoxide, which produces the potent and toxic oxidant peroxynitrite *(6)*. However, most of the nonlytic effects of NO are mediated by cGMP. In the NO/cGMP signaling pathway, released NO helps to regulate blood flow and blood pressure through actions on vascular smooth muscle; it is also involved in inhibition of platelet aggregation and adhesion and probably in inhibition of vascular smooth muscle proliferation *(5)*.

The use of NOS antagonists, such as *N*-monomethyl-L-arginine, helps to elucidate some of the physiological effects of NO. Inhibition of NO synthesis with an NOS antagonist increases total peripheral resistance and mean arterial pressure and decreases heart rate and cardiac index *(22–24)*. Interestingly, in earlier studies using animal models, small doses of NOS inhibitors inhibited erections *(25)*.

Guanylyl Cyclases

Guanylyl cyclases are a family of membrane-bound or soluble enzymes that catalyze the conversion of GTP to cGMP *(3,4)*. They respond to diverse signals, including peptide ligands and changes in intracellular calcium concentrations. However, NO is the chief activator of sGC (Fig. 1; *26*). sGC is found in the cytoplasm of almost all mammalian cells, and NO binds directly to the heme group of sGC to form a ferrous-nitrosyl-heme complex (Fig. 2; *2*). cGMP and pyrophosphate are the sole products of catalysis of GTP *(27)*.

Cyclic Guanosine Monophosphate

CELL SIGNALING

cGMP interacts with cGMP-dependent protein kinases (PKGs), cGMP-regulated ion channels, and cGMP-regulated PDEs (Fig. 1; *1*). Increased availability of intracellular cGMP has different physiological and functional outcomes depending on the type, combination, and intracellular localization of cGMP targets and on the cGMP-metabolizing activity of PDEs *(2)*. This complex interaction of cellular processes involves multiple intracellular signaling pathways, "crosstalk" between pathways, and feedback loops, which gives rise to a great diversity of responses that can be cell and tissue specific. cGMP signaling to protein kinases and ion channels is discussed below, and the interaction of cGMP with PDEs is discussed in "Substrate Selectivity."

Protein kinases catalyze the phosphorylation of target proteins, and PKG is the principal mediator of cGMP signals. Phosphorylation has been demonstrated in vitro for many proteins, but only a few have been recognized clearly as physiological substrates, indicating the importance of intracellular localization or compartmentalization.

The principal family of cyclic nucleotide-gated ion channels regulates the influx of Ca^{2+} and Na^+ into cells. All are regulated by intracellular and/or extracellular Ca^{2+} and are activated by both cGMP and cAMP, although certain isotypes are more sensitive to one or the other of the cyclic nucleotides *(2)*. Cyclic nucleotide-gated ion channels are involved in the physiology of vascular smooth muscle relaxation. They are also the means by which cGMP regulates retinal phototransduction in rod and cone photoreceptors and by which cGMP and cAMP regulate olfaction *(28)*.

PHYSIOLOGICAL EFFECTS

Intracellular levels of cGMP affect numerous cellular functions, including extent of smooth muscle relaxation, intestinal fluid and electrolyte homeostasis, initiation of visual signal phototransduction, neutrophil degranulation, and inhibition of platelet aggregation *(29)*. Regulation of vascular smooth muscle motility is a major function of cGMP generated via the NO/cGMP signaling pathway.

Chapter 6 / Sildenafil and NO/cGMP

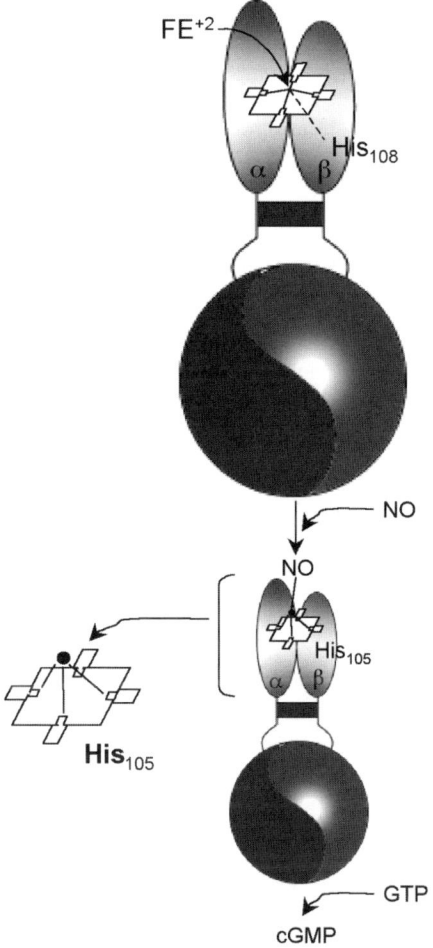

Fig. 2. Soluble guanylyl cyclases are heterodimers that possess a heme prosthetic group with a pentacoordinated ferrous (Fe^{2+}) core that forms an imidazole axial bond with His_{105} of the β-subunit. NO activates sGC by directly binding to the sixth position of the ferrous core, breaking the bond between iron and histidine, dissociating it from the axial imidazole ligand, and displacing the iron from the plane of the porphyrin ring. NO, nitric oxide; sGC, soluble guanylyl cyclase; cGMP, cyclic guanosine monophosphate; GTP, guanosine triphosphate. Reproduced with permission from Lucas et al. *(2)*.

cGMP mediates vascular smooth muscle relaxation via reduction of, and desensitization to, intracellular Ca^{2+}. Reduction of intracellular Ca^{2+} is mediated by PKG phosphorylation of proteins associated with Ca^{2+}-gated channels. Desensitization of the contractile apparatus to

Table 1
PDE Nomenclature and Families

PDE family	Subfamily (no. of splice variants)	Substrate
1	A (4), B (1), C (5)	cAMP/cGMP
2	A (3)	cAMP/cGMP
3	A (1), B (1)	cAMP/cGMP
4	A (8), B (3), C (4), D (5)	cAMP
5	A (3)	cGMP
6	A (1), B (1), C (1)	cGMP
7	A (3), B (1)	cAMP
8	A (5), B (1)	cAMP
9	A (6)	cGMP
10	A (2)	cAMP/cGMP
11	A (4)	cAMP/cGMP

PDE, phosphodiesterase; cAMP, cyclic adenosine monophosphate; cGMP, cyclic guanosine monophosphate.

Ca^{2+} is effected via cGMP-dependent protein kinase I α, which interacts with myosin light chain phosphatase to dephosphorylate myosin light chain *(30)*.

PDEs and PDE5

PDEs are intracellular enzymes that are of critical importance for regulating the levels of cyclic nucleotides (cAMP and cGMP) in the cell. They constitute a large superfamily, are highly regulated by several signaling pathways, exert their inhibitory activity mainly via hydrolysis of the 5′-nucleoside monophosphate (but may also function as a means of sequestration of cGMP), and are targeted by many drugs *(29,31)*.

DESCRIPTION, CLASSIFICATION, AND NOMENCLATURE

The PDE superfamily contains two classes, but all mammalian PDEs are contained in Class I *(31)*. Class I contains 11 families and 21 subfamilies, each from separate genes, among which there are more than 59 variations/isoforms (Table 1). The individual PDEs are differentiated by their substrate selectivities (cGMP and/or cAMP), mechanisms of regulation, tissue distribution, inhibitor selectivity, and subcellular localization (Table 2; *32*).

PDE5 was first purified two decades ago by Francis et al. *(33)*. This group has undertaken much of the subsequent work on this enzyme

Table 2
Physiological and/or Functional Roles of PDEs

PDE family	Role(s)	Evidence (31,35,43–45,115,116)
1	Vascular smooth muscle proliferation; Ca^{2+} modulation of olfaction.	Broad distribution, but highest levels in proliferating vascular smooth muscle cells, testes, heart, and neural tissues (e.g., olfactory epithelial cells); binding and inactivation by Ca^{2+}/calmodulin.
2	Regulation of Ca^{2+} channels, olfaction, platelet aggregation, and aldosterone secretion.	Broad distribution, but highest levels in brain and adrenal cortex.
3	Cardiac contractility, insulin secretion, and lipolysis	Broad distribution, but particular abundance in adipose tissue, liver, cardiac muscle, vascular smooth muscle, and platelets; inhibited by drugs with cardiotonic, vasodilatory, thrombolytic, and antiplatelet aggregation properties; stimulated by insulin, leptin, and insulin-like growth factor.
4	Immunological and inflammatory signaling processes; smooth muscle tone; depression	Broad distribution, highest levels in neural and endocrine tissue; inflammatory cells to participate in the pathogenesis of inflammatory diseases (i.e., asthma and chronic obstructive pulmonary disease), preferentially express PDE4.
5	Penile erection; smooth muscle tone of vasculature, airways, and gastrointestinal tract.	Abundant distribution in smooth muscle; clinical efficacy of the PDE5-specific inhibitor, sildenafil, for treatment of ED.
6	Vision	Distribution in rod and cone photoreceptor cells; some visual defects related to PDE6 mutations.
7	T-lymphocyte activation and proliferation; skeletal muscle metabolism.	Distribution is predominantly in T-lymphocytes (PDE7A1); PDE7 mRNA is abundant in skeletal muscle tissue, T-lymphocytes, and B-lymphocytes, but protein and activity are readily measurable only in T-lymphocytes.
8	T-cell activation.	PDE8A mRNA widely expressed (highest in testis); PDE8B is specific to thyroid gland *(117)*.
9	Possibly maintains basal intracellular cGMP levels or natriuresis and vascular tone.	mRNA widely expressed, particularly in spleen, intestine, kidney, heart, and brain.
10	Unknown.	Human PDE10 widely distributed.
11	Sperm capacitation; other functions unknown.	mRNA occurs at highest levels in skeletal muscle, prostate, kidney, liver, pituitary and salivary glands, and testis; protein localized to vascular smooth muscle cells, cardiac myocytes, corpus cavernosum of the penis, prostate, and skeletal muscle *(118,119)*.

PDE, phosphodiesterase; cGMP, cyclic guanosine monophosphate.

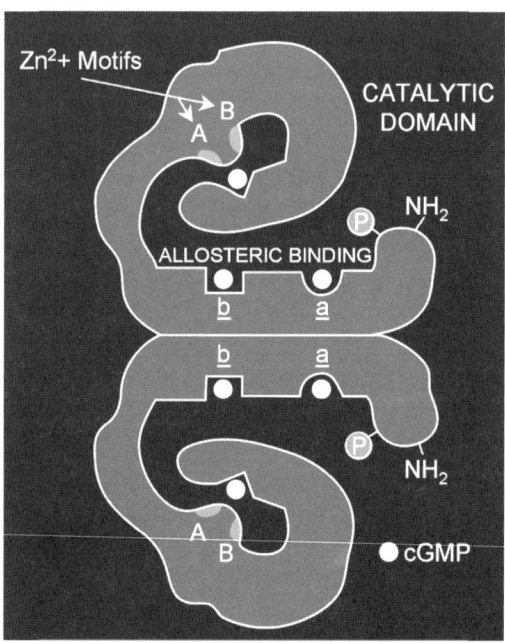

Fig. 3. Working model of PDE5: The regulatory domain in the amino-terminal portion contains a phosphorylation site and two allosteric cGMP-binding sites, a and b, that are theorized to be involved in a cGMP negative-feedback loop. The catalytic domain in the carboxyl-terminal portion contains 2 Zn^{2+}-binding motifs, A and B, and a cGMP-binding substrate site. cGMP, cyclic guanosine monophosphate; PDE5, phosphodiesterase type-5. Reproduced with permission from Corbin and Francis *(29)*.

and has published several excellent reviews *(29,31)*. Their working model of PDE5 illustrates the dimeric structure common to all mammalian PDEs (Fig. 3).

Substrate Selectivity

Certain PDEs are specific for cGMP (PDEs 5, 6, and 9), and others are specific for cAMP (PDEs 4, 7, and 8); both cAMP and cGMP are substrates for the "dual-specificity" PDEs (PDEs 1, 2, 3, 10, and 11), as measured in vitro (Table 1). PDE5 is a cGMP-binding, cGMP-specific PDE *(34)* that is particularly abundant in smooth muscle. The PDE5 catalytic site has a significantly higher affinity for cGMP (K_m approximately 1–5 μM) than for cAMP (K_m approximately 300 μM), but cAMP can be hydrolyzed if the concentration is artificially maintained high enough and it is the only in vitro substrate available *(31)*.

However, under normal physiological conditions, only cGMP is hydrolyzed by PDE5. PDE11 is the most similar to PDE5 based on amino acid sequence analysis (50% identity in the catalytic domain; *35*). However, PDE5 is cGMP-binding and cGMP-specific, whereas PDE11 is a dual-specificity PDE. Three splice variants of the PDE5A family have been identified. PDE5A1, PDE5A2, and PDE5A3 have similar cGMP catalytic activities, with binding rate constants for the catalytic site of 6.2, 5.75, and 6.06 μM, respectively *(36)*.

Mechanisms of Regulation

Various mechanisms regulate PDE activity, and most of these are known to be active with PDE5. As theorized by Corbin and Francis *(29)*, several specific mechanisms appear to interact in a complex manner to regulate PDE5 through negative feedback: (a) increased intracellular cGMP concentration stimulates increased cGMP catalysis by PDE5 because of mass action (increased substrate availability); (b) binding of cGMP at the PDE5 catalytic site enhances cGMP binding at PDE5 allosteric sites, inducing a conformational change in PDE5; (c) cGMP binding at PDE5 allosteric binding sites increases phosphorylation of PDE5 by PKG, which leads to (d) further increases in cGMP catalysis. Compartmentalization between cells can physically segregate different cyclic nucleotide signaling pathways and prevent crosstalk, for example, between PDE3, which is expressed within the cardiac myocyte, and PDE5, which is not *(37,38)*. Furthermore, compartmentalization within the cell can also serve to limit crosstalk between signaling pathways involving PDEs, as has been recently and well characterized for PDE4 *(39)*.

Tissue Distribution and Intracellular Localization

Intracellular localization of PDEs can affect their ability to influence or be influenced by other components of cyclic nucleotide signaling pathways *(37)* and, therefore, can determine the physiological and functional role of a PDE. Some PDEs are localized primarily in either the particulate fraction (PDEs 6 and 7A2) or the cytoplasmic fraction (PDEs 5 and 8) of the cell, whereas others are distributed more evenly in both compartments (e.g., PDEs 3 and 4; *31*), which is determined by the isoform in question. Certain PDEs appear to be expressed selectively in different tissues, and PDE5 is relatively less widely distributed compared with many other PDEs *(31)*. PDE5 is abundant in vascular smooth muscle of all tissues, including penis and lung. It is also present in platelets and visceral smooth muscle (gastrointestinal and urogenital tracts; *33,40–43)*. Recent PDE localization studies using immunohistochemistry have confirmed that PDE5 is highly expressed in vascular medial smooth muscle and smooth muscle bundles *(38, 44,45)*. Among cardiovascular tissues, PDE5 activity was found in the saphenous vein (along with activity for PDEs 1 and 4), the mesenteric artery (along with activity for PDEs 1, 2, 3, and 4), and coronary vascular smooth muscle tissue but not in the cardiac ventricle or cardiac myocytes *(38,46)*. Two PDE5 isoforms, PDE5A1 and PDE5A2, have been isolated from penile and nonpenile tissues, whereas PDE5A3 has been reported to be detected only in tissues with substantial amounts of smooth muscle *(36)*. Parums et al. *(38,46)*, using a specific polyclonal antibody against PDE5 and immunohistochemistry techniques, have not been able to detect PDE5 in human cardiac myocytes. However, there have been reports of PDE5 in cardiac myocytes in the dog *(47)*. Senzaki et al. used chemifluorescent immunohistochemistry to demonstrate PDE5A expression in both the vasculature and myocytes of normal and failing dog hearts, but the possibility of a false positive signal caused by epifluorescence in cardiac tissue cannot be discounted *(47)*.

INHIBITOR SELECTIVITY

Competitive inhibitors of PDE are analogs of cyclic nucleotides that bind to the substrate-binding site and directly decrease the rate of substrate catalysis. Noncompetitive inhibitors bind to different, nonactive sites and, therefore, indirectly decrease the rate of substrate catalysis, perhaps by effecting conformational changes in the PDE molecule. Inhibitors do not interact with the cGMP-binding allosteric sites *(33)*.

Some nonselective PDE inhibitors, for example, zaprinast *(35)*, may exhibit inhibitory effects on multiple PDE families, but others are quite selective for a specific PDE (Table 3). Selectivity is dependent on how the inhibitor molecule fits into the catalytic site of the PDE enzyme molecule, which will vary between PDE families and will be dependent upon inhibitor structure. Therefore, structurally related molecules generally will have similar selectivity profiles, for example, sildenafil and vardenafil, which are potent PDE5 inhibitors with moderate selectivity over PDE6 (Table 3). In contrast, structurally unrelated molecules may have different selectivity profiles. For example, although sildenafil and tadalafil are both potent PDE5 inhibitors, only tadalafil has moderate selectivity over PDE11. The specific role that PDE5 plays in controlling vascular smooth muscle relaxation in the corpus cavernosum of the penis has now become apparent with the demonstration that sildenafil selectively increases penile levels of cGMP *(48)*.

Table 3
PDE Inhibition and Selectivity

Geometric mean IC_{50} values (μM)
(fold selectivity vs PDE5 in brackets)

Compound	PDE1	PDE2	PDE3	PDE4	PDE5	PDE6 (rod)
Sildenafil	0.281 (80)	>30 (>8570)	16.2 (4630)	7.68 (2190)	0.00350	0.037 (11)
Tadalafil	>30 (>4450)	>100 (>14,800)	>100 (>14,800)	>100 (>14,800)	0.00674	1.26 (187)
Vardenafil	0.070 (500)	6.20 (44,290)	>1.0 (>7140)	6.10 (43,570)	0.00014	0.0035 (25)

	PDE6 (cone)	PDE7A	PDE8A	PDE9A	PDE10A	PDE11A
Sildenafil	0.034 (10)	21.3 (6090)	29.8 (8510)	2.61 (750)	9.80 (2800)	2.73 (780)
Tadalafil	1.30 (193)	>100 (>14,800)	>100 (>14,800)	>100 (>14,800)	>100 (>14,800)	0.037 (5)
Vardenafil	0.0006 (4)	>30 (>214,000)	>30 (>214,000)	0.581 (4150)	3.0 (21,200)	0.162 (1160)

IC_{50}s were determined using either native enzyme purified from human tissue (PDE1, heart; PDEs 2, 3, and 5, corpus cavernosum; PDE4, skeletal muscle; PDE6, retina) or using recombinant human enzymes expressed in Sf9 cells (PDEs 7–11) and purified by anion-exchange chromatography.

PDE, phosphodiesterase; IC_{50}, drug concentration necessary to inhibit 50% of enzyme activity.

Adapted from Gbekor et al. *(50)*.

PDE5 INHIBITION BY SILDENAFIL

Chemistry and Pharmacology of Sildenafil

Sildenafil is a highly selective competitive inhibitor of PDE5 (Fig. 4). The pyrazolopyrimidinone nucleus of sildenafil is similar to the guanosine base of cGMP, the endogenous ligand of PDE5. The propyl, methyl, and ethoxyl groups of the pyrazolopyrimidinone nucleus enhance the specificity of sildenafil for PDE5 compared with PDEs 1 and 3 *(49)*. Substitution of a polar sulfonamide group off the ethoxyphenyl moiety also increases the specificity of sildenafil for PDE5 and increases solubility of the drug *(49)*.

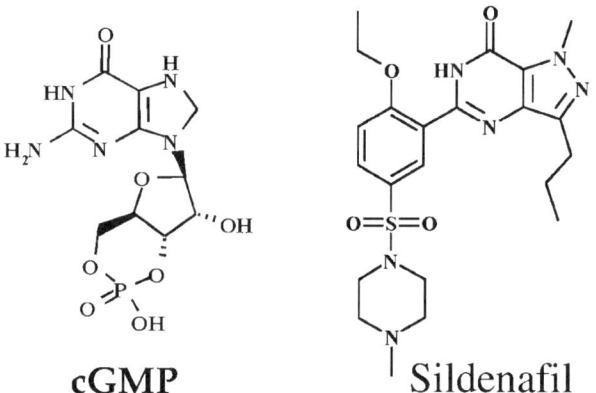

Fig. 4. Comparison of the structure of the competitive PDE5 inhibitor, sildenafil, with that of native substrate, cGMP. cGMP, cyclic guanosine monophosphate; PDE5, phosphodiesterase type-5.

The cGMP catalytic activity of all three isoforms of PDE5 is inhibited by sildenafil, with essentially identical 50% inhibitory concentrations (IC_{50}) for isoforms cloned from human penile tissues *(36)*. In an attempt to define the complete biochemical selectivity profile of sildenafil, molecular cloning techniques and enzyme activity assays in the presence and absence of sildenafil and other competitive PDE5 inhibitors were used to determine the IC_{50} for PDEs 1 through 11 (Table 3; *50*). The results indicate that sildenafil exerts a high degree of selectivity for PDE5 and a minor inhibitory action against PDE6. PDE6 is present exclusively in rod and cone photoreceptors, and sildenafil has about 10-fold less inhibitory activity against it than PDE5 *(42,51)*. This lower inhibitory action of sildenafil against PDE6 can result in a transient blue tinge to vision or an increased perception of light in a small minority of patients, most often when taken at higher doses (*see* "Vision"). Based on the selectivity of sildenafil for PDE5, doses approved for treating ED have little or no clinically significant effect on physiological processes mediated by other PDEs.

Relevance to Erectile Function

Penile erectile tissue consists of the corpus cavernosum and the corpus spongiosum, which are composed of sponge-like, interconnected trabecular spaces lined by vascular epithelium and smooth muscle and surrounded by a thick fibrous sheath, the tunica albuginea. Relaxation of the smooth muscle cells allows increased blood flow into, and expansion of, the penis *(52)*. Pressure of the expanded corpus cavernosum against the inflexible tunica albuginea reduces the outflow of venous blood and causes further pressure increase, resulting in erection.

During sexual stimulation, noncholinergic, nonadrenergic, autonomic nerve endings, and also endothelial cells in the arteries and sinusoids of the corpus cavernosum, release NO, which diffuses into the vascular smooth muscle cells. The generation of neurally derived NO, leading to formation of cGMP, relaxes penile vessels and corpus cavernosum and mediates penile erections *(25)*. Although neurally derived NO is important in initiating erection, endothelial release of NO is important in maintaining erection *(53)*. The main cGMP-hydrolyzing PDE activity detected in human corpus cavernosum is PDE5, with PDEs 2 and 3 also being detected at lower levels; PDE9 and PDE11 also have been detected by reverse transcriptase polymerase chain reaction and immunohistochemistry, respectively *(45,48,51,54,55)*.

In vitro studies in rabbits demonstrated that sildenafil increases cGMP levels in corpus cavernosum, and the increase is augmented in the presence of sodium nitroprusside, an NO donor *(48)*. Furthermore, in vivo studies in dogs with sildenafil demonstrated a dose-dependent enhancement of corpus cavernosum relaxation and intracavernosal pressure, and hence penile erection, in response to endogenously released NO after cavernous nerve stimulation *(56)*. This indicates involvement of PDE5 in the NO-mediated relaxation pathway and enhancement of nitrergic relaxation of corpus cavernosum by sildenafil. Sildenafil enhanced the electrical field-stimulated relaxation of human corpus cavernosum in a concentration-dependent manner (Fig. 5; ref. *51*). Despite the coexpression of PDE11 with PDE5 in the vascular smooth muscle and smooth muscle bundles of corpus cavernosum, PDE11 has been shown to play no role in NO-mediated relaxation of corpus cavernosum *(45)*.

Sildenafil is rapidly absorbed after oral administration, achieving maximum plasma concentrations (C_{max}) within 1 h; concentrations decline in a biexponential manner with a mean terminal half-life of 3–5 h *(55)*. Approximately 95% of absorbed sildenafil is bound to plasma protein, leaving the remainder circulating in plasma as unbound free drug available for interaction with PDE5 at its intracellular receptor *(57,58)*. Administration of a 100-mg dose of sildenafil achieves a C_{max} of unbound free sildenafil of approximately 40 nM *(55,58)*, which is well below the IC_{50} values of sildenafil for most PDEs but is sufficient to achieve greater than 95% inhibition of the PDE5 catalytic site if equilibration occurs between the plasma and the cell (Table 3).

Modulating cGMP levels have a rapid effect on erectile function, and the window of opportunity for use of sildenafil in men with ED is

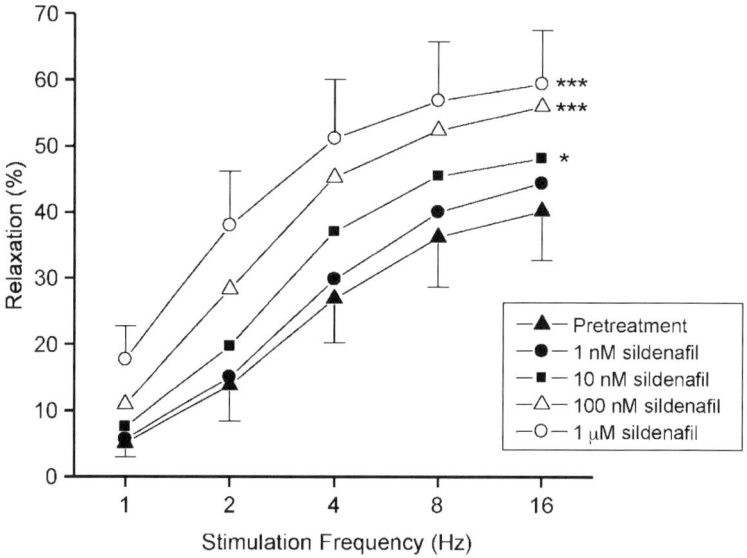

Fig. 5. Effect of sildenafil on electrical field stimulation-induced relaxation of contracted human corpus cavernosal tissue strips. Tissues were contracted with phenylephrine (10 μM) before electrical field stimulation (1–16 Hz). Effects of sildenafil at 10 nM and higher were significantly different from those of control groups. *p <0.05; ***p <0.001. Reproduced with permission from Ballard et al. *(51)*.

consistent with its pharmacokinetic profile. This was demonstrated in randomized, double-blind studies using penile rigidity monitoring devices in a controlled laboratory environment to quantify the magnitude, time to onset, and duration of the erectile response to sildenafil treatment *(59,60)*. Within 30 min of receiving sildenafil 50 mg, 71% of 17 men experienced onset of erection in response to visual sexual stimulation. In a second study, erections rigid enough for penetration occurred at least 4 h after sildenafil administration, which is consistent with the mean drug elimination half-life of 3–5 h. Further studies have indicated that a significant proportion of patients can obtain erections for up to 12 h after taking an oral dose of sildenafil *(60)*.

Clinical Utility of Sildenafil in the Treatment of ED

Sildenafil improves erectile function in a high percentage of individuals with ED *(59,61)*. Sildenafil is well-tolerated and effectively enhances the penile erectile response to sexual stimulation, improving the satisfaction and quality of life of patients and their partners *(62–65)*. A brief overview of the current state of knowledge of the clinical properties of sildenafil follows. Some of the information will be highlighted for the insight it provides on the actions of sildenafil on the NO/cGMP pathway.

PREREGISTRATION

At the time of regulatory submission in September 1997 in the United States, the pharmacokinetics, efficacy, and safety of sildenafil had been studied in greater than 60 clinical trials, which enrolled over 5000 men *(66)*. Phase III trials, most of which incorporated a double-blind treatment period lasting for 12 or 24 wk, showed sildenafil to be an effective, on-demand treatment of ED in men with various associated medical conditions. The main exclusion criteria were recent onset of serious cardiovascular disease (>6 month) and use of nitrates, but patients with stable cardiovascular disease (e.g., controlled hypertension, previous myocardial infarction, stable exertional angina) were not excluded.

Men in whom the cause of dysfunction was thought to be predominantly psychogenic had the highest response rates to the global efficacy question, "Did treatment improve your erections?" (sildenafil 84%; placebo 24%). Among patients with predominantly organic causes of ED, the overall response rate was 68% (vs 19% for placebo), but the rate was 59% (vs 16% for placebo) in patients with diabetes mellitus and 43% (vs 15% for placebo) in a nonselected group of patients post prostatectomy. In numerous long-term studies (lasting 36–52 wk), only 5% of patients discontinued sildenafil treatment because of lack of efficacy.

The main adverse events were headache and facial flushing, followed by indigestion and nasal congestion *(61)*; given the selectivity of sildenafil over all human PDEs (Table 3), these events are almost certainly PDE5 mechanism related. Transient visual symptoms, mainly disturbances of color vision, occurred predominantly with the 100-mg dose and at the time of peak plasma concentrations and are almost certainly caused by transient inhibition of PDE6 in rods and cones. Across the whole clinical trial database, serious adverse events occurred in a similar incidence with sildenafil and placebo, and none were considered related to sildenafil therapy. The main contraindication to sildenafil therapy is coadministration with nitrates, because, as described, both nitrates and sildenafil act on the NO/cGMP pathway and the combination can lead to excessive vasodilatory effects *(67,68)*.

POSTMARKETING

Since its launch in the United States in April 1998 for treatment of ED, sildenafil has received regulatory approval in more than 110 countries. The postmarketing clinical experience is extensive: over 100 million prescriptions issued to over 20 million patients and over 500 million tablets distributed worldwide. In addition, preclinical and clinical study of sildenafil has continued, with new publications relating to sexual medicine as well as to cardiology, respiratory medicine, and reproductive medicine *(69–88)*. Documentation of efficacy in the treatment of ED has now been extended to patients with multiple sclerosis *(89)*, Parkinson's disease *(90)*, untreated symptoms of minor depression *(91)*, spina bifida *(92)*, and in patients with prostate cancer treated with radiotherapy (external beam or local; *93–95*). Encouraging data indicate efficacy of sildenafil in the treatment of patients following major surgery: prostatectomy *(96,97)*, heart transplant *(98)*, and renal transplant *(99)*. Although a recent publication suggested that some patients might experience loss of efficacy with prolonged use *(100)*, other reports indicate that the efficacy of sildenafil is maintained over periods of a year or longer *(101,102)*.

INSIGHTS INTO THE NO/cGMP SYSTEM

It is interesting to consider the clinical profile as summarized above in the light of current knowledge of sildenafil's action on the NO/cGMP system. The subjectively assessed efficacy of sildenafil is significantly greater than that of placebo regardless of whether ED is organic or psychogenic in origin (Table 4; *62*). The high response rates (84%) in patients without recognized organic disease indicates that amplification of cGMP levels is an efficient way of treating ED of predominantly psychogenic cause in individuals with relatively healthy vascular and neurologic systems. In patients with organic illnesses such as hypertension and CAD, response rates are only slightly lower (60–70%), indicating that amplification of cGMP can be effective in overcoming the effects of vascular disease and associated medications in impairing the relaxation of the corpus cavernosum smooth muscle. The lower response rates in diabetics (approximately 50–60%) than for most other organic diseases may reflect pathological processes at multiple sites (large vessels, small vessels, peripheral nerves).

Clinical data indicate the importance of a neural pathway that is at least partially intact for the therapeutic action of sildenafil. Provided there is some innervation, sildenafil can often be very effective. For example, response rates of approximately 80% have been observed in patients with spinal cord injury *(103)*. Many patients with spinal cord injury have high level cord lesions and experience reflexogenic erections induced by various stimuli. Reflexogenic erections occur because there is an intact sensory and autonomic pathway below the cord lesion

Table 4
Mean Scores of Responses to Questions 3 and 4 of the International Index of Erectile Function and Global Efficacy Question Responses for Men Receiving Sildenafil or Placebo in a Randomized, Double-Blind, 12-Wk Flexible-Dose-Escalation Study

Pathophysiology of ED

Treatment group	Baseline	End-of-treatment	Percent change	p value
IIEF[a] question 3 (ability to achieve)				
Organic				
Placebo (n = 90)	2.0 ± 0.2	2.0 ± 0.2	0	
Sildenafil (n = 81)	1.8 ± 0.2	3.6 ± 0.2	100	<0.001
Psychogenic				
Placebo (n = 24)	2.2 ± 0.2	2.3 ± 0.4	5	
Sildenafil (n = 19)	2.0 ± 0.2	4.3 ± 0.4	115	<0.001
Mixed				
Placebo (n = 24)	2.3 ± 0.3	2.8 ± 0.3	22	
Sildenafil (n = 38)	2.3 ± 0.3	3.6 ± 0.3	57	0.08
IIEF[a] question 4 (Ability to maintain)				
Organic				
Placebo (n = 90)	1.4 ± 0.1	1.4 ± 0.2	0	
Sildenafil (n = 80)	1.4 ± 0.1	3.3 ± 0.2	136	<0.001
Psychogenic				
Placebo (n = 24)	1.7 ± 0.2	1.9 ± 0.3	12	
Sildenafil (n = 19)	1.6 ± 0.2	3.8 ± 0.4	138	<0.001
Mixed				
Placebo (n = 24)	1.8 ± 0.3	2.3 ± 0.4	28	
Sildenafil (n = 38)	1.6 ± 0.2	3.7 ± 0.4	131	0.005
GEQ (Did the treatment improve your erections?)				
Placebo (n = 118)		19%		
Sildenafil (n = 136)		74%		<0.001

[a]Based on a scale of 1 (almost never or never) to 5 (almost always or always), with 0 representing "did not attempt intercourse." Values are means ±SE. Percent differences are between the final and baseline mean scores. *p* values are calculated according to analysis of covariance (ordered categorical variable), with baseline score, age, smoking, and duration and cause of ED as covariates. IIEF, International Index of Erectile Function; GEQ, Global Efficacy Question.

Adapted from Goldstein et al. *(62)*.

(via the sacral segments of the spinal cord) but generally are short-lived and insufficient for sexual intercourse. Administration of sildenafil amplifies the signal leading to a reflexogenic erection and, in many patients, allows this to be maintained for intercourse. The partially intact innervation of the penis is also the reason why sildenafil is effective in patients with spina bifida and other neurological conditions such as multiple sclerosis *(89,92)*.

An intact neural pathway is also key to the efficacy of sildenafil in patients who have had radical prostatectomy. A review of early clinical trials determined that only 43% of 87 patients with ED after radical retropubic prostatectomy responded to sildenafil therapy *(61)*. The low response rate is thought to reflect surgical damage to the cavernous nerves, resulting in an inability to activate the NO/cGMP signaling pathway *(62)*. If, during surgery, no attempt is made to spare the microscopic cavernous nerves that course round the prostate, then sildenafil is completely ineffective, consistent with the complete disruption of the nitrergic innervation of the penis. However, if nerve-sparing surgery is undertaken, then sildenafil can be effective, although patients generally have to wait several months to a year or more after surgery before an acceptable response is obtained. This is consistent with some degree of nerve damage during surgery and slow recovery of neural supply postsurgery. In men with ED after radical retropubic prostatectomy, sildenafil response rates as high as 80% were reported if the surgery incorporated bilateral nerve-sparing procedures, 50% for unilateral nerve-sparing surgery, and 15% for non-nerve-sparing surgery *(104)*.

Actions of Sildenafil on the NO/cGMP Pathway in Other Systems

Sildenafil is a highly potent and selective inhibitor of PDE5 and a weak inhibitor of PDE6. Thus, in addition to the fact that PDE5 inhibition underlies the therapeutic effect, virtually all of the adverse effects attributed to the drug can be explained in terms of PDE5 or PDE6 inhibition. The adverse events most commonly associated with sildenafil treatment in clinical trials were headache, flushing, dyspepsia, nasal congestion, and mild transient visual effects in a small number of patients *(105)*. These reflect PDE5 inhibition in the systemic vasculature, esophagogastric sphincter, and the nasal mucosa and transient inhibition of PDE6 in the retinal photoreceptor cells. For vision and for the cardiovascular system, the molecular basis for potential sildenafil effects is discussed briefly below.

VISION

As noted previously (*see* "Chemistry and Pharmacology of Sildenafil"), sildenafil exerts a minor inhibitory action against PDE6, which is present exclusively in rod and cone photoreceptors. Sildenafil PDE6 IC$_{50}$s were 37 nM (rods) and 34 nM (cones) compared with a

PDE5 IC_{50} of 3.5 (Table 3). Peak plasma concentrations of free sildenafil achieved with the maximum therapeutic dose of 100 mg may reach the PDE6 IC_{50}, which may result in a mild, transient blue tinge to vision or an increased perception of light in a small minority of patients *(105,106)*. However, rapid elimination of sildenafil (half-life of 3–5 h) limits systemic drug exposure, so adverse effects are usually transient, lasting minutes to a few hours. There have been no long-term consequences of prolonged PDE5/6 inhibition in animals exposed to very high doses of sildenafil. In long-term clinical and postmarketing studies, there was no consistent pattern of adverse events to suggest that intermittent partial inhibition of PDE5 or PDE6 by sildenafil can induce changes to the retina or other structures of the eye *(104,107)*.

CARDIOVASCULAR

In the systemic vasculature, endothelial release of NO is important in modulating smooth muscle activity. Consistent with the presence of PDE5 in vascular smooth muscle and the role of the NO/cGMP signaling pathway in the regulation of blood pressure *(108,109)*, sildenafil has modest transient vasodilatory effects *(88)*. Although the effects of sildenafil alone are modest, it potentiates the hypotensive effects of nitrates via its effect on the NO/cGMP signaling pathway *(68)*. Although there appears to be a limit to the degree of vasodilation that can be achieved by inhibiting PDE5, when the NO/cGMP pathway is also augmented by endogenous sources of NO, the coadministration of sildenafil can result in excessive vasodilation. Thus, administration of sildenafil to patients using organic nitrates, either regularly or intermittently, in any form, is contraindicated. Although amplification of the NO/cGMP system via PDE5 inhibition appears to have only modest effects on the systemic circulation (in the absence of an exogenous source of NO), the same may not be true in the pulmonary circulation and in localized areas of the systemic circulation affected by various disease processes. For example, in certain forms of pulmonary arterial hypertension, where there is considerable hypertrophy of the smooth muscle of the pulmonary arteries and arterioles, PDE5 inhibition appears to show tremendous promise as a treatment to improve symptoms and functional capacity of severely disabled patients. A more extensive review of the hemodynamics of PDE5 inhibition is provided in Chapter 8.

PDE3 is present in cardiac muscle and PDE3 inhibitors such as milrinone potentiate the cardiac contractile response by augmenting cAMP levels in the cardiac myocytes *(110)*. PDE3 is a dual-specificity PDE (catalyzes both cAMP and cGMP), and cGMP exerts feedback inhibition on PDE3 *(111)*. A report that supratherapeutic levels of sildenafil stimulate the production of cAMP in isolated human cardiac muscle raised some questions that PDE5 inhibition by sildenafil could indirectly increase myocyte contractility via elevation of cGMP levels and consequent inhibition of PDE3 *(112)*. However, this theory has been refuted by in situ hybridization and immunohistochemistry studies, which did not find PDE3 and PDE5 colocalization in cardiac myocytes *(38,46)*, ruling out the potential for crosstalk in the cardiac myocyte. More importantly, preclinical and clinical studies show that sildenafil does not have a direct positive inotropic action on the human heart *(113,114)*. The safety of PDE5 inhibition in cardiac patients is reviewed in Chapter 9.

CONCLUSION

Regulation of vascular smooth muscle tone is the major function of cGMP generated via the NO/cGMP signaling pathway. This pathway controls relaxation of penile vessels and corpus cavernosum and mediates penile erections. The central role of PDE5 in regulating the availability of cGMP in the NO/cGMP signaling pathway, and the less broad tissue distribution of PDE5 compared with other PDEs, makes it an ideal target for pharmacological intervention. The selectivity of sildenafil for PDE5 further contributes to a high degree of specificity, resulting in an effective and well-tolerated treatment for ED.

REFERENCES

1. Pfeifer A, Ruth P, Dostmann W, et al. Structure and function of cGMP-dependent protein kinases. Rev Physiol Biochem Pharmacol 1999;135:105–149.
2. Lucas KA, Pitari GM, Kazerounian S, et al. Guanylyl cyclases and signaling by cyclic GMP. Pharmacol Rev 2000;52:375–414.
3. Wedel BJ, Garbers DL. New insights on the functions of the guanylyl cyclase receptors. FEBS Lett 1997;410:29–33.
4. Wedel B, Garbers D. The guanylyl cyclase family at Y2K. Annu Rev Physiol 2001;63:215–233.
5. Moncada S, Palmer RM, Higgs EA. Nitric oxide: physiology, pathophysiology, and pharmacology. Pharmacol Rev 1991;43:109–142.
6. McDonald LJ, Murad F. Nitric oxide and cyclic GMP signaling. Proc Soc Exp Biol Med 1996;211:1–6.
7. Parker JD, Parker JO. Nitrate therapy for stable angina pectoris. N Engl J Med 1998;338:520–531.
8. Campbell SF. Science, art and drug discovery: a personal perspective. Clin Sci (Lond) 2000;99:255–260.
9. Ignarro LJ, Bush PA, Buga GM, et al. Nitric oxide and cyclic GMP formation upon electrical field stimulation cause relaxation of corpus cavernosum smooth muscle. Biochem Biophys Res Commun 1990;170:843–850.

10. Bush PA, Aronson WJ, Buga GM, et al. Nitric oxide is a potent relaxant of human and rabbit corpus cavernosum. J Urol 1992;147:1650–1655.
11. Azadzoi KM, Kim N, Brown ML, et al. Endothelium-derived nitric oxide and cyclooxygenase products modulate corpus cavernosum smooth muscle tone. J Urol 1992;147:220–225.
12. Marsh N, Marsh A. A short history of nitroglycerine and nitric oxide in pharmacology and physiology. Clin Exp Pharmacol Physiol 2000;27:313–319.
13. Arnold WP, Mittal CK, Katsuki S, et al. Nitric oxide activates guanylate cyclase and increases guanosine 3':5'-cyclic monophosphate levels in various tissue preparations. Proc Natl Acad Sci USA 1977;74:3203–3207.
14. Furchgott RF, Zawadzki JV. The obligatory role of endothelial cells in the relaxation of arterial smooth muscle by acetylcholine. Nature 1980;288:373–376.
15. Ignarro LJ, Buga GM, Wood KS, et al. Endothelium-derived relaxing factor produced and released from artery and vein is nitric oxide. Proc Natl Acad Sci USA 1987;84:9265–9269.
16. Palmer RM, Ferrige AG, Moncada S. Nitric oxide release accounts for the biological activity of endothelium-derived relaxing factor. Nature 1987;327:524–526.
17. Rakhit RD, Marber MS. Nitric oxide: an emerging role in cardioprotection? Heart 2001;86:368–372.
18. Buchwalow IB, Podzuweit T, Bocker W, et al. Vascular smooth muscle and nitric oxide synthase. FASEB J 2002;16:500–508.
19. Rajasekaran M, Mondal D, Agrawal K, et al. Ex vivo expression of nitric oxide synthase isoforms (eNOS/iNOS) and calmodulin in human penile cavernosal cells. J Urol 1998;160(6 Pt 1):2210–2215.
20. Bloch W, Klotz T, Sedlaczek P, et al. Evidence for the involvement of endothelial nitric oxide synthase from smooth muscle cells in the erectile function of the human corpus cavernosum. Urol Res 1998;26:129–135.
21. Stanarius A, Uckert S, Machtens SA, et al. Immunocytochemical distribution of nitric oxide synthase in the human corpus cavernosum: an electron microscopical study using the tyramide signal amplification technique. Urol Res 2001;29:168–172.
22. Haynes WG, Noon F, Walker B, et al. Inhibition of nitric oxide synthesis increases blood pressure in healthy humans. J Hypertens 1995;13:709–710.
23. Clarkson PB, Lim PO, MacDonald TM. Influence of basal nitric oxide secretion on cardiac function in man. Br J Clin Pharmacol 1995;40:299–305.
24. Castellano M, Rizzoni D, Beschi M, et al. Relationship between sympathetic nervous system activity, baroreflex and cardiovascular effects after acute nitric oxide synthesis inhibition in humans. J Hypertens 1995;13:1153–1161.
25. Burnett AL, Lowenstein CJ, Bredt DS, et al. Nitric oxide: a physiologic mediator of penile erection. Science 1992;257:401–403.
26. Stone JR, Marletta MA. Soluble guanylate cyclase from bovine lung: activation with nitric oxide and carbon monoxide and spectral characterization of the ferrous and ferric states. Biochemistry 1994;33:5636–5640.
27. Tsai SC, Shindo H, Manganiello VC, et al. Products of reaction catalyzed by purified rat liver guanylate cyclase determined by 31p NMR spectroscopy. Proc Natl Acad Sci USA 1980;77:5734–5737.
28. Biel M, Zong X, Hofmann F. Cyclic nucleotide gated channels. Adv Second Messenger Phosphoprotein Res 1999;33:231–250.
29. Corbin JD, Francis SH. Cyclic GMP phosphodiesterase-5: target of sildenafil. J Biol Chem 1999;274:13,729–13,732.

30. Surks HK, Mochizuki N, Kasai Y, et al. Regulation of myosin phosphatase by a specific interaction with cGMP-dependent protein kinase I alpha. Science 1999; 286:1583–1587.
31. Francis SH, Turko IV, Corbin JD. Cyclic nucleotide phosphodiesterases: relating structure and function. Prog Nucleic Acid Res Mol Biol 2001;65:1–52.
32. Beavo J, Conti M, Heaslip R. Multiple cyclic nucleotide phosphodiesterases. Mol Pharmacol 1994;46:399–405.
33. Francis SH, Lincoln TM, Corbin JD. Characterization of a novel cGMP binding protein from rat lung. J Biol Chem 1980;255:620–626.
34. Lincoln TM, Cornwell TL. Intracellular cyclic GMP receptor proteins. FASEB J 1993;7:328–338.
35. Fawcett L, Baxendale R, Stacey P, et al. Molecular cloning and characterization of a distinct human phosphodiesterase gene family: PDE11A. Proc Natl Acad Sci USA 2000;97:3702–3707.
36. Lin CS, Lau A, Tu R, et al. Expression of three isoforms of cGMP-binding cGMP-specific phosphodiesterase (PDE5) in human penile cavernosum. Biochem Biophys Res Commun 2000;268:628–635.
37. Pelligrino DA, Wang Q. Cyclic nucleotide crosstalk and the regulation of cerebral vasodilation. Prog Neurobiol 1998;56:1–18.
38. Parums DV, Charlton RG, Johnson N, et al. Immunohistochemical (IHC), in situ hybridisation (ISH) and biochemical characterisation of phosphodiesterase type 5 (PDE5) in normal and ischaemic human cardiac tissue (PDE5). Eur Heart J 2000;21:616.
39. Houslay MD, Sullivan M, Bolger GB. The multienzyme PDE4 cyclic adenosine monophosphate-specific phosphodiesterase family: intracellular targeting, regulation, and selective inhibition by compounds exerting anti-inflammatory and antidepressant actions. Adv Pharmacol 1998;44:225–342.
40. Hamet P, Coquil JF. Cyclic GMP binding and cyclic GMP phosphodiesterase in rat platelets. J Cyclic Nucleotide Res 1978;4:281–290.
41. Kuthe A, Stief C, Magert J. Molecular biological characterization of phosphodiesterases 3A and 5 in human corpus cavernosum penis. Eur Urol 1999;35 (Suppl 2):102.
42. Beavo JA. Cyclic nucleotide phosphodiesterases: functional implications of multiple isoforms. Physiol Rev 1995;75:725–748.
43. Dousa TP. Cyclic-3′,5′-nucleotide phosphodiesterase isozymes in cell biology and pathophysiology of the kidney. Kidney Int 1999;55:29–62.
44. Baxendale R, Phillips SC. Human PDE11: a distinct, dual-substrate phosphodiesterase expressed in vascular smooth muscle and cardiac myocytes. Circulation 2000;102:320.
45. Baxendale RW, Wayman CP, Turner L, et al. Cellular localisation of phosphodiesterase type 11 (PDE11) in human corpus cavernosum and the contribution of PDE11 inhibition on nerve-stimulated relaxation. J Urol 2001;165:223.
46. Wallis RM, Corbin JD, Francis SH, et al. Tissue distribution of phosphodiesterase families and the effects of sildenafil on tissue cyclic nucleotides, platelet function, and the contractile responses of trabeculae carneae and aortic rings in vitro. Am J Cardiol 1999;83(Suppl 5A):3C–12C.
47. Senzaki H, Smith CJ, Juang GJ, et al. Cardiac phosphodiesterase 5 (cGMP-specific) modulates beta-adrenergic signaling in vivo and is down-regulated in heart failure. FASEB J 2001;15:1718–1726.

48. Jeremy JY, Ballard SA, Naylor AM, et al. Effects of sildenafil, a type-5 cGMP phosphodiesterase inhibitor, and papaverine on cyclic GMP and cyclic AMP levels in the rabbit corpus cavernosum in vitro. Br J Urol 1997;79:958–963.
49. Terrett N, Bell A, Brown D, et al. Sildenafil (Viagra), a potent and selective inhibitor of type 5 cGMP phosphodiesterase with utility for the treatment of male erectile dysfunction. Bioorganic Medicinal Chem Lett 1996;6:1819–1824.
50. Gbekor EG, Bethell SB, Fawcett LF, et al. Selectivity of sildenafil and other phosphodiesterase type 5 (PDE5) inhibitors against all human phosphodiesterase families. Eur Urol 2002;(Suppl 1):63.
51. Ballard SA, Gingell CJ, Tang K, et al. Effects of sildenafil on the relaxation of human corpus cavernosum tissue in vitro and on the activities of cyclic nucleotide phosphodiesterase isozymes. J Urol 1998;159:2164–2171.
52. Andersson KE. Pharmacology of penile erection. Pharmacol Rev 2001;53: 417–450.
53. Hurt KJ, Musicki B, Palese MA, et al. Akt-dependent phosphorylation of endothelial nitric-oxide synthase mediates penile erection. Proc Natl Acad Sci USA 2002;99:4061–4066.
54. Kuthe A, Wiedenroth A, Magert HJ, et al. Expression of different phosphodiesterase genes in human cavernous smooth muscle. J Urol 2001;165:280–283.
55. Boolell M, Allen MJ, Ballard SA, et al. Sildenafil: an orally active type 5 cyclic GMP-specific phosphodiesterase inhibitor for the treatment of penile erectile dysfunction. Int J Impot Res 1996;8:47–52.
56. Carter AJ, Ballard SA, Naylor AM. Effect of the selective phosphodiesterase type-5 inhibitor sildenafil on erectile function in the anesthetized dog. J Urol 1998;160:242–246.
57. Walker DK, Ackland MJ, James GC, et al. Pharmacokinetics and metabolism of sildenafil in mouse, rat, rabbit, dog and man. Xenobiotica 1999;29:297–310.
58. Purvis K, Muirhead GJ, Harness JA. The effects of sildenafil on human sperm function in healthy volunteers. Br J Clin Pharmacol 2002;53(Suppl 1): 53S–60S.
59. Eardley I, Ellis P, Boolell M, et al. Onset and duration of action of sildenafil citrate for the treatment of erectile dysfunction. Br J Clin Pharmacol 2002; 53:61S–65S.
60. Gingell C, Gepi-Attee S, Sultana SR, et al. Duration of action of sildenafil citrate among men with erectile dysfunction of no known organic cause. Presented at: 9th World Meeting on Impotence Research; Nov 27–29, 2000; Perth, Australia.
61. Steers WD. Viagra—after one year. Urology 1999;54:12–17.
62. Goldstein I, Lue TF, Padma-Nathan H, et al. Oral sildenafil in the treatment of erectile dysfunction. N Engl J Med 1998;338:1397–1404.
63. Dinsmore WW, Hodges M, Hargreaves C, et al. Sildenafil citrate (VIAGRA) in erectile dysfunction: near normalization in men with broad-spectrum erectile dysfunction compared with age-matched healthy control subjects. Urology 1999; 53:800–805.
64. McMahon CG, Samali R, Johnson H. Efficacy, safety and patient acceptance of sildenafil citrate as treatment for erectile dysfunction. J Urol 2000;164:1192–1196.
65. Marks LS, Duda C, Dorey FJ, et al. Treatment of erectile dysfunction with sildenafil. Urology 1999;53:19–24.
66. Osterloh IH, Riley A. Clinical update on sildenafil citrate. Br J Clin Pharmacol 2002;53:219–223.

67. Webb DJ, Freestone S, Allen MJ, et al. Sildenafil citrate and blood-pressure-lowering drugs: results of drug interaction studies with an organic nitrate and a calcium antagonist. Am J Cardiol 1999;83(Suppl 5A):21C–28C.
68. Webb DJ, Muirhead GJ, Wulff M, et al. Sildenafil citrate potentiates the hypotensive effects of nitric oxide donor drugs in male patients with stable angina. J Am Coll Cardiol 2000;36:25–31.
69. Halcox JP, et al. Sildenafil: effects on human vascular function, platelet activation and myocardial ischaemia. Heart 2001;85(Suppl 1):24.
70. Jackson G. Phosphodiesterase 5 inhibition: effects on the coronary vasculature. Int J Clin Pract 2001;55:183–188.
71. Przyklenk K, Kloner RA. VIAGRA® does not exacerbate ischemia, but renders platelets refractory to the inhibitory effects of adenosine. Circulation 2000;102 (Suppl II):254.
72. Traverse J, Chen YJ, Du R, et al. Cyclic nucleotide phosphodiesterase type 5 activity limits blood flow to ischemic myocardium during exercise. Circulation 2000;102:2997–3002.
73. Chen Y, Du R, Traverse JH, et al. Effect of sildenafil on coronary active and reactive hyperemia. Am J Physiol Heart Circ Physiol 2000;279:H2319–H2325.
74. Ishikura F, Beppu S, Hamada T, et al. Effects of sildenafil citrate (Viagra) combined with nitrate on the heart. Circulation 2000;102:2516–2521.
75. Herrmann HC, Chang G, Klugherz BD, et al. Hemodynamic effects of sildenafil in men with severe coronary artery disease. N Engl J Med 2000;342:1622–1626.
76. Vardi Y, Bulus M, Reisner S, et al. Ergometric studies for evaluating sildenafil effect in cardiac patients. J Urol 2000;163(Suppl 4):200.
77. Pelliccia F, Leonardo F, Pagnotta P, et al. Effects of phosphodiesterase-5 inhibition on myocardial ischemia in patients with chronic stable angina in therapy with beta-blockers. J Am Coll Cardiol 2000;35(Suppl A):339.
78. Bocchi E, Guimaraes G, Belloti G, et al. Beneficial effects of a phosphodiesterase type 5 inhibitor (sildenafil) on exercise, neurohormonal activation, and erectile dysfunction in patients with congestive heart failure-a double-blind placebo-controlled cross-over randomised study. J Am Coll Cardiol 2001;37(Suppl A):163A.
79. Herbert K, Arcement LM, Ferguson TG. Is sildenafil (Viagra®) safe and effective for the treatment of erectile dysfunction in patients with heart failure? Circulation 2000;102(Suppl II):413.
80. Katz SD, Balidemaj K, Homma S, et al. Acute type 5 phosphodiesterase inhibition with sildenafil enhances flow-mediated vasodilation in patients with chronic heart failure. J Am Coll Cardiol 2000;36:845–851.
81. Kloner RA, Brown M, Prisant LM, et al. Efficacy and safety of Viagra (sildenafil citrate) in patients with erectile dysfunction taking concomitant antihypertensive therapy. Am J Hypertens 2000;14:70–73.
82. Jackson G. Sildenafil (Viagra) and cardiac patients: an open outpatient study. Heart 2001;85(Suppl I):P42.
83. Vlachopoulos C, O'Rourke MF, Hirata K. Sildenafil (Viagra®) improves the elastic properties of the aorta. Am J Hypertens 2001;14:6A.
84. Olsson AM, Persson CA. Efficacy and safety of sildenafil citrate for the treatment of erectile dysfunction in men with cardiovascular disease. Int J Clin Pract 2001;55:171–176.
85. Agelink MW, Majewski T, Schmitz T, et al. Effects of sildenafil (VIAGRA®) on cardiovascular autonomic function (CAF) in man: preliminary results. Eur Psychiatry 2000;15(Suppl):396S.

86. Shakir SAW, Wilton LV, Boshier A, et al. Cardiovascular events in users of sildenafil: results from first phase of prescription event monitoring in England. BMJ 2001;922:651–652.
87. Jackson G. The use of sildenafil in heart disease. Hosp Med 2000;61:526–527.
88. Jackson G, Benjamin N, Jackson N, et al. Effects of sildenafil citrate on human hemodynamics. Am J Cardiol 1999;83(Suppl 5A):13C–20C.
89. Fowler C, Miller J, Sharief M. Viagra (sildenafil citrate) for the treatment of erectile dysfunction in men with multiple sclerosis. Ann Neurol 1999;46:497.
90. Hussain IF, Brady CM, Swinn MJ, et al. Treatment of erectile dysfunction with sildenafil citrate (Viagra) in parkinsonism due to Parkinson's disease or multiple system atrophy with observations on orthostatic hypotension. J Neurol Neurosurg Psychiatry 2001;71:371–374.
91. Seidman SN, Roose SP, Menza MA, et al. Treatment of erectile dysfunction in men with depressive symptoms: results of a placebo-controlled trial with sildenafil citrate. Am J Psychiatry 2001;158:1623–1630.
92. Palmer JS, Kaplan WE, Firlit CF. Erectile dysfunction in patients with spina bifida is a treatable condition. J Urol 2000;164:958–961.
93. Zelefsky MJ, McKee AB, Lee H, et al. Efficacy of oral sildenafil in patients with erectile dysfunction after radiotherapy for carcinoma of the prostate. Urology 1999;53:775–778.
94. Incrocci L, Koper PC, Hop WC, et al. Sildenafil citrate (Viagra) and erectile dysfunction following external beam radiotherapy for prostate cancer: a randomized, double-blind, placebo-controlled, cross-over study. Int J Radiat Oncol Biol Phys 2001;51:1190–1195.
95. Merrick GS, Butler WM, Lief JH, et al. Efficacy of sildenafil citrate in prostate brachytherapy patients with erectile dysfunction. Urology 1999;53:1112–1116.
96. Hong EK, Lepor H, McCullough AR. Time dependent patient satisfaction with sildenafil for erectile dysfunction (ED) after nerve-sparing radical retropubic prostatectomy (RRP). Int J Impot Res 1999;11(Suppl 1):S15–S22.
97. Zagaja GP, Mhoon DA, Aikens JE, et al. Sildenafil in the treatment of erectile dysfunction after radical prostatectomy. Urology 2000;56:631–634.
98. Wren FJ, Jarowenko MV, Burg J, et al. Incidence of erectile dysfunction and efficacy of sildenafil in the cardiac transplantation patient. J Heart Lung Transpl 2001:246.
99. Prieto Castro RM, Anglada Curado FJ, Regueiro Lopez JC, et al. Treatment with sildenafil citrate in renal transplant patients with erectile dysfunction. BJU Int 2001;88:241–243.
100. El-Galley R, Rutland H, Talic R, et al. Long-term efficacy of sildenafil and tachyphylaxis effect. J Urol 2001;166:927–931.
101. Steers W, Guay AT, Leriche A, et al. Assessment of the efficacy and safety of Viagra (sildenafil citrate) in men with erectile dysfunction during long-term treatment. Int J Impot Res 2001;13:261–267.
102. Hackett GI, Milledge D. A 12-month follow-up of 260 consecutive patients treated with sildenafil following attendance at a NHS erectile dysfunction clinic from July 1999 to June 2000. Presented at the European Society for Sexual and Impotence Research; September 30–October 3, 2001; Rome, Italy.
103. Schmid DM, Schurch B, Hauri D. Sildenafil in the treatment of sexual dysfunction in spinal cord-injured male patients. Eur Urol 2000;38:184–193.
104. Sadovsky R, Miller T, Moskowitz M, et al. Three-year update of sildenafil citrate (Viagra) efficacy and safety. Int J Clin Pract 2001;55:115–128.

105. Morales A, Gingell C, Collins M, et al. Clinical safety of oral sildenafil citrate (VIAGRA) in the treatment of erectile dysfunction. Int J Impot Res 1998;10: 69–74.
106. Laties AM, Zrenner E. Viagra® (sildenafil citrate) and ophthalmology. Prog Ret Eye Res 2002;21:485–506.
107. Marmor MF, Kessler R. Sildenafil (Viagra) and ophthalmology. Surv Ophthalmol 1999;44:153–162.
108. Rees DD, Palmer RMJ, Moncada S. Role of endothelium-derived nitric oxide in the regulation of blood pressure. Proc Natl Acad Sci USA 1989;86:3375–3378.
109. Vallance P, Chan N. Endothelial function and nitric oxide: clinical relevance. Heart 2001;85:342–350.
110. Cone J, Wang S, Tandon N, et al. Comparison of the effects of cilostazol and milrinone on intracellular cAMP levels and cellular function in platelets and cardiac cells. J Cardiovasc Pharmacol 1999;34:497–504.
111. Rascon A, Lindgren S, Stavenow L, et al. Purification and properties of the cGMP-inhibited cAMP phosphodiesterase from bovine aortic smooth muscle. Biochim Biophys Acta 1992;1134:149–156.
112. Stief CG, Uckert S, Becker AJ, et al. Effects of sildenafil on cAMP and cGMP levels in isolated human cavernous and cardiac tissue. Urology 2000;55:146–150.
113. Corbin JD, Francis SH, Osterloh IH. Effects of sildenafil on cAMP and cGMP levels in isolated human cavernous and cardiac tissue [letter]. Urology 2000; 56:545.
114. Sugiyama A, Satoh Y, Shiina H, et al. Cardiac electrophysiologic and hemodynamic effects of sildenafil, a PDE5 inhibitor, in anesthetized dogs. J Cardiovasc Pharmacol 2001;38:940–946.
115. Hayashi M, Matsushima K, Ohashi H, et al. Molecular cloning and characterization of human PDE8B, a novel thyroid-specific isozyme of 3′,5′-cyclic nucleotide phosphodiesterase. Biochem Biophys Res Commun 1998;250: 751–756.
116. Soderling SH, Bayuga SJ, Beavo JA. Cloning and characterization of a cAMP-specific cyclic nucleotide phosphodiesterase. Proc Natl Acad Sci USA 1998;95: 8991–8996.
117. Glavas NA, Ostenson C, Schaefer JB, et al. T cell activation up-regulates cyclic nucleotide phosphodiesterases 8A1 and 7A3. Proc Natl Acad Sci USA 2001;98: 6319–6324.
118. Baxendale RW, Burslem F, Phillips SC. Phosphodiesterase type 11 (PDE11) cellular localisation: progress towards defining a physiological role in testis and/or reproduction. J Urol 2001;165(Suppl):340.
119. Lunny C, Baxendale R, Fawcett L, et al. Ablation of phosphodiesterase type 11 (PDE11) in mice by gene knockout induces changes in spermatozoa function. Int J Impot Res 2002;14(Suppl 3):B5.9.

7 Phosphodiesterase-5 Inhibition
Importance to the Cardiovascular System

*Jackie D. Corbin, PhD,
Stephen R. Rannels, PhD,
and Sharron H. Francis, PhD*

CONTENTS

>PDE5 AND OTHER PHOSPHODIESTERASE FAMILIES
>PDE5 CATALYTIC DOMAIN
>PDE5 IN VASCULAR SMOOTH MUSCLE
>SELECTIVITY OF PDE5 INHIBITORS FOR PDE5
>>AND POTENTIAL SIDE EFFECTS
>
>COULD PDE5 INHIBITORS AFFECT THE HEART?
>CROSS-TALK
>ROLE OF THE REGULATORY DOMAIN OF PDE5
>>IN NEGATIVE FEEDBACK CONTROL OF THE CYCLIC
>>GMP PATHWAY
>
>NEGATIVE FEEDBACK CONTROL OF PDE5 ENGENDERS
>>GREATER PDE5 INHIBITOR EFFICACY
>
>ACKNOWLEDGMENTS
>REFERENCES

PDE5 AND OTHER PHOSPHODIESTERASE FAMILIES

Mammalian cyclic nucleotide phosphodiesterases (PDE) are a superfamily of enzymes that currently consists of 11 families named PDE1–PDE11 (Fig. 1; ref. *1*). Some of these families contain multiple

From: *Contemporary Cardiology: Heart Disease and Erectile Dysfunction*
Edited by: R. A. Kloner © Humana Press Inc., Totowa, NJ

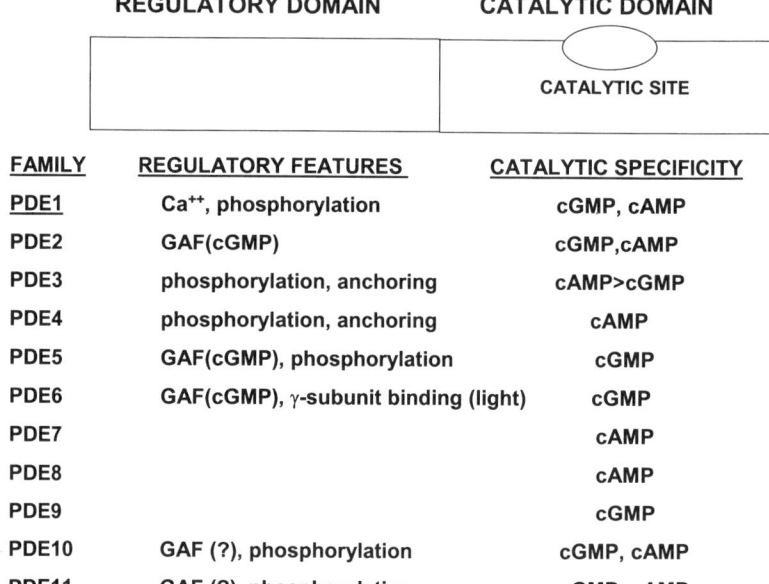

Fig. 1. Model for domain structure, regulatory features, and catalytic specificities of PDE families. cGMP, cyclic GMP; cAMP, cyclic AMP; GAF, cyclic GMP-Anabaena adenylyl cyclase-*Escherchia coli* FhIA, a domain present in many proteins that binds various ligands.

genes so that now there are known to be more than 20 PDE genes, and splicing variation of most of the genes yields even more PDEs with a final total of more than 50 isoforms *(2)*. Some of the PDEs degrade cyclic guanosine monophosphate (cGMP), some degrade cyclic adenine monophosphate (cAMP), and some degrade both cyclic nucleotides. These enzymes vary in tissue distributions and are believed to have different physiological roles. PDE1, PDE2, PDE3, PDE4, and PDE7 are present in cardiac tissue, and PDE1, PDE2, PDE3, PDE4, PDE5, and PDE11 are present in vascular smooth muscle.

The domain structure of each PDE is represented by the generic diagram shown in Fig. 1 *(1)*. Most PDEs are dimers containing two of these structures, but the functions of the dimeric structure are unknown. For some of the PDEs, the monomeric form retains all of the salient functions of the dimeric form in vitro *(3)*. Each PDE contains a regulatory domain in the more amino terminal portion of the protein and a catalytic domain located in the more carboxyl terminal portion. The regulatory domains vary widely among the PDEs. These domains can contain Ca^{2+}/calmodulin-binding sites, GAF (named for c<u>G</u>MP-binding PDEs, *Anabaena* <u>a</u>denylyl cyclase, *Escherichia coli* <u>F</u>hlA; ref. 4) domains that bind cGMP or perhaps other ligands, and phosphorylation sites; all of these can contribute to regulation of the respective PDE. The regulatory domains may also contain a component that provides for selective intracellular anchoring and localization of the PDE in a particular region of the cell. As will be described below, although the regulatory domains are not directly involved in interaction with PDE inhibitors, they may have profound impacts on PDE inhibitor effects.

The catalytic domains contain the molecular components for binding cGMP and cAMP and then degrading these nucleotides. The catalytic domains are homologous, that is, evolutionarily related, in all of the PDEs, which means that all of the PDE catalytic domains have similar amino acid sequences and similar modes of action. However, they also exhibit much dissimilarity, as exemplified by the aforementioned differences in cyclic nucleotide specificities. These differences have been exploited by the pharmaceutical industry, which has designed and synthesized specific PDE inhibitors for several PDE families. Prominent among these inhibitors are milrinone for PDE3, rolipram or Ariflo™ (Bayer, GlaxoSmithKline) for PDE4, and sildenafil (Viagra™, Pfizer, Inc., New York, NY), vardenafil (Levitra, Bayer, Germany; GlaxoSmithKline, UK), or tadalafil (Cialis, Lilly, Indianapolis; ICOS Bethel, WA) for PDE5. In general, these inhibitors have structural similarity to cGMP or cAMP and compete with the cyclic nucleotide for the catalytic domain of the respective PDE. Sildenafil, tadalafil, and vardenafil are relatively specific for inhibiting PDE5. Because this enzyme degrades cGMP, its inhibition fosters cGMP elevation in tissues where this enzyme is present in sufficient amounts and where cGMP synthesis is stimulated.

PDE5 CATALYTIC DOMAIN

The PDE5 catalytic domain is believed to contain a single site for interaction with cGMP (Fig. 2). Once cGMP is bound to the catalytic site, the catalytic machinery surrounding the molecule breaks the cyclic phosphate bond to form linear 5'-GMP, which is then released. The catalytic machinery includes at least one bound Zn^{2+} *(5)* and possibly other divalent cations, as well as key amino acids involved in the catalytic process *(6,7)*. Because PDE5 inhibitors such as sildenafil, vardenafil, and tadalafil have molecular features resembling those of cGMP, they can occupy the site, but unlike cGMP they are not

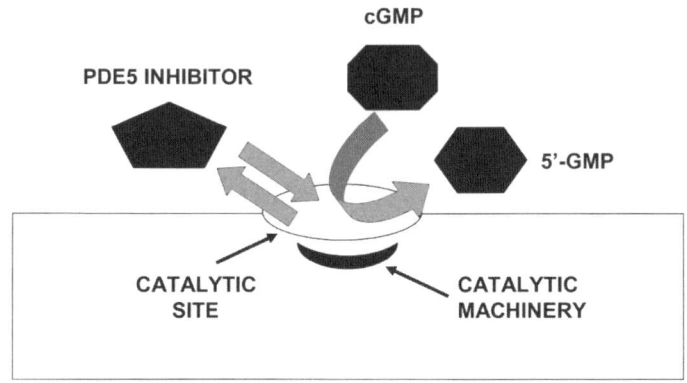

PDE5 CATALYTIC DOMAIN

Fig. 2. Model for physiological function of PDE5 catalytic domain.

degraded during occupation of the site. In other words, they are nonhydrolyzable competitive inhibitors of cGMP. Their potencies in occupying the site (IC_{50}s approximately 0.1–6 nM) can be compared with the potency of cGMP in occupying the site (K_m approximately 1 µM). Therefore, potent PDE5 inhibitors such as these possess about 1000–10,000 times higher affinity for the catalytic site than does the natural substrate cGMP (ref. *8*; Corbin et al., in press). This is the molecular basis of their efficacy to enhance tumescence in men with erectile dysfunction (ED) *(9,10)*. When PDE5 inhibitors occupy the catalytic site, cGMP cannot enter the site to be degraded by the catalytic machinery. This effect synergizes with increased cGMP synthesis because of stimulation by nitric oxide (NO) release in the penis, and results in penile erection. A similar synergism can occur in vascular smooth muscle outside the penile corpus cavernosum, which is the reason that combination of PDE5 inhibitor and nitrates is contraindicated.

PDE5 IN VASCULAR SMOOTH MUSCLE

Cyclic GMP and PDE5 have important roles in vascular smooth muscle (Fig. 3; refs. *11–14*). NO diffuses into smooth muscle cells to stimulate soluble guanylyl cyclase, an enzyme that synthesizes cGMP from GTP. Atrial natriuretic factor, a hormone derived mainly from cardiac tissue, stimulates a membrane-bound guanylyl cyclase to increase cGMP in this tissue. Elevation of cGMP by either agent acti-

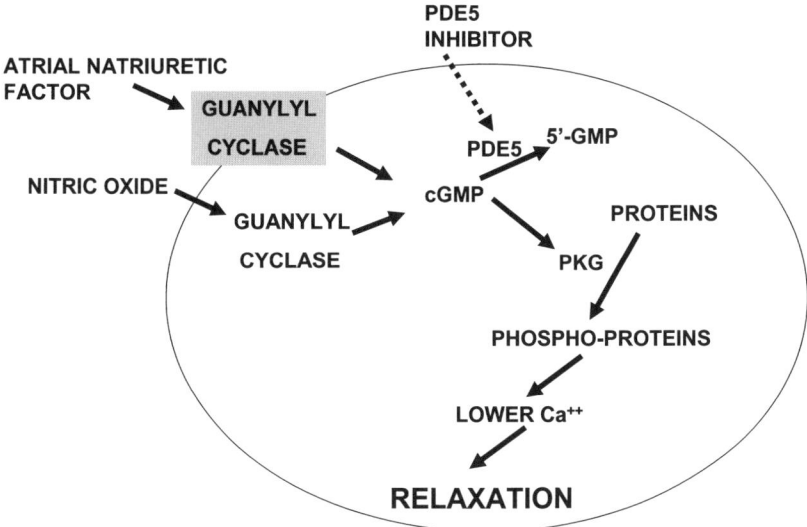

Fig. 3. cGMP pathway for regulation of vascular smooth muscle relaxation.

vates cGMP-dependent protein kinase (PKG), which phosphorylates several proteins to cause lowering of the intracellular Ca^2 or reduction in Ca^{2+} sensitivity. Because smooth muscle contraction is dependent on the Ca^{2+} level, lowering of Ca^{2+} produces relaxation of the muscle, resulting in dilation of the vessel. This can enhance local blood flow, decrease heart filling and work, or reduce systemic blood pressure. The effect increases coronary artery blood flow as well.

With regard to the penile vasculature, relaxation of smooth muscle caused by cGMP elevation increases blood flow into the cavernosal sinusoids, and causes sinusoidal expansion and venous occlusion, which together cause penile erection (8). Therefore, cGMP is the molecular trigger for penile erection. Activation of the cGMP-signaling pathway in the penis may be insufficient to elicit an erection when nerve stimulation, blood flow, or other functions are compromised. Because PDE5 degrades cGMP, this enzyme is normally responsible for dampening or terminating the pathway, meaning that penile erection is inhibited. PDE5 inhibitors, provided to the cavernosal smooth muscle cell by the blood flow, penetrate into these cells and inhibit PDE5. When cGMP synthesis is also increased, these two processes together potentiate cGMP elevation and penile erection. cGMP elevation brought about by PDE5 inhibitors is almost entirely dependent on concomitant stimulation of synthesis of cGMP, which explains why sildenafil efficacy requires simultaneous stimulation of cGMP synthesis by penile NO release caused by sexual arousal. The reasons that sildenafil selectively affects penile vascular smooth muscle over that of extra-penile tissues could be because (a) sexual arousal selectively provides the local NO stimulus with which PDE5 inhibition is synergistic in penis, and (b) PDE5 is highly abundant in penile corpus cavernosum *(15)*.

SELECTIVITY OF PDE5 INHIBITORS FOR PDE5 AND POTENTIAL SIDE EFFECTS

Most of the reported side effects of sildenafil, tadalafil, and vardenafil (headaches, flushing, lowering of blood pressure) can probably be explained by the presence of PDE5 in vascular smooth muscle outside the penile corpus cavernosum *(16)*. PDE5 and the other components of the cGMP pathway described earlier for the penis are known to be present in most vascular smooth muscle, including that of coronary vessels. These PDE5 inhibitors may cross-react to some extent with other PDEs or other proteins to produce side effects in patients. The potency of a PDE inhibitor is referred to as IC_{50} (inhibitor concentration 50%), which is the concentration of inhibitor that inhibits the respective PDE by 50% in vitro, not in vivo. It should be emphasized that the lower the IC_{50}, the more potent the inhibitor. Sildenafil and tadalafil have similar IC_{50} values, and vardenafil has a significantly lower value *(16)*. Efficacy of a PDE5 inhibitor in producing penile erection is dependent in part on its IC_{50}, but it is also strongly influenced by other factors including its pharmacokinetic properties. Selectivity of an inhibitor for one PDE over another PDE can be assessed by comparing IC_{50} of the inhibitor for these two PDEs. Absolute values for IC_{50} reported in the literature vary widely apparently because of the use of different sources of enzymes and conditions for assays *(16)*. Sildenafil IC_{50} ranges from 1 to 6 nM. This drug has more than 1000 times lower IC_{50} for PDE5 than for PDE2, PDE3, PDE4, PDE7, PDE8, PDE9, PDE10, or PDE11. It is very unlikely that sildenafil would cross-react with these PDEs to produce side effects in patients. Sildenafil has 100 times lower IC_{50} for PDE5 than for PDE1, so cross-reaction with this enzyme is also unlikely. However, this value is only 10 times lower for PDE5 than for retinal rod PDE6. Retinal PDE6 is a direct mediator of vision, and it is likely that cross-reaction of sildenafil with the PDE6 family could explain visual disturbances reported by some patients *(16)*. Newly described PDE5 inhibitors such as vardenafil and tadalafil may have less cross-reaction with PDE6. Cross-reaction of tadalafil with PDE11 is possible, but the functions of this enzyme are not clear at this time.

COULD PDE5 INHIBITORS AFFECT THE HEART?

During the first years after launch of sildenafil, and contrary to lack of effects of this drug on heart rate or cardiac index during clinical tests *(17)*, there was some speculation that this drug could have deleterious effects on the heart. Some of the concern was the result of the clinical history of milrinone, a PDE3 inhibitor known to produce heart complications *(18)*. Effects of several positive inotropic and chronotropic agents, such as adrenergic compounds, are mediated by elevation of cAMP in myocardial cells. Conversely, effects of negative inotropic and chronotropic agents, such as acetylcholine, are mediated by lowering of cAMP. Because milrinone inhibits PDE3 in myocardial cells, and this enzyme degrades cAMP, continual synthesis of cAMP in the absence of degradation causes cAMP elevation, which produces a positive inotropic effect. This effect is believed to underlie the heart complications that are sometimes seen with milrinone. However, it should be emphasized that PDE5, not PDE3, is the target of sildenafil in men. Despite common evolutionary origins of PDE3 and PDE5, these enzymes are quite distinct in several features. PDE5 degrades only cGMP, and PDE3 is believed to degrade mainly cAMP in cells. PDE3 can hydrolyze cGMP, albeit weakly, and cGMP competes with and inhibits cAMP hydrolysis. Sildenafil is selective for PDE5 over PDE3 by more than 4000-fold *(16)*, and it does not seem possible that there could be any cross-reaction on PDE3 at recommended doses of sildenafil. Thus, there is no scientific basis to consider sildenafil as a substitute for milrinone in its clinical effects. This should also apply to other PDE5 inhibitors if they exhibit a high selectivity for PDE5 over PDE3.

Although the physiological role of cGMP in myocardial cells is still debated, most studies suggest that elevation of this cyclic nucleotide causes a negative inotropic effect *(19)*, that is, opposite to that of cAMP. Based on this, it seems unlikely that PDE5 inhibitors could produce milrinone-like effects in the heart. It has been proposed that the negative inotropic effect of cGMP elevation is caused by the lowering of myocardial cell Ca^{2+} *(20)*, which is the same overall mechanism for cGMP-induced relaxation of vascular smooth muscle cells. The latter effect is believed to be responsible for the increased coronary artery flow seen with sildenafil.

Some studies have tested sildenafil effect on isolated dog *(21,21a)* or human cardiac muscle in organ baths. In neither case was there a significant effect on contractility at concentrations of the drug higher than the free sildenafil concentration would be in plasma of men after a 100-mg dose. In these experiments, either epinephrine, milrinone, or a nonspecific PDE inhibitor (3-isobutyl-1-methylxanthine) was used as a positive control to establish that the tissue was responding to positive inotropic agents.

CROSS-TALK

Another mechanism that has been mentioned as a route of potential effect of sildenafil or other PDE5 inhibitor on the heart is through a phenomenon called cross-talk. In this case, cross-talk refers to an interaction between PDE3 and PDE5. Most of the evidence for this interaction is derived from studies using platelets *(22)*. Elevation of either cAMP or cGMP in platelets inhibits aggregation. Agents that cause cGMP elevation may block platelet aggregation directly through activation of PKG, or they may do so indirectly through cross-talk or cross-activation of PKA. Elevated cGMP interacts with PDE3 to inhibit the hydrolysis of cAMP, leading to cAMP elevation, which directly blocks platelet aggregation by cAMP activation of PKA. In summary, cross-talk results in elevation of cAMP after elevation of cGMP. The process necessitates that both PDE3 and PDE5 reside in the same cell because cAMP and cGMP are not believed to pass from one cell to another in significant amounts. There is no doubt that PDE3 is present in myocardial cells, and PDE1, PDE2, PDE4, and PDE7 have also been reported to be present in this tissue. Most studies report the absence of PDE5 or presence of very low levels of this enzyme in these cells. Some *(21,23–27)* of these studies have utilized Northern analysis, which is an indirect method because it measures the mRNA coding for PDE5. The actual amount of a particular protein often does not correlate well with the amount of mRNA for that protein. More direct methods are Western analysis, which uses antibodies against the PDE5 protein, and measurement of enzyme activity. In most reported Western analyses, actual quantification of enzyme protein was not done. By the enzyme activity approach, we have detected very low levels of PDE5 in heart muscle homogenates *(21a)*. We could not rule out that the activity observed was derived from cell types other than myocardial cells, particularly since this preparation would also contain the smooth

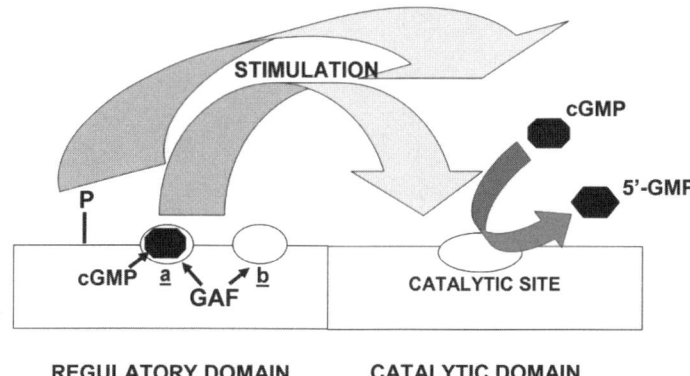

Fig. 4. Mechanisms for physiological activation of the PDE5 catalytic domain by the regulatory domain.

muscle from coronary vessels. This criticism would also apply to most studies using mRNA analysis.

ROLE OF THE REGULATORY DOMAIN OF PDE5 IN NEGATIVE FEEDBACK CONTROL OF THE CYCLIC GMP PATHWAY

The regulatory domain of PDE5 contains two GAF domains, at least one of which, GAFa, functions as a highly selective allosteric site for cGMP binding (Fig. 4; refs. *28,29*). Cyclic GMP stimulates PDE5 catalytic activity by binding to this site, but the bound cGMP is not degraded as it is when bound to the catalytic site. Sildenafil and possibly other PDE5 inhibitors do not interact directly with this site and produce their salient effects by interacting with the catalytic domain of the enzyme as discussed earlier. Four other PDE families (PDE2, PDE6, PDE10, and PDE11) also possess GAF domains *(1,30–34)*. In addition to PDE5, two other PDE families (PDE2, PDE6) have been shown to bind cGMP *(35,36)*. Binding of cGMP to the GAF domains of PDE2 stimulates catalytic activity of this enzyme by increasing affinity of the catalytic site for the substrate, cAMP or cGMP *(37)*. The regulatory domain of PDE5 is phosphorylated by cGMP-dependent protein kinase (PKG) at Ser-92 (bovine) both in vitro and in intact cells *(38–42)*. Regulation of phosphorylation of this site is substrate-directed because occupation of a GAF domain by cGMP is required for phosphorylation by PKG. Phosphorylation causes stimulation of both catalytic activity and cGMP binding to the GAF domain *(43,43a)*. It has been proposed that these effects are responsible for negative feedback regulation of active cGMP levels in cells.

Elevation of cGMP has been shown to cause increased PDE5 activity that is associated with cGMP-sensitive phosphorylation *(39–41)*. Elevation of cGMP is required for phosphorylation of PDE5 by PKG, and this process stimulates degradation of cGMP by the catalytic site as well as sequestration of cGMP in the GAF domain *(43)*, both of which represent negative feedback on the cGMP pathway. Negative feedback regulation of cGMP would be enhanced if cGMP binding to the GAF domain also directly stimulates the catalytic domain. This was predicted earlier from the principle of reciprocity *(44)*, which states that if a ligand allosterically stimulates binding of a second ligand molecule, then binding of the second ligand should stimulate binding of the first ligand *(45,46)*. Binding of 3-isobutyl-1-methylxanthine or a PDE5 inhibitor, such as sildenafil to the catalytic domain, has been shown to stimulate binding of cGMP to a GAF domain, and direct evidence that binding of cGMP to a GAF domain stimulates the catalytic domain has recently been presented. Okada and Asakawa recently reported that cGMP stimulates PDE5 catalytic activity when measured using a fluorescent cGMP analog that is specific for the catalytic site of the enzyme *(47)*. They suggested that this stimulation occurs through cGMP binding to the GAF domains. This suggestion is supported by studies in our laboratory showing that cGMP binding to the GAF domains stimulates radiolabeled sildenafil binding to the catalytic domain *(48)*. This observation has profound implications for PDE5 inhibitor efficacy as will be described later.

The consequence of negative feedback control of the cGMP pathway in the penis would be to dampen or terminate penile erection. The existence of such an intricate concert of mechanisms for this feedback implies that the cGMP elevation that produces penile erection is tightly limited. Apparently, vascular smooth muscle cells cannot readily tolerate excessive or persistent elevation of cGMP. Moreover, the feedback mechanism would theoretically potentiate reversal of erection, that is flaccidity.

NEGATIVE FEEDBACK CONTROL OF PDE5 ENGENDERS GREATER PDE5 INHIBITOR EFFICACY

From a physiological viewpoint, the negative feedback system described earlier would be inhibitory for penile erection because cGMP levels would be lowered by this process. From a pharmacological viewpoint, the efficacy of PDE5 inhibitors should theoretically be enhanced by this system (Fig. 5). This would occur because PDE5

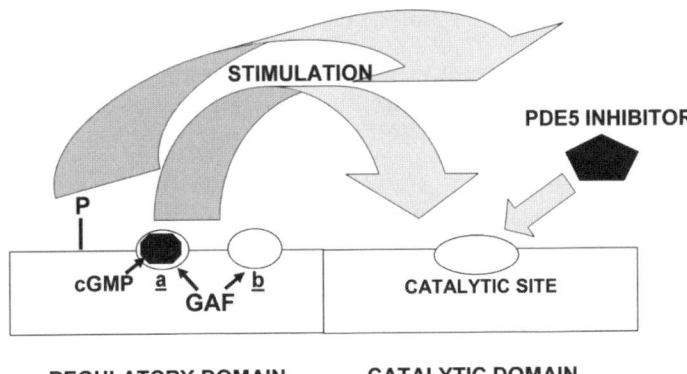

Fig. 5. Proposed mechanisms by which a PDE5 inhibitor stimulates its own affinity and efficacy through elevation of cGMP.

inhibitors increase the cGMP level, and there would be increased cGMP binding to the GAF domain. This, in turn, would increase the catalytic domain binding affinity for sildenafil or presumably other PDE5 inhibitors. The improved affinity for the inhibitor is fostered by the feedback mechanisms initiated by cGMP elevation. As these PDE5 inhibitors bind to the catalytic domain to cause cGMP elevation, this elevation causes further inhibitor binding and higher cGMP elevation, which stimulates further penile erection. In other words, were it not for the presence of negative feedback control of the cGMP pathway, much higher doses of the inhibitors would be required to produce penile erections.

ACKNOWLEDGMENTS

This work was supported by NIH DK58277, DK40029, and a grant from Pfizer.

REFERENCES

1. Francis SH, Turko IV, Corbin JD. Cyclic nucleotide phosphodiesterases: relating structure and function. Prog Nucleic Acid Res Mol Biol 2001;65:1–52.
2. Conti M, Jin SL. The molecular biology of cyclic nucleotide phosphodiesterases. Prog. Nucleic Acid Res Mol Biol 1999;63:1–38.
3. Fink TL, Francis SH, Beasley A, et al. Expression of a fully active, monomeric catalytic domain of the cGMP-binding cGMP-specific phosphodiesterase (PDE5). J Biol Chem 1999;274:34,613–34,620.
4. Aravind L, Ponting CP. The GAF domain: an evolutionary link between diverse phototransducing proteins. Trends Biochem Sci 1997;22:458–459.

5. Francis SH, Colbran JL, McAllister-Lucas LM, et al. Zinc interactions and conserved motifs of the cGMP-binding cGMP-specific phosphodiesterase suggest that it is a zinc hydrolase. J Biol Chem 1994;269:22,477–22,480.
6. Turko IV, Francis SH, Corbin JD. Potential roles of conserved amino acids in the catalytic domain of the cGMP-binding cGMP-specific phosphodiesterase. J Biol Chem 1998;273:6460–6466.
7. Xu RX, Hassell AM, Vanderwall D, et al. Atomic structure of PDE4: insights into phosphodiesterase mechanism and specificity. Science 2000;288: 1822–1825.
8. Corbin JD, Francis SH. Cyclic GMP phosphodiesterase-5: target of sildenafil. J Biol Chem 1999;274:13,729–13,732.
9. Boolell M, Allen MJ, Ballard SA, et al. Sildenafil: an orally active type 5 cyclic GMP-specific phosphodiesterase inhibitor for the treatment of penile erectile dysfunction. Int J Impotence Res 1996; 8:47–52.
10. Uckert S, Kuthe A, Stief CG, et al. Phosphodiesterase isoenzymes as pharmacological targets in the treatment of male erectile dysfunction. World J Urol 2001; 19:14–22.
11. Waldman SA, Murad F. Biochemical mechanisms underlying vascular smooth muscle relaxation: the guanylate cyclase-cyclic GMP system. J Cardiovasc Pharmacol 1988;12(Suppl 5):S115–S118.
12. Jiang H, Colbran JL, Francis SH, et al. Direct evidence for cross-activation of cGMP-dependent protein kinase by cAMP in pig coronary arteries. J Biol Chem 1992;267:1015–1019.
13. Lincoln TM, Cornwell TL. Towards an understanding of the mechanism of action of cyclic AMP and cyclic GMP in smooth muscle relaxation. Blood Vessels 1991;28:129–137.
14. Walter U. Physiological role of cGMP and cGMP-dependent protein kinase in the cardiovascular system. Rev Physiol Biochem Pharmacol 1989;113:41–88.
15. Gopal VK, Francis SH, Corbin JD. Allosteric sites of phosphodiesterase-5 (PDE5). A potential role in negative feedback regulation of cGMP signaling in corpus cavernosum. Eur J Biochem 2001;268:3304–3312.
16. Corbin JD, Francis SH. Pharmacology of phosphodiesterase-5 inhibitors. Int J Clin Pract 2002;56:453–459.
17. Jackson G, Benjamin N, Jackson N, et al. Effects of sildenafil citrate on human hemodynamics. Am J Cardiol 1999;83:13C–20C.
18. Lynch JJ Jr., Uprichard AC, Frye JW, et al. Effects of the positive inotropic agents milrinone and pimobendan on the development of lethal ischemic arrhythmias in conscious dogs with recent myocardial infarction. J Cardiovasc Pharmacol 1989;14:585–597.
19. Nawrath H. Does cyclic GMP mediate the negative inotropic effect of acetylcholine in the heart? Nature 1977;267:72–74.
20. Hartzell HC, Fischmeister R. Opposite effects of cyclic GMP and cyclic AMP on Ca^{2+} current in single heart cells. Nature 1986;323:273–275.
21. Wallis RM, Corbin JD, Francis SH, et al. Tissue distribution of phosphodiesterase families and the effects of sildenafil on tissue cyclic nucleotides, platelet function, and the contractile responses of trabeculae carneae and aortic rings in vitro. Am J Cardiol 1999;83:3–12.
21a. Corbin J, Rannels S, Neal D, et al. Sildenafil citrate does not affect cardiac contractility in human or dog heart. Curr Med Res Opin 2003;19:747–752.

22. Maurice DH, Haslam RJ. Molecular basis of the synergistic inhibition of platelet function by nitrovasodilators and activators of adenylate cyclase: inhibition of cyclic AMP breakdown by cyclic GMP. Mol Pharmacol 1990;37:671–681.
23. Loughney K, Hill TR, Florio VA, et al. Isolation and characterization of cDNAs encoding PDE5A, a human cGMP-binding cGMP-specific 3′,5′-cyclic nucleotide phosphodiesterase. Gene 1998;216:137–147.
24. Yanaka N, Kotera J, Ohtsuka A, et al. Expression, structure and chromosomal localization of the human cGMP-binding cGMP-specific phosphodiesterase PDE5A gene. Eur J Biochem 1998;255:391–399.
25. Kotera J, Fujishige K, Akatsuka H, et al. Novel alternative splice variants of cGMP-binding cGMP-specific phosphodiesterase. J Biol Chem 1998;273: 26,982–26,990.
26. Kotera J, Fujishige K, Imai Y, et al. Genomic origin and transcriptional regulation of two variants of cGMP-binding cGMP-specific phosphodiesterases. Eur J Biochem 1999;262:866–872.
27. Senzaki H, Smith CJ, Juang GJ, et al. Cardiac phosphodiesterase 5 (cGMP-specific) modulates beta-adrenergic signaling in vivo and is down-regulated in heart failure. FASEB J 2001;15:1718–1726.
28. McAllister-Lucas LM, Sonnenburg WK, Kadlecek A, et al. The structure of a bovine lung cGMP-binding, cGMP-specific phosphodiesterase deduced from a cDNA clone. J Biol Chem 1993;268:22,863–22,873.
29. Liu L, Underwood T, Li H, et al. Specific cGMP binding by the cGMP binding domains of cGMP-binding cGMP-specific phosphodiesterase. Cell Signalling 2001;13:1–7.
30. Charbonneau H, Prusti RK, LeTrong H, et al. Identification of a noncatalytic cGMP-binding domain conserved in both the cGMP-stimulated and photoreceptor cyclic nucleotide phosphodiesterases. Proc Natl Acad Sci USA 1990;87: 288–292.
31. Charbonneau H. Structure-function relationships among cyclic nucleotide phosphodiesterases. In: Beavo J, Houslay MD, eds. Cyclic Nucleotide Phosphodiesterases: Structure, Regulation and Drug Action. Wiley, New York, 1990, pp. 267–296.
32. Soderling SH, Bayuga SJ, Beavo JA. Isolation and characterization of a dual-substrate phosphodiesterase gene family: PDE10A. Proc Natl Acad Sci USA 1999;96:7071–7076.
33. Fujishige K, Kotera J, Michibata H, et al. Cloning and characterization of a novel human phosphodiesterase that hydrolyzes both cAMP and cGMP (PDE10A). J Biol Chem 1999;274:18,438–18,445.
34. Fawcett L, Baxendale R, Stacey P, et al. Molecular cloning and characterization of a distinct human phosphodiesterase gene family: PDE11A. Proc Natl Acad Sci USA 2000;97:3702–3707.
35. Stroop SD, Beavo JA. Structure and function studies of the cGMP-stimulated phosphodiesterase. J Biol Chem 1991;266:23,802–23,809.
36. Yamazaki A, Sen I, Bitensky MW, et al. Cyclic GMP-specific, high affinity, noncatalytic binding sites on light-activated phosphodiesterase. J Biol Chem 1980; 255:11,619–11,624.
37. Beavo JA, Hardman JG, Sutherland EW. Stimulation of adenosine 3′,5′-monophosphate hydrolysis by guanosine 3′,5′-monophosphate. J Biol Chem 1971;246:3841–3846.

38. Thomas MK, Francis SH, Corbin JD. Substrate- and kinase-directed regulation of phosphorylation of a cGMP-binding phosphodiesterase by cGMP. J Biol Chem 1990;265:14,971–14,978.
39. Wyatt TA, Naftilan AJ, Francis SH, et al. ANF elicits phosphorylation of the cGMP phosphodiesterase in vascular smooth muscle cells. Am J Physiol Heart Circ Physiol 1998;274:H448–H455.
40. Murthy KS. Activation of phosphodiesterase 5 and inhibition of guanylate cyclase by cGMP-dependent protein kinase in smooth muscle. Biochem J 2001;360: 199–208.
41. Mullershausen F, Russwurm M, Thompson WJ, et al. Rapid nitric oxide-induced desensitization of the cGMP response is caused by increased activity of phosphodiesterase type 5 paralleled by phosphorylation of the enzyme. J Cell Biol 2001;155:271–278.
42. Rybalkin SD, Rybalkina IG, Feil R, et al. Regulation of cGMP-specific phosphodiesterase (PDE5) phosphorylation in smooth muscle cells. J Biol Chem 2002;277:3310–3317.
43. Corbin JD, Turko IV, Beasley A, et al. Phosphorylation of phosphodiesterase-5 by cyclic nucleotide-dependent protein kinase alters its catalytic and allosteric cGMP-binding activities. Eur J Biochem 2000;267:2760–2767.
43a. Francis SH, Bessay EP, Kofera J, et al. Phosphorylation of isolated human phosphodiesterase-5 regulatory domain induces an apparent conformational change and increases cGMP binding affinity. J Biol Chem 2002;277:47,581–47,587.
44. Thomas MK, Francis SH, Corbin JD. Characterization of a purified bovine lung cGMP-binding cGMP phosphodiesterase. J Biol Chem 1990;265:14,964–14,970.
45. Weber G. Energetics of ligand binding to protein. Adv Protein Chem 1975; 29:1–83.
46. Francis SH, Thomas MK, Corbin JD. Cyclic GMP-binding cyclic GMP-specific phosphodiesterase from lung. In: Beavo, J., Houslay, M. D., eds.Cyclic Nucleotide Phosphodiesterases: Structure, Regulation, and Drug Action. Wiley, New York, 1990, pp. 117–140.
47. Okada D, Asakawa S. Allosteric activation of cGMP-specific, cGMP-binding phosphodiesterase (PDE5) by cGMP. Biochemistry 2002; 41:9672–9679.
48. Corbin J, Blount MA, Weeks JL, et al. [^{3}H] sildenafil binding to phosphodiesterase-5 is specific, kinetically heterogeneous, and stimulated by cGMP. Mol Pharmacol 2003;63:1364–1372.

8 The Hemodynamics of Phosphodiesterase-PDE5 Inhibitors

Graham Jackson, FRCP, FESC, FACC, FAHA

CONTENTS
INTRODUCTION
HEMODYNAMIC STUDIES (SILDENAFIL)
TADALAFIL AND VARDENAFIL
NITRATE INTERACTION
ARTERIAL STIFFNESS
HEMODYNAMIC PROPERTIES AND CLINICAL USE
CONCLUSION
REFERENCES

INTRODUCTION

Sildenafil citrate (Viagra™; Pfizer, Inc., New York, NY) is the first of a series of orally active phosphodiesterase (PDE) type-5 inhibitors that have and will continue to transform the treatment of erectile dysfunction (ED) *(1)*. Initially advocated as a potential alternative to oral nitrates for the treatment of stable angina pectoris, sildenafil's short half-life and its modest nitrate-like hemodynamic properties were not seen as a clinical advance. Sildenafil's role in the treatment of ED follows from erections in healthy volunteers being recorded as "adverse events." The subsequent recognition that vascular disease accounts for greater than 70% of ED cases and that cardiac disease, either documented or silent, is a frequent cause of ED refocused attention on silde-

From: *Contemporary Cardiology: Heart Disease and Erectile Dysfunction*
Edited by: R. A. Kloner © Humana Press Inc., Totowa, NJ

nafil's hemodynamic properties, initially in the context of safety but more recently as a form of therapy (2). Therefore, because PDE5 is present in smooth muscle cells throughout the vasculature, the potential for PDE5 inhibition reducing the degradation of guanosine monophosphate has widespread implications throughout the vascular system.

HEMODYNAMIC STUDIES (SILDENAFIL)

Coronary Disease Patients

As part of the original anginal protocol, an intravenous hemodynamic study was performed in eight men with stable angina and proven severe coronary disease at angiography (3). Intravenous sildenafil at a cumulative dose of 40 mg was administered over a 60-min interval between two supine bicycle exercise tests.

All antianginal medications, including vasodilating drugs and also diuretics, were uneventfully withdrawn 48 h before the study. A pulmonary artery catheter and arterial line were inserted for pressure monitoring. An initial bicycle exercise test determined the workload to angina and whether exercise could be maintained for 4 min. A baseline hemodynamic data set was recorded during a second 4-min bicycle exercise test. After a 20-min rest period, additional baseline resting hemodynamic recordings were made over a 15-min period. Sildenafil was then infused over four 15-min periods at doses of 5, 5, 10, and 20 mg. After the final infusions, resting hemodynamics were recorded and then repeated after a 4-min bicycle exercise test (supine as before). Plasma levels of sildenafil taken after the final infusion ranged from 950–2023 ng/mL—similar to 100–200 mg of oral sildenafil.

Sildenafil, in effect, behaved like a nitrate (Table 1). At rest, there was a small fall in wedge pressure (1.6 mmHg), pulmonary artery pressure (4.6 mmHg), and systolic (9 mmHg) and diastolic (8 mmHg) arterial pressure compared with baseline. Heart rate was unchanged as was cardiac output measured using thermodilution techniques. On exercise, the falls in wedge and pulmonary artery pressure increased as would be predicted (vasodilatory response) with also a 12/5 mmHg fall in arterial pressure and a small (7%) reduction in cardiac output. The study identified a modest decrease in central filling pressures with a reduction in peripheral blood pressure in keeping with mixed vasodilatory properties. There were no adverse events.

Healthy Volunteers

Numerous studies have been performed in healthy volunteers (age range 18–81 yr) evaluating the effects of sildenafil on heart rate and

Table 1
Effects of Sildenafil on Mean Hemodynamic Parameters at Rest and During Exercise in Patients With Stable Ischemic Heart Disease

Parameter	At Rest		After 4-Min Exercise Test	
	Baseline (n = 7)	Sildenafil (40 mg, IV) (n = 8)	Baseline (n = 8)	Sildenafil (40 mg, IV) (n = 8)
PAOP (mm Hg)	8.1 ± 5.1	6.5 ± 4.3	36.0 ± 13.7	27.8 ± 15.3
PAP (mm Hg)	16.7 ± 4.0	12.1 ± 3.9	39.4 ± 12.9	31.7 ± 13.2
RAP (mm Hg)	5.7 ± 3.7	4.1 ± 3.7	NR	NR
Systolic SAP (mm Hg)	150 ± 12	141 ± 16	200 ± 37	188 ± 30
Diastolic SAP (mm Hg)	74 ± 8	66 ± 10	85 ± 10	80 ± 9
Cardiac output (L/min)	5.6 ± 0.9	5.2 ± 1.1	11.5 ± 2.4	10.2 ± 3.5
Heart rate (beats/min)	67 ± 11	67 ± 12	102 ± 12	99 ± 20

Values represent the mean ± 2D.

IV, intravenous; NR, not recorded; PAP, pulmonary acterial pressure; PAOP, pulmonary arterial occluded pressure; RAP, right artrial pressure; SAP, systemic arterial pressure.

blood pressure *(1,3)*. In a single-blind four-way crossover trial, eight healthy volunteers were randomly assigned to receive three escalating single doses of 20, 40, and 80 mg of sildenafil *(3)*. In a second study, eight healthy male volunteers were evaluated in a single-blind four-way crossover dose-escalation study of 100, 150, and 200 mg sildenafil and randomly selected placebo *(3)*. There was no evidence of a dose–response effect on cardiovascular variables with the mean maximum reduction in supine blood pressure (8/6 mmHg) occurring 1–2 h after oral dosing and at the end of the infusion period. There were no orthostatic effects recorded. Blood pressure readings were back to baseline within 5 h of receiving sildenafil. In the oral study, there was a 5 beats/min reduction in heart rate after 100 mg sildenafil, but no changes were noted in the intravenous study. In these studies, sildenafil was again seen to be a modest vasodilator with a balanced effect on arterial resistance and venous compliance.

Comment

The data from hemodynamic studies in volunteers and those with coronary disease are compatible with the original concept of sildenafil having nitrate-like properties, which could be advantageous to the ischemic patient. A modest vasodilator affecting both preload and afterload with no significant effect on heart rate cardiac output or systemic or pulmonary vascular resistance, sildenafil, in this population, is not surprisingly associated with no increased hemodynamic risks. The possibility of these properties being used in specific treatment groups (e.g., pulmonary hypertension and cardiac failure) has led to considerable scientific interest, which has translated into clinical benefit (*see* Chapter 13).

TADALAFIL AND VARDENAFIL

Tadalafil differs from vardenafil and sildenafil in having a longer half-life (17 h), which may delay safe subsequent nitrate use *(5,6)*. Both drugs, as a result of their mechanism of action, have mild vasodilating properties similar to sildenafil. Tadalafil has been evaluated in more detail (10 and 20 mg) in both healthy volunteers and phase III trials, and no statistically significant hemodynamic effects were recorded in comparison with placebo *(7)*.

NITRATE INTERACTION

The synergistic effect between sublingual and oral nitrates is well documented and applies to all PDE5 inhibitors. It is unpredictable and not inevitable, but, because the scale of pressure drop can be substantial, the contraindication to simultaneous use is without exception *(1,7,8)*.

ARTERIAL STIFFNESS

In the early original hemodynamic studies, forearm blood flow and venous compliance was evaluated *(3)*. A placebo-controlled trial was performed using escalating brachial artery infusions of sildenafil up to 300 µg/min in 12 healthy volunteers.

Mean ratios of cannulated to noncannulated forearm blood flow increased with the infusion rate of sildenafil compared to placebo equating to a reduction in forearm vascular resistance (Fig. 1). From a baseline of 1.1%, a cuff pressure of 20 mmHg produced a maximum increase in forearm volume of 1.4% (26% increase), and at 40 mmHg the volume increased from baseline 1.9% to 2.3% (23% increase). No changes occurred during placebo infusions.

Subsequent studies have identified benefits on brachial arterial flow both acutely and chronically (Chapter 13), suggesting potential long-term benefits on endothelial function *(9)*. Arterial stiffness predicts mortality in hypertension and can be evaluated using pulse wave velocity studies *(10,11)*. In stiff arteries, whether atherosclerotic hyper-

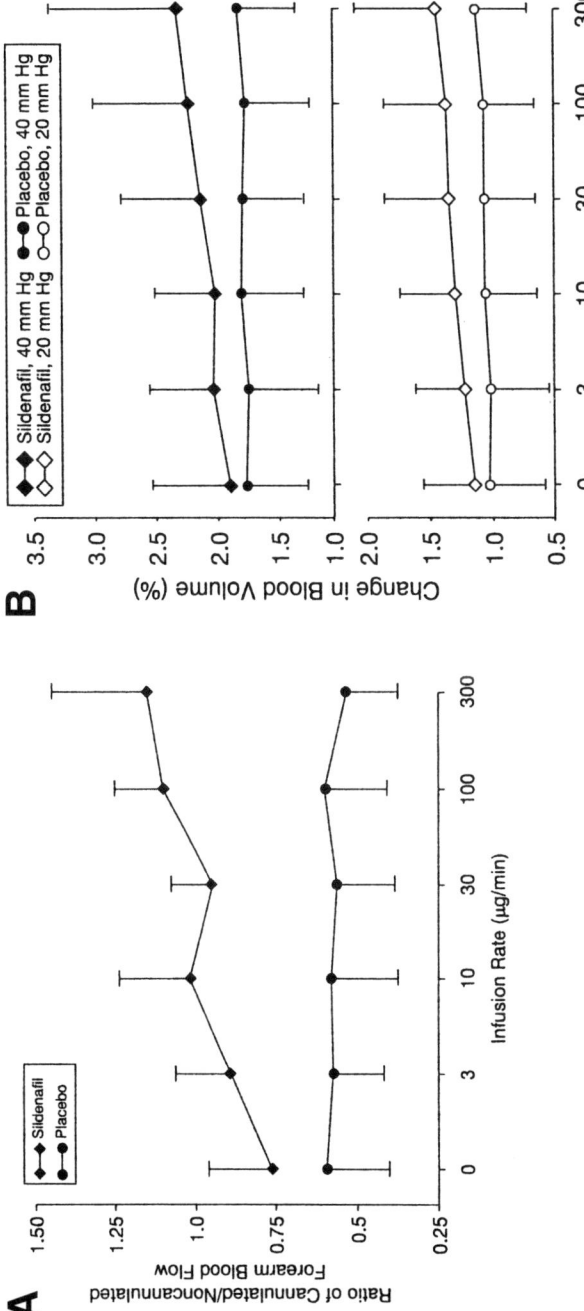

Fig. 1. Changes in forearm blood flow and venous compliance during intraarterial infusion of sildenafil and placebo in healthy men. (**A**) represents the ratio of cannulated-to-noncannulated forearm blood flow in subjects administered increasing doses of sildenafil. (**B**) represents percent changes in forearm volume in subjects treated with increasing doses of sildenafil and using two different cuff pressures, 20 mm Hg or 50 mm Hg. The baseline infusion (0) consisted of dextrose (5%) norepinephrine and mannitol (5%). Data are presented as mean values ± SD; $n = 8$ per group. Reproduced with permission from ref. 3.

tensive or both, the pulse wave velocity is faster than in more compliant arteries. Central aortic pressure waveforms can be derived from the radial artery. A forward wave occurs during systole and is followed by a reflected wave returning to the central circulation. In health, the reflected wave is in diastole, but with stiffness the wave is more proximal and the pulse wave velocity increases. A second augmented systolic peak may occur and the pulse pressure widen. The augmentation index (AI) represents the pressure difference between the two peaks with the pulse pressure as the denominator and is expressed as a percentage.

Sildenafil significantly lowers the AI in hypertensive patients as well as those with risk factors for ED *(11)*. Systolic aortic and diastolic pressures fell by 14.4 and 9.6 mmHg, respectively, with the AI reduced 13% *(12)*. Although this effect could be a blood pressure-lowering effect, it could also be explained by sildenafil having a direct effect on endothelial function, which would be in keeping with its mechanism of action and the initial forearm, flow studies. Furthermore, brachial arterial flow mediated dilatation was improved in diabetics who were not hypertensive after both acute (25 mg) and chronic oral sildenafil therapy *(9)*.

HEMODYNAMIC PROPERTIES AND CLINICAL USE

In hypertensive patients there is a blood pressure-lowering effect that is greater the higher the baseline blood pressure when sildenafil vs placebo is added to background hypertensive therapy *(11)*. The maximum reductions were 24 ± 10 vs 6 ± 8 mmHg ($p < 0.05$) in systolic and 8 ± 5 vs 3 ± 2 mmHg ($p < 0.05$) in diastolic pressure, readings comparable with the expected response from conventional hypertensive therapy.

Effects in pulmonary hypertension and cardiac failure are reviewed in Chapter 13. The overall impression is of a potent and potentially important new class of drugs for managing cardiovascular disease.

CONCLUSION

Hemodynamically, the PDE5 inhibitors are balanced nitrate-like vasodilators. Their use in patients with ED (not taking nitrates) is safe and potentially beneficial for the cardiovascular patient *(1)*. In disease states where the nitric oxide–cyclic guanosine monophosphate pathway (cGMP) is impaired, by preventing degradation cGMP PDE5 inhibitors may be a mechanistic and functional solution (part or full) to the clinical endpoint problem. This might include patients with hypertension, cardiac failure, pulmonary hypertension, and arterial stiffness.

Sildenafil, the original oral PDE5 inhibitor, has come full circle from cardiac drug to ED therapy and back to cardiac drug. ED stands for endothelial as well as erectile dysfunction, and PDE5 inhibitors may turn out to be therapy for both. The mode of action of PDE inhibitors with reference to endothelial function might translate into a role chronically in preventative vascular disease.

REFERENCES

1. Padma-Nathan H, Eardley I, Kloner R, et al. A 4-year update on the safety of sildenafil citrate (Viagra). Urology 2002;60(Suppl 2B):67–90.
2. Jackson G. Erectile dysfunction and cardiovascular disease. Int J Clin Pract 1999;53:363–368.
3. Jackson G, Benjamin N, Jackson N, et al. Effects of sildenafil citrate on human hemodynamics. Am J Cardiol 1999;83:13C–20C.
4. Gillies HC, Roblin D, Jackson G. Coronary and systemic haemodynamic effects of sildenafil citrate: from basic science to clinical studies in patients with cardiovascular disease. Int J Cardiol 2002;86:131–141.
5. Giuliano F, Varanese L. Tadalafil: a novel treatment for erectile dysfunction. Eur Heart J 2002;4(Suppl H):H24–H31.
6. Thadani U, Smith W, Nash S, et al. The effect of vardenafil, a potent and highly selective phosphodiesterase-5 inhibitor for the treatment of erectile dysfunction, on the cardiovascular response to exercise in patients with coronary artery disease. J Am Coll Cardiol 2002;40:2006–2012.
7. Emmick JT, Stuewe SR, Mitchell M. Overview of the cardiovascular effects of tadalafil. Eur Heart J 2002;4(Suppl H):H32–H47.
8. Webb DJ, Freestone S, Allen MJ, et al. Sildenafil citrate and blood-pressure-lowering-drugs; results of drug interaction studies with an organic nitrate and a calcium antagonist. Am J Cardiol 1999;83:21C–28C.
9. DeSouza C, Parulkar A, Lumpkin D, et al. Acute and prolonged effects of sildenafil on brachial artery flow-mediated dilatation in type 2 diabetes. Diabetes Care 2002;25:1336–1339.
10. Laurent S, Boutouyrie R, Asmar R, et al. Aortic stiffness is an independent predictor of all-cause mortality in hypertensive patients. J Hypertens 2000;18:582.
11. Mahmud A, Hennessey M, Freely J. Effect of sildenafil on blood pressure and arterial wave reflection in treated hypertensive men. J Human Hypertens 2001;15:707–713.
12. Vlachopoulos C, Hirata K, O'Rourke M. Effects of sildenafil (Viagra®) on wave reflection: a new insight into its cardiovascular effects. J Am Coll Cardiol 2001;37(Suppl A):260A.

9 Cardiovascular Safety of Phosphodiesterase-5 Inhibitors

Robert A. Kloner, MD, PhD

CONTENTS
INTRODUCTION
HOW DO PDE5 INHIBITORS WORK?
SILDENAFIL (VIAGRA)
TADALAFIL (CIALIS)
VARDENAFIL (LEVITRA)
POTENTIAL NEW THERAPEUTIC OPTIONS
   FOR PDE5 INHIBITORS
CONCLUSION
REFERENCES

INTRODUCTION

Oral phosphodiesterase-5 (PDE5) inhibitors have been shown to be effective oral agents for the treatment of organic, psychogenic, and mixed erectile dysfunction (ED). There are numerous PDE isoforms throughout the body *(1)*. PDE5 is concentrated in genitalia but is also found in systemic arteries and veins throughout the body as well as in smooth muscle cells in the gastrointestinal tract and platelets *(2–4)*.

HOW DO PDE5 INHIBITORS WORK?

During sexual stimulation, nitric oxide (NO) is released from nerve cells and endothelial cells in the corpus cavernosum of the penis

From: *Contemporary Cardiology: Heart Disease and Erectile Dysfunction*
Edited by: R. A. Kloner © Humana Press Inc., Totowa, NJ

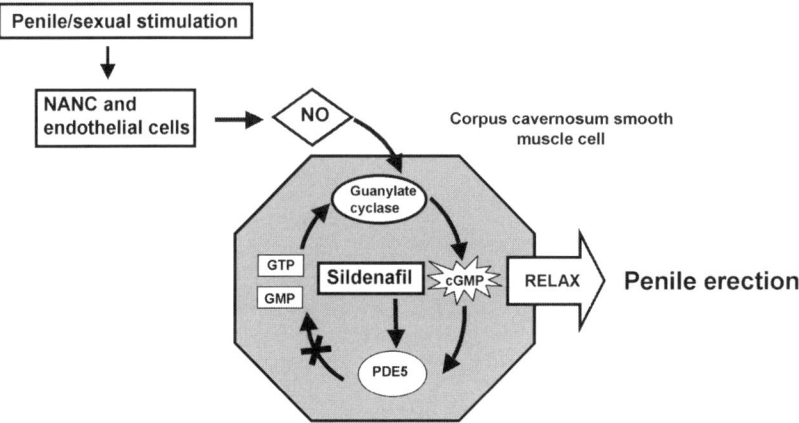

Fig. 1. Nitric oxide (NO)-cyclic guanosine monophosphate (cGMP) mechanism of penile erection and the NO-enhancing effect of the phosphodiesterase type-5 (PDE5) inhibitor sildenafil. GTP, guanosine triphosphate; NANC, nonadrenergic-noncholinergic neurons. From Zusman (16); used with permission.

(Figs. 1 and 2). NO stimulates the enzyme guanylate cyclase to catalyze the formation of cyclic guanosine monophosphate (cGMP) (5–7). By reducing influx of calcium into smooth muscle cells, cGMP eventually results in relaxation of smooth muscle cells of the arteries, arterioles, and sinusoids of the corpus cavernosum (6). The vascular structures relax and sinusoids fill up with blood, much like a sponge filling with water. Corporal blood pressure approaches or exceeds mean arterial pressure. The subtunica venous plexus becomes compressed under the tunica albuginea, resulting in a venous–occlusive mechanism that maintains penile erection. PDE5 degrades intracellular cGMP, terminating its smooth muscle-relaxing effects. PDE5 inhibitors, such as sildenafil, tadalafil, vardenafil, and others in development, prevent the breakdown of cGMP by PDE5 (8). cGMP levels increase and allow better vasodilation of the vascular structure of the corpus cavernosum. These agents have been shown in randomized, placebo-controlled, multicenter trials to improve ED in a high percentage of men with ED (9–12). They are effective in men with ED on the basis of atherosclerosis (vascular), neurogenic, endocrine, and psychogenic causes (13). They are effective in men with ED who have hypertension and are on antihypertensive medicines (14). Their efficacy rates are somewhat lower in men with diabetes or in men who have undergone radical prostate surgery without nerve sparing.

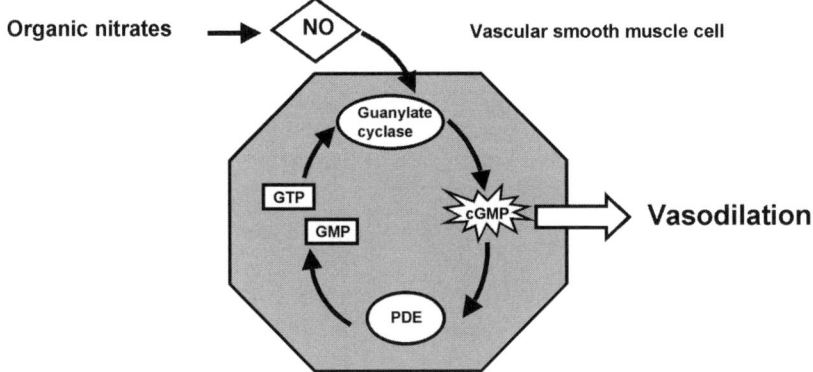

Fig. 2. Mechanism of endothelium-dependent vasodilation and the effect of organic nitrates and nitric oxide (NO) donors. cGMP, cyclic guanosine monophosphate; PDE, phosphodiesterse. From Zusman *(16)*; used with permission.

SILDENAFIL (VIAGRA)

Sildenafil was the first of the oral PDE5 inhibitors approved for ED. This agent has been studied in greatest detail regarding cardiovascular safety *(15,16)*. Sildenafil was studied initially as a potential antianginal agent because its hemodynamic profile resembles that of a weak nitrate. As mentioned, the enzyme PDE5 is found not only in the corpus cavernosum of the penis but also in the smooth muscle cells of arteries and veins throughout the body. Hence, administration of a PDE5 inhibitor will result in some degree of systemic vasodilation of arteries and veins. Intravenous sildenafil at 80 mg reduced systolic blood pressure by –9.2 mmHg and diastolic blood pressure by –6.7 mmHg in healthy men *(3)*. Reductions in blood pressure were transient with return of blood pressure within 5 h. Sildenafil reduced systemic vascular resistance but, interestingly, had no effect on heart rate. In another study, oral doses of sildenafil (100, 150, and 200 mg) were administered to healthy men *(3)*. Mean maximal blood pressure decrease was –10/–7 mmHg occurring 3 h after dosing (Fig. 3A). Of note, decrease in blood pressure did not correlate with dose, in that the 200-mg oral dose did not decrease pressure to a greater extent than the two lower doses. There was no orthostatic drop in blood pressure compared with placebo. Cardiac index increased slightly but transiently after the 100 and 200 mg doses of sildenafil but did not change significantly vs placebo from 1–12 h after oral therapy (Fig. 3B). Other studies documented similar small

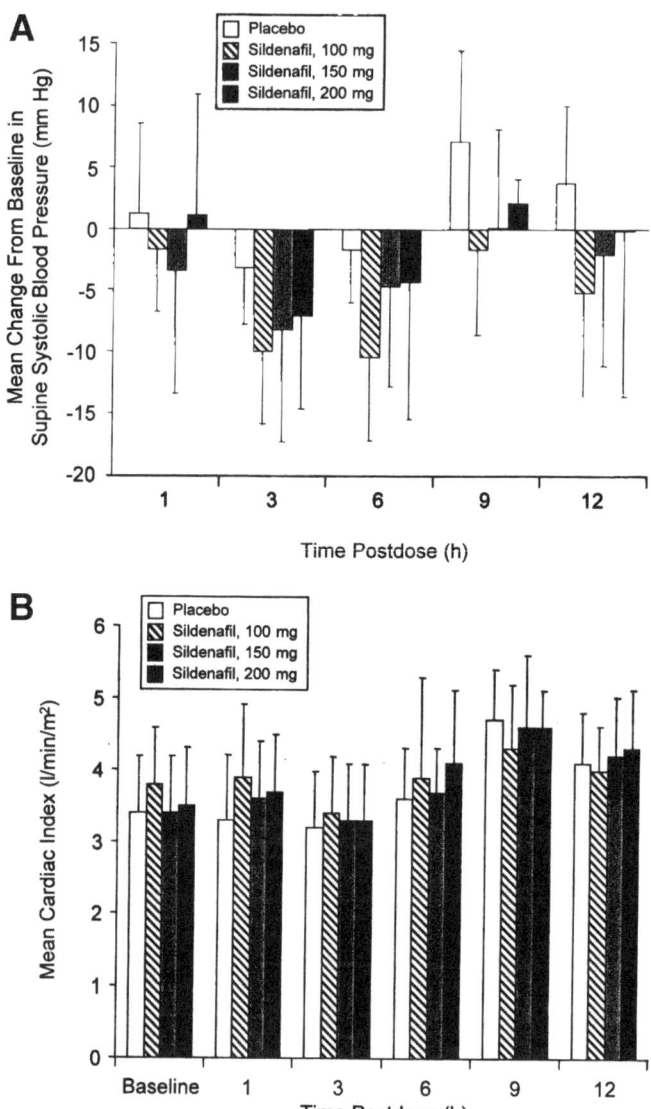

Fig. 3. Hemodynamic changes after the administration of increasing oral doses of sildenafil in healthy men. **A**, Supine systolic blood pressure changes from baseline; **B**, mean supine cardiac index. Values are mean ± SD; $n = 8$ per group. From ref. *3*; used with permission.

falls in blood pressure in middle-age volunteers receiving sildenafil (ref. *16*; Fig. 4).

Thus, sildenafil is a weak vasodilator, and, because its hemodynamic effects resemble to some extent a weak nitrate, it initially was tested as

Chapter 9 / Cardiovascular Safety of PDE5 Inhibitors

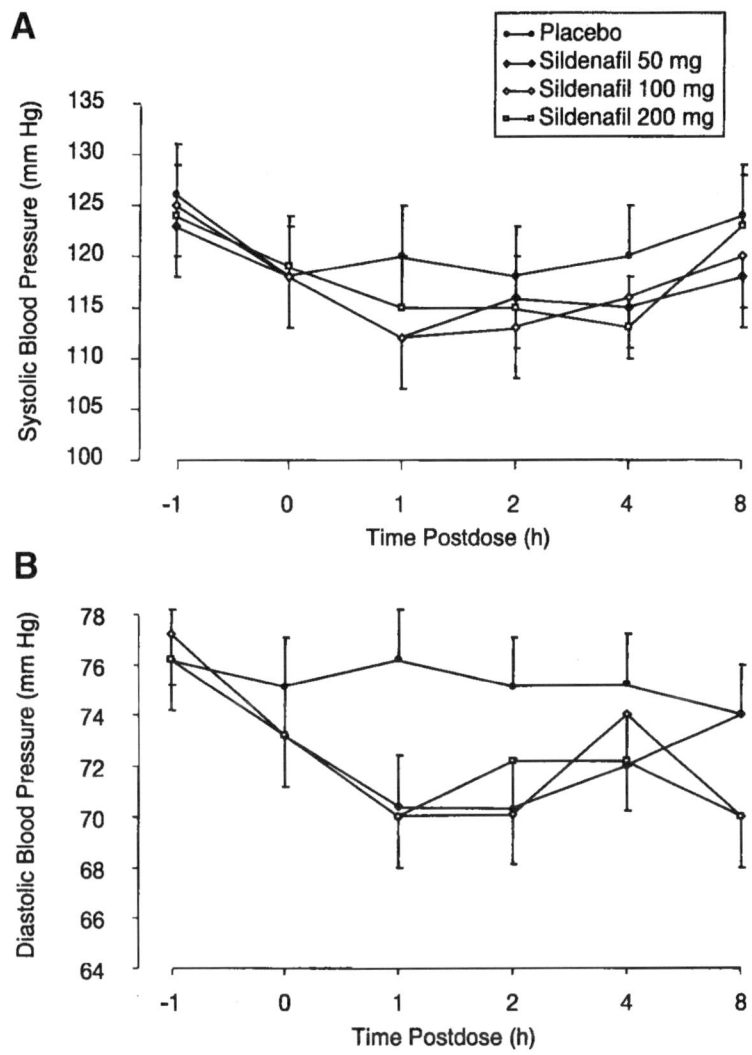

Fig. 4. Mean decreases in supine systolic (**A**) and diastolic (**B**) blood pressure over time in middle-aged volunteers. Values represent the mean ± SD, $n = 16$ per group; $p < 0.05$ for overall treatment effect of sildenafil groups compared with placebo group. There were no significant differences among the groups receiving different sildenafil doses. From ref. *16*; used with permission.

an antianginal agent. Sildenafil was not effective as an antianginal agent, but during clinical trials testing its efficacy, the interesting side effect of improved erections was discovered and this finding eventually became the indication for the drug.

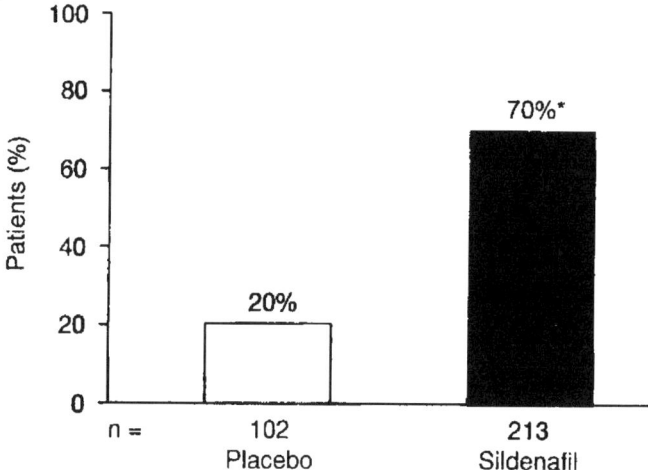

Fig. 5. Percentage of patients with erectile dysfunction and ischemic heart disease reporting improved erections after treatment with placebo or sildenafil in nine double-blind, placebo-controlled studies. *$p < 0.0001$ for the comparison with placebo. From ref. *17;* used with permission.

Sildenafil has been shown to be effective in men with ED who have either coronary artery disease (CAD) or hypertension. In one study, sildenafil improved erections in 70% of men with ED who had chronic CAD (Fig. 5; ref. *17*). In another study, sildenafil improved erections in 72% of men with hypertension *(14)*. It was effective in men on and not on antihypertensive medicines.

As reviewed in detail elsewhere in this volume, sildenafil was shown to have no deleterious effects on coronary artery blood flow, coronary artery diameter, or coronary vascular resistance in both experimental and clinical trials, including one clinical trial of patients studied in the catheterization laboratory *(18)*. Of note, sildenafil did improve coronary artery vasodilator reserve in response to adenosine. Sildenafil was shown to have no deleterious effects when it was administered to patients undergoing exercise stress tests *(19,20)*. In one study, sildenafil actually improved exercise tolerance in patients with CAD *(19)*. In none of these studies did sildenafil appear to induce ischemia or shorten the time from onset of exercise to ischemia or worsen ST segment or echocardiographic evidence of ischemia.

Because sildenafil is a mild vasodilator, some physicians have expressed concern about administering the drug to patients already on antihypertensive medicines. However, the data available to date suggest that sildenafil is safe in patients on antihypertensive medicines. In one study, Zusman and coworkers *(21)* analyzed changes in blood pressure in men who were already on usual antihypertensive medicines (diuretics, β-blockers, α-blockers, calcium channel blockers, angiotensin converting enzyme inhibitors). Patients received either placebo or sildenafil on top of their usual antihypertensive medicines. The mean drops in systolic blood pressure and diastolic pressure were modest at –3.6/–1.9 mmHg with sildenafil vs –2.2/–2.0 mmHg in the placebo arm. There was no clinically significant change in heart rate in either group. In a double-blind, placebo-controlled, crossover study patients took their usual dose of the long-acting dihydropyridine calcium channel blocker amlodipine (5 or 10 mg/d) and 2 h later took a single oral dose of sildenafil (100 mg) vs placebo *(22)*. The sildenafil–amlodipine combination was associated with a greater decrease in mean maximum supine and standing blood pressure compared with placebo–amlodipine. Mean maximal changes from baseline in standing systolic blood pressure/diastolic blood pressure were –19.8/–11.1 mmHg for amlodipine plus sildenafil vs –9.9/–3.5 mmHg for placebo–amlodipine alone. Thus, the declines in blood pressure observed when sildenafil was given to patients already on antihypertensive medicines were similar to the drops in blood pressure observed in patients that received sildenafil who were not on antihypertensive medicines.

There were no increases in sildenafil-related side effects (flushing, hypotension, dizziness) in patients taking antihypertensive medicines vs patients not taking antihypertensive medicines *(14)*. Syncope and hypotension were seen infrequently in patients taking sildenafil plus antihypertensive drugs, and there was no increase in these events even when patients were taking two or three or more antihypertensive medicines. A very important observation in this recent analysis was that patients on sildenafil plus 1, 2, or ≥3 antihypertensive medicines did not demonstrate any increase in angina, myocardial infarction, or coronary death *(14)*.

Thus, although an early consensus statement from the American College of Cardiology (ACC) and the American Heart Association (AHA) recommended caution in prescribing sildenafil to patients on multiple or complicated antihypertensive regimens *(23)*, the available data suggest that, in most cases, sildenafil is quite safe in these patients. However, common sense dictates that if a patient is frankly hypotensive or frankly hypovolemic then it would not be prudent to administer any type of vasodilator, including a PDE5 inhibitor.

In 2003, there was a change in the package insert regarding sildenafil and α-blockers. A label precaution was added suggesting that sildenafil doses greater than 25 mg not be given within a 4-h period of α-blockers. This was owing to a study in which some patients who simultaneously received 4 mg of doxazosin plus 50 or 100 mg of sildenafil had symptomatic hypotension. The 25 mg dose of sildenafil, when coadministered with 4 mg doxazosin, was not associated with hypotension.

Shortly after release of sildenafil, there were reports that some men who used the drug died. The concern became whether sildenafil per se was inducing cardiac events. A recent analysis by the Food and Drug Administration (FDA) of these early reports suggests that the number of cardiac events in patients on sildenafil was well within, if not below, expected rates for this population of men *(24)*. A small number of these early deaths were likely associated with the concomitant use of organic nitrates, an issue that is addressed in more detail later.

In a 1998 meta-analysis by Morales et al. *(15)*, safety data from 18 double-blind, placebo-controlled studies of 2722 sildenafil and 1552 placebo patients were reported. There were no increased rates of myocardial infarction (MI) or other serious cardiovascular events in the sildenafil group compared with the placebo group. Mild vasodilator side effects, such as headache, were more common in the sildenafil group (16%) vs the placebo group (4%); flushing was more common in the sildenafil group (10%) than the placebo group (1%). MI, angina, and coronary artery disorder occurred in about 6% of both groups.

In another analysis, Zusman et al. *(16)* showed that the incidence of MI was 1.7 per 100 patient-years exposure to sildenafil in double-blind studies vs 1.4 per 100 patient-years of placebo, whereas the incidence of MI in patients on sildenafil as part of open-label studies was 0.7 per 100 patient-years (Fig. 6). Of note, the timing of onset of strokes and MIs did not reveal a pattern suggesting a close temporal relationship to the last dose of sildenafil. Most cardiac events occurred days after sildenafil was taken.

A more recent analysis by Mittleman et al. *(25)* reported data from 30 double-blind, placebo-controlled studies and 23 open-label studies (6884 patient-years of sildenafil exposure) in which rates of MI and all-cause death per 100 patient-years were low and did not differ from placebo.

An important recent analysis is the Prescription Even Monitoring Study of the English National Health Service, reported by Shakir et al. *(26)*. This study looked at the incidence of fatal MI or ischemic heart disease among men in the United Kingdom on sildenafil vs men not on sildenafil. Of 5600 men on sildenafil, (15% of whom had diabetes) the all-cause mortality rate was 30% lower than that of the general population of English men. The rate of fatal and nonfatal MI was also low in men who were taking sildenafil at 0.6 per 100 patient-years. Importantly, the age distribution of men taking sildenafil (mean age:

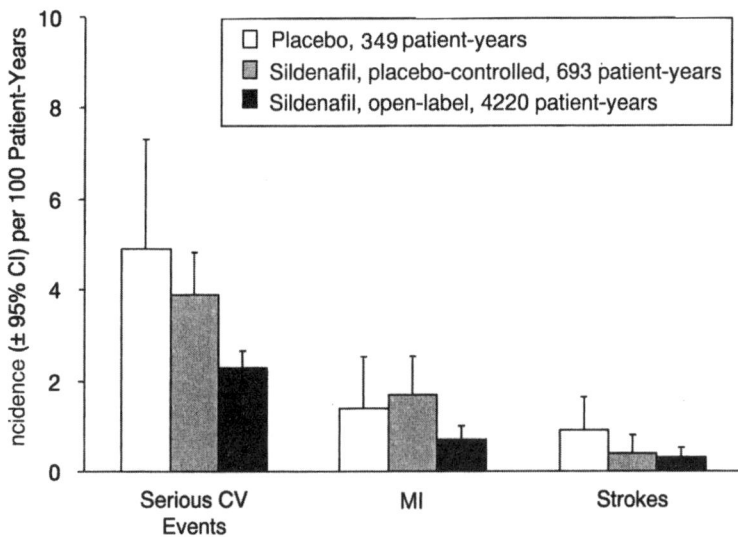

Fig. 6. Incidence of serious cardiovascular (CV) adverse events in patients with sildenafil or placebo in phase II/III studies. Incidence is expressed as the rate per 100 patient-years of treatment ± 95% confidence interval (CI). Serious CV events include any CV event resulting in death or permanent disability or considered to be life-threatening or causing hospitalization or prolongation of a hospital stay, and include MI, angina, and other coronary artery disorders. From ref. *16*; used with permission.

57.4 yr) was similar to that of men in clinical trials of sildenafil in the United States.

Thus, despite some anecdotal reports that have suggested that sildenafil may be associated with cardiac events, analysis of placebo-controlled studies, open-label studies, prescription event-monitoring studies, and even the FDA's own spontaneous event-reporting studies have not suggested a causal role sildenafil in precipitating cardiac events *(27–29)*. Finally, a 4-yr update on the safety of sildenafil again showed no evidence for an increase in death or cardiac events among patients taking sildenafil *(30)*.

Nitrates and Sildenafil

The one contraindication to the use of the PDE5 inhibitor, sildenafil, and probably the other PDE5 inhibitors in development is the use of organic nitrates. Organic nitrates include the antianginal medicines, such as nitroglycerin (sublingual, spray, patch, paste, oral buccal, intravenous, virtually all preparations), long-acting nitrates, such as isosorbide mononitrate and isosorbide dinitrate, and also so-called "poppers" (amyl nitrite or amyl nitrate) that are used recreationally to enhance vasodilation during sexual activity. These organic nitrates are NO donors and thus catalyze the formation of cGMP (Fig. 2). Recall that PDE5 inhibitors prevent the breakdown of cGMP. By using the two types of substances together (NO donor plus PDE5 inhibitor), there may be a large build up of cGMP and marked vasodilation of the systemic arteries and veins (again PDE5 is found in the smooth muscle cells of the systemic arteries and veins). Sildenafil given alone to healthy young men causes mild vasodilation with a slight decrease in systemic arterial pressure (–8.0 mmHg/–5.5 mmHg). However, in one study, when these men received a sublingual dose of nitroglycerin on top of sildenafil, there was a synergistic fall in systolic pressure (–26 to –51 mmHg) and diastolic pressure, and men developed vasodilator side effects of dizziness, headache, and nausea, resulting in their "spitting-out" of the sublingual nitroglycerin tablet *(22)*. Similar findings were observed when sildenafil was administered to men taking isosorbide mononitrate. Sildenafil plus isosorbide mononitrate decreased standing mean maximal systolic blood pressure by 52 mmHg vs a 25 mmHg change with placebo. The combination of sildenafil plus isosorbide mononitrate decreased standing diastolic pressure by 29 mmHg vs 15 mmHg with placebo–isosorbide mononitrate *(31)*. Therefore, these studies suggest that PDE5 inhibition plus organic nitrate results in a synergistic drop in blood pressure (Fig. 7). Because of this finding, sildenafil is absolutely contraindicated in patients taking organic nitrates. In an early FDA report of men who died on sildenafil, a small number of the deaths occurred in men who took sildenafil while on organic nitrates *(24)*. Pfizer Pharmaceuticals sent letters to emergency rooms notifying them of the problem with the combination of sildenafil plus nitrates. Guidelines issued by the ACC/AHA recommend that patients who complain of angina that have used sildenafil not be treated with a nitrate within 24 h of sildenafil use *(23)*. In these circumstances, a non-nitrate antianginal/anti-ischemic agent should be used. These include β-blockers, calcium channel blockers, oxygen, aspirin, morphine heparin, and, if indicated, lipid-lowering agents such as statins. Patients that have a full-blown acute MI while on sildenafil may receive usual and standard therapy, except for nitroglycerin, including intravenous nitroglycerin. Thrombolytics and antiplatelet agents can be used as well as angioplasty and/or stenting but not nitroglycerin *(23)*.

An early theoretical concern regarding sildenafil and cardiac patients was that it might have a milrinone-like effect on the heart that could

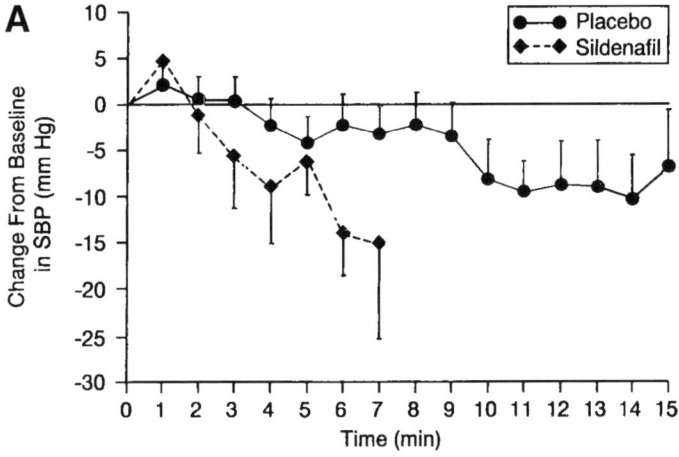
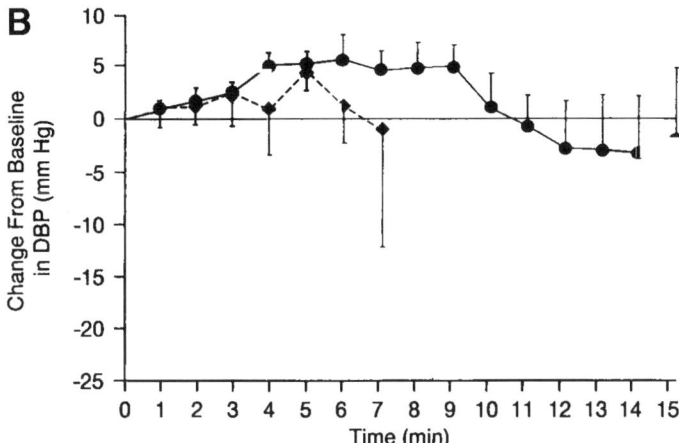

Fig. 7. Mean changes from baseline (±SE) in systolic blood pressure (**A**) and diastolic blood pressure (**B**) on d 5 after sublingual administration of a 500-µg tablet of glyceryl trinitrate (GTN) to healthy men who had received sildenafil (25 mg, three times a day) or placebo for 4 d and a 25-mg dose of sildenafil or placebo on d 5. During placebo treatment, 8 of 12 men completed the 15-min GTN challenge compared with 0 of 12 men during treatment with sildenafil. DBP, diastolic blood pressure; SBP, systolic pressure. From ref. *22*; used with permission.

induce cardiac arrhythmias. Milrinone is a PDE3 inhibitor that increases ventricular contractility and is a vasodilator. However, it also can exacerbate arrhythmias. PDE5 has not been observed within human cardiomyocytes, whereas PDE3 is present in cardiac myocytes. Theoretically, if both PDE5 and PDE3 were present within a cardiomyocyte, then there could be "cross-talk" between them. If PDE5 were inhibited (for example by sildenafil), then there would be an increase in cGMP, which is a known inhibitor of PDE3. Inhibition of PDE3 results in an increased accumulation of cyclic adenosine monophosphate (cAMP), which can increase contractility and stimulate arrhythmias, that is, a milrinone effect *(27)*. However, careful immunohistochemistry results show that PDE5 is contained within vasculature and microvasculature of the heart but not within the cardiomyocytes *per se*. Because cGMP and cAMP do not cross the cell membrane, then the concept of cross talk between PDE5 and PDE3 is unlikely to be an issue in the heart. Furthermore, in experimental studies, we did not observe an increase in cardiac arrhythmias during ischemia when sildenafil was present *(32,33)*. Finally, sildenafil did not exhibit an increase in contractility of isolated cardiac muscle whereas milrinone (through a PDE3 inhibitor effect) did *(4)*.In summary, sildenafil is a highly effective oral PDE5 inhibitor that improves erectile function in men with ED, including men with vascular disease, such as CAD and hypertension. Because PDE5 is found in smooth muscle cells of systemic arteries and veins, sildenafil is a mild afterload and preload reducer. The drug results in mild falls in systolic and diastolic blood pressure and has minimal adverse effects (flushing, headache, nasal congestion, dyspepsia) related to relaxation of smooth muscle cells. In general, the drug's effects on coronary flow are neutral, and the drug does not exacerbate ischemia or prolong the QT interval. Sildenafil is safe to administer to patients with hypertension and is effective in these patients even when they are receiving antihypertensive medicines. Data from placebo-controlled and open-label trials do not suggest an increase in adverse cardiovascular events in patients receiving sildenafil. Finally, sildenafil (and newer PDE5 inhibitors) are contraindicated in patients receiving nitrates.

TADALAFIL (CIALIS)

Tadalafil is a potent and selective PDE5 inhibitor. Like sildenafil, it has been shown to be highly effective in treating ED because of various causes *(34)*. The molecular structure of tadalafil differs substantially from that of sildenafil or vardenafil. It has a half-life of 17.5 h and, therefore, is considerably longer acting than either sildenafil or vardenafil. In healthy volunteers, tadalafil had little effect on blood pressure. The mean maximal changes from baseline in standing blood pressure vs placebo after a 20-mg dose of tadalafil was −4.6 mmHg in standing diastolic blood pressure and −0.2 mmHg in standing systolic blood pressure. There was no change in heart rate *(35)*.

In patients with CAD, who typically had higher baseline blood pressures than normal volunteers, standing systolic blood pressure decreased by 2 mmHg on placebo vs approx 7–8 mmHg on 10 mg of tadalafil *(36)*. Standing diastolic blood pressure decreased 2 mmHg on placebo and 4 mmHg for 10 mg of tadalafil at T_{max} (2 h after drug administration). Thus, tadalafil was associated with small decreases in standing systolic and diastolic blood pressure in patients with chronic stable angina, a group known to be at risk for developing ED. In general, the fall in diastolic pressures reported in these studies was similar to those observed with sildenafil, whereas the reductions in systolic blood pressure with tadalafil tended to be less marked. Changes in diastolic blood pressure tended to be less marked in the supine position. These observations are consistent with known mild vasodilator effects of PDE5 inhibitors.

A series of studies were performed to determine whether there was a tadalafil–organic nitrate interaction similar to that reported with sildenafil. Again, the one contraindication to the use of sildenafil is in men who are taking organic nitrates.

In one study, chronic stable angina patients received sublingual nitroglycerin 2 h after tadalafil 5 mg or 10 mg or placebo *(36,37)*. On the following day the patients received a repeat dose of nitroglycerin to evaluate the possibility of a prolonged interaction because of tadalafil's long half-life. Mean maximum changes from prenitrate baseline were −28 mmHg in standing systolic blood pressure of patients that received placebo plus 0.4 nitroglycerin, −36 mmHg on tadalafil 5 mg plus nitroglycerin; and −31 mmHg on tadalafil 10 mg plus nitrate. The −36 mmHg was significant regarding a noninferiority analysis. Changes in standing diastolic blood pressure after nitrate plus placebo, 5 mg of tadalafil, and 10 mg of tadalafil were −13, −18, and −17, respectively. On the second day (nitrate alone) there were no differences compared to placebo. There also were no significant differences among placebo or tadalafil after nitroglycerin in sitting systolic or diastolic blood pressure or heart rates on d 1 or d 2. Although the change in mean maximal pressure in standing systolic blood pressure was not that impressive in tadalafil (−36, −31 mmHg) vs placebo (−28 mmHg:) groups, additional analyses were performed to better characterize outliers.

An outlier who might demonstrate a clinically significant fall in blood pressure was defined as a patient who demonstrated a decrease in systolic pressure of >30 mmHg from baseline, an absolute systolic blood pressure of <85 mmHg, a decrease in diastolic blood pressure of >20 mmHg from baseline, or an absolute diastolic blood pressure of <45 mmHg. On d 1, the incidence of outliers was greater for tadalafil 5 mg and 10 mg vs placebo for standing systolic blood pressure <85 mmHg: 13 (26%) and 11 (22%) patients in the tadalafil 5 mg plus nitrate and tadalafil 10 mg plus nitrate groups vs placebo plus nitrate 1 (2%) patient ($p \leq 0.001$ and $p \leq 0.01$ for tadalafil 5 mg vs placebo and 10 mg vs placebo, respectively). Also for the category change from baseline in standing diastolic blood pressure >20 mmHg, 19 (38%) of the tadalafil 5 mg plus nitrate (≤ 0.001 vs placebo) and 15 (30%) tadalafil 10 mg plus nitrate patients (≤ 0.01) achieved this vs 4 (8%) of placebo patients. There were no significant differences in the other outlier criteria in standing blood pressure among groups. On d 2 there were no statistically significant differences in patients reaching outlier criteria among the treatment groups (36,37).

This study suggested that tadalafil was associated with minimal-to-small effects on further decreasing mean blood pressure in the setting of sublingual nitroglycerin. However, on d 1, the frequency of outliers was greater with tadalafil vs placebo, indicating that, in some patients, tadalafil will augment the decrease in blood pressure associated with nitrates. Therefore, tadalafil, like sildenafil, carries an organic nitrate contraindication.

A second study (36,37) in which tadalafil was given to patients on the long-acting nitrate isosorbide mononitrate showed more outliers than placebo, but the results were less dramatic than with sublingual nitroglycerin. A third study (38) was a placebo-controlled three-way crossover study examining the hemodynamic effects of 0.4 mg sublingual nitroglycerin administered after placebo, tadalafil 10 mg, or sildenafil 50 mg in healthy men and women ages 55 yr and older. Nitroglycerin was administered at expected time of C_{max} for tadalafil (2 h) and sildenafil (1 h). Subjects were re-evaluated on day 2 at which time they received repeat nitroglycerin but no PDE5 inhibitor, to evaluate for potential of any prolonged interaction.

On d 1 the mean maximal drop in standing systolic blood pressure was 25 mmHg for tadalafil, 25 mmHg for placebo, and 29 mmHg for sildenafil (sildenafil was significantly different vs placebo). However, the frequency of outliers on d 1 was higher for both tadalafil and sildenafil vs placebo. For example, standing systolic blood pressure was <85 mmHg in 23 (47%) tadalafil 10 mg patients, 23 (46%) sildenafil 50 mg patients vs 12 (24%) of placebo patients ($p < 0.05$ for both tadalafil and sildenafil vs placebo). Supine systolic blood pressure on d 1 was <85 mmHg in 18 (36%) patients on 50 mg sildenafil ($p < 0.05$ vs placebo) vs 9 (18%) tadalafil and 3 (6%) placebo patients. On d 2, the number of outliers in both the tadalafil and sildenafil treatment groups was lower than on d 1. Subjects in the supine position on d 2 did not show an excess of outliers in either the tadalafil or sildenafil group compared with placebo. A recent analysis suggested that tadalafil augmented the blood pressure-lowering effect of sublingual nitroglycerin when nitroglycerin was administered at timepoints to 24 h following the last dose of tadalafil. However, this interaction was no longer detectable when nitroglycerin was administered 48 h or beyond, after tadalafil administration *(38a)*. Electrocardiographic analysis of patients on tadalafil did not show a prolongation of the QT interval. Also, QTC was not prolonged *(35,37)*.

In the placebo-controlled phase III studies 291 of 1328 (21.9%) of patients had an underlying cardiovascular disorder *(35)*. About 10% had evidence of ischemic CAD. Also, 58.9% had at least one cardiovascular risk factor including diabetes in 34% of patients, hypertension in 30%, and hyperlipidemia in 21% of patients. Compared with placebo, tadalafil did not significantly increase the incidence of adverse cardiovascular events. The overall safety database for tadalafil included over 4000 participants and over 2700 patients who were in phase II, phase III, and open-label studies. There were six reports of MI in the tadalafil-treated patients for an incidence rate of 0.39 MIs per 100 patient-years in the tadalafil-treated patients vs 1.1 per 100 patient-years in the placebo patients. The incidence rate of MI in a similar age-standardized British male population is 0.6 per 100 patient-years. Thus, there was no signal in these data suggesting that tadalafil was increasing rates of MI *(35)*. During the tadalafil trials there were six deaths; three of these were reported as cardiac deaths. The calculated cardiac mortality in tadalafil-treated patients was less than 2.0 per 1000 patient-years, which is similar to the cardiac mortality rates reported in an age-standardized general population of British males (2.6 per 1000 patient-years).

In a recent analysis, tadalafil was administered to men with CAD undergoing exercise tolerance tests. Tadalafil had no adverse effects on exercise duration or development of ST change *(39)*.

In conclusion, tadalafil in healthy individuals caused no or minimal drops in mean maximal systolic and diastolic blood pressure. Tadalafil did cause small decreases in standing mean systolic and diastolic blood pressure in patients with CAD, consistent with known systemic vasodilating effects of PDE5 inhibition. Nitrate interaction studies showed that there were modest additive effects of tadalafil on nitrate-induced reductions in mean blood pressure. Because a subset of patients were outliers in that, in general, they dropped their blood pressure to clinically unacceptable levels when tadalafil was given with organic nitrates, as with sildenafil, tadalafil should not be used in combination with nitrates. Overall safety database for tadalafil from a large number of participants in clinical studies showed that morbidity and mortality rates from serious cardiovascular events in patients with tadalafil were similar to placebo as well as similar to rates reported for the population of men with ED.

A series of cardiovascular safety studies were carried out in patients taking various antihypertensive agents plus tadalafil (40). The addition of tadalafil to patients on enalapril, metoprolol, or bendrofluazide was associated with little or no further drop in blood pressure compared to placebo. For example, mean difference between tadalafil 10 mg and placebo in standing systolic blood pressure in patients on enalapril was −3 mmHg; and difference between these in change in standing diastolic pressure was −4 mmHg. Mean difference between tadalafil 10 mg and placebo in patients on metoprolol was −7 mmHg for standing systolic blood pressure and −4 mmHg for standing diastolic blood pressure. For patients on the diuretic bendrofluazide, the mean difference between tadalafil 10 mg and placebo was −6 mmHg for standing systolic blood pressure and −4 mmHg standing for diastolic blood pressure. In these interaction studies with enalapril, metoprolol, and bendrofluazide, there no deaths or serious cardiovascular adverse events associated with tadalafil.

A randomized, double-blind, placebo-controlled, crossover study was performed assessing the effects of a single dose of tadalafil 20 mg with placebo in health volunteers who were receiving amlodipine. Ambulatory blood pressure monitoring was used. No significant interaction was observed between tadalafil and amlodipine. There was no difference in outlier drops in blood pressure between placebo and tadalafil (40).

In a group of patients with difficult to control hypertension who were taking angiotensin receptor blockers, tadalafil administration was associated with lower systolic blood pressure than placebo. The mean difference between tadalafil 20 mg and placebo in maximum change in systolic blood pressure was −8 mmHg; the maximum change in diastolic blood pressure was −4 mmHg. There were more outliers in the tadalafil plus angiotensin receptor blocker group vs the placebo plus angiotensin receptor blocker group. However, tadalafil was well tolerated, and there were no reports of serious or severe adverse events related to drop in blood pressure. Mean blood pressure measures taken in these patients (not necessarily temporally related to tadalafil use) did not show significant differences between patients on placebo vs tadalafil.

Mean maximal post-baseline drops in standing systolic blood pressure and standing and supine diastolic blood pressures were greater following administration of tadalafil 20 mg vs placebo during treatment with doxazosin 8 mg. There was a difference from placebo of –4/–3 mmHg in the supine position and –10/–5 mmHg in the standing position. In healthy subjects, administration of tadalafil and tamsulosin 0.4 mg resulted in blood pressure reductions that were not dose-related or clinically meaningful. The use of tadalafil with α-blockers is contrainindicated except for 0.4 mg tamsulosin.

In placebo-controlled phase III studies 272 (28.7%) of tadalafil-treated patients and 105 (27.7%) of placebo-treated patients were receiving antihypertensive therapy. Incidence rates of treatment-emergent cardiovascular events were similar between patients who did and did not receive concomitant antihypertensive therapy. Most cardiovascular events were infrequent and occurred in less than 1% of patients. Flushing was more common with tadalafil (3.4–4.4%) compared with placebo (2.2–0%) as expected. Flushing was similar for tadalafil patients who were taking antihypertensives (4.4%) vs those were not (3.4%). Dizziness occurred in 1.8% of patients on tadalafil plus an antihypertensive agent vs 2.7% of patients on tadalafil who were not on antihypertensive therapy. Syncope was reported in two placebo patients on antihypertensive medicines but no tadalafil patients on antihypertensive medicines. Importantly, tadalafil with or without antihypertensive therapy was not associated with an increase in MI, hypotension, postural hypotension, heart failure, angina, or arrhythmia compared with placebo.

In summary, in patients taking concomitant antihypertensive therapy, tadalafil administration may result in no or, in general, mild additional reduction in blood pressure, which is not likely to be clinically meaningful. This small additive drop in blood pressure, observed in some patients, is consistent with the vasodilator properties of PDE5 inhibition. Analysis of placebo-controlled phase III studies did not show a difference in adverse events in patients taking tadalafil with or without the concomitant use of antihypertensives. Appropriate clinical advice should be given when prescribing tadalafil to patients educating them of a possible additional decrease in blood pressure when taking it with concomitant antihypertensive medications. Except for tamsulosin, tadalafil should not be used in patients on α-blockers.

VARDENAFIL (LEVITRA)

Vardenafil is a new PDE5 inhibitor that, like sildenafil and tadalafil, is highly effective in the treatment of ED *(11)*. Its molecular structure is similar to sildenafil, and it has a half-life that is similar to sildenafil at about 4 h. There are less cardiovascular data available for vardenafil vs sildenafil or vardenafil. Its effect on blood pressure and heart rate in normal volunteers is minimal. One preliminary study done in normal healthy volunteers in the sitting position suggested that there was no nitrate interaction *(41)*. However, whether this would be true in patients with cardiovascular disease or risk factors for cardiovascular disease in the standing position is not known. When vardenafil was released in the United States, it received a nitrate contrainindication, as will be likely for the entire class of PDE5 inhibitors.

In patients with hypertension, who usually start out with a higher baseline blood pressure than normal volunteers, vardenafil was associated with a small fall in blood pressure and small increase in heart rate compared to placebo. In all hypertensive patients, vardenafil reduced mean standing systolic blood pressure by –4.6 mmHg and mean standing diastolic blood pressure by –3.1 mmHg; it increased heart rate by 2 beats/min *(42)*. In contrast, placebo reduced mean standing systolic blood pressure by –0.1 mmHg, mean standing diastolic blood pressure by –0.02 mmHg, and heart rate by –0.2 beats/min. There was no difference in response to vardenafil in patients on or not on antihypertensive medicines (which included angiotensin converting enzyme inhibitor, calcium blocker, β- or α-blockers, diuretics, and angiotensin receptor blocker). In patients not on antihypertensive medicines, vardenafil reduced standing systolic blood pressure by –4.2 mmHg, mean standing diastolic blood pressure by –2.6 mmHg, and increased heart rate by 2.0 beats/min. In patients taking one or more antihypertensive medicines, vardenafil reduced mean standing systolic blood pressure by –5.1 mmHg, mean standing diastolic blood pressure by –3.7 mmHg, and increased heart rate by 1.9 beats/min. Importantly the incidence of adverse cardiovascular events—angina, arrhythmia, MI, or syncope—was low and similar in placebo vs vardenafil-treated patients with or without concomitant use of antihypertensive medicines *(42,43)*. The conclusion of this study was that concomitant antihypertensive medicines plus vardenafil use did not result in changes in blood pressure or elevations of heart rate of clinical concern compared to changes observed with vardenafil alone. In another study it was observed that vardenafil was well tolerated in men with ED on antihypertensive medicines and was highly effective in improving erectile function *(44)*. Vardenafil (5, 10, and 20 mg) significantly improved erectile function domain, penetration, and maintenance of erection rates in these men.

However, vardenafil is contrainindicated in patients taking α-blockers based on hypotension that occurred when vardenafil was administered to patients on terazosin and to a lesser extent on tamsulosin in one study.

Vardenafil caused small increases in QT interval in healthy men at both therapeutic (10 mg) and supratherapeutic (80 mg) doses. It is recommended that patients with congenital QT prolongation and patients receiving class IA (quinidine, procainamide) antiarrhythmic agents or class II (amiodarone, sotalol) antiarrhythmic agents avoid vardenafil.

In a double-blind, crossover, single-dose study of men with CAD who had reproducible exercise tolerance tests, either vardenafil 10 mg or placebo was given 1 h prior to an exercise treadmill test (5–10 METS; ref. *45*). Vardenafil did not alter total treadmill exercise time or time to angina pectoris. However, vardenafil did significantly prolong the time to ST-segment depression ≥ 1 mm (381 ± 108 s with vardenafil vs 334 ± 108 with placebo; $p = 0.0004$). Vardenafil was well tolerated in these men. Facial flushing and headache were the most common side effects reported. Changes in heart rate and blood pressure were similar between vardenafil and placebo. The study concluded that vardenafil did not impair the ability of patients with stable CAD to exercise at levels that were similar to those for sexual activity.

In general, then, vardenafil, like sildenafil and tadalafil, is a mild vasodilator, is, in general, safe to administer in patients on antihypertensive medicines (except α-blockers), and does not exacerbate ischemia. None of the PDE5 inhibitors have been shown to definitely precipitate MI. However, as reviewed elsewhere in this book, there is a small but finite increased risk of a cardiovascular event with sexual activity and any drug or therapy that enables men with ED to now engage in sexual activity will expose them to that risk. In general, PDE5 inhibitors are withheld from unstable cardiac patients or those on organic nitrates. The Princeton Consensus Statement *(46)* and Guidelines of the ACC/AHA *(23)* serve as useful general approaches to the management of sexual dysfunction in the cardiac patient. These guidelines, which are reviewed elsewhere in this volume, should be kept in mind when physicians are considering prescribing PDE5 inhibitors for ED.

POTENTIAL NEW THERAPEUTIC OPTIONS FOR PDE5 INHIBITORS

The PDE5 inhibitor sildenafil was developed initially as a cardiovascular agent, that is, an antianginal agent. As mentioned earlier, it was not a useful antianginal medicine, but the serendipitous find of improved erections became the focus of the drug. Recently, therapies for cardiovascular disorders again have become a focus of research regarding the PDE5 inhibitors. Several studies have suggested that sildenafil may be a useful treatment option for the condition of pulmonary hypertension. Lung tissue is rich in PDE5. Sildenafil reduced hypoxia-induced increases in pulmonary artery pressure without significantly affecting systemic blood pressure *(47)*. A recent case report of a 21-yr-old man with pulmonary hypertension illustrated the potential benefit of sildenafil in patients with this entity. The young man received up to 100 mg of sildenafil five times a day. After 3 months of sildenafil therapy, his pulmonary artery pressure fell from 120 mmHg to 90 mmHg *(48)*.

In one clinical trial of patients with pulmonary hypertension, pulmonary artery pressure fell by 9.4 ± 1.3 mmHg with administration of the prostacyclin analogue iloprost but fell to a significantly greater level (by 13.8 ± 1.4, $p < 0.009$) when sildenafil was coadministered with iloprost *(49)*. As pulmonary hypertension, especially primary pulmonary hypertension, is such a difficult entity to treat, new effective therapy with an agent such as sildenafil would be a welcome addition.

PDE5 inhibitors may have a potential role in the treatment of congestive heart failure. It is known that in patients with congestive heart failure there may be impaired endothelium-dependent, NO-mediated vasodilation. Patients with impaired endothelium-dependent vasodilation and congestive heart failure demonstrated improved brachial arterial flow-mediated vasodilation after transient blood pressure cuff occlusion with 25 or 50 mg of sildenafil vs placebo *(50)*.

Another potential use of PDE5 inhibitors in cardiovascular medicine is antihypertensive therapy. Studies to date suggest that these agents induce mild-to-moderate reductions in blood pressure in patients with hypertension. It is conceivable that this group of drugs, which work through a unique mechanism of action compared with existing antihypertensive agents, could be a useful add-on therapy.

CONCLUSION

In conclusion, PDE5 inhibitors, such as sildenafil, tadalafil, and vardenafil, are highly effective oral agents for the treatment of ED. They appear to be effective in men with underlying cardiovascular disease, including chronic stable angina and hypertension. These agents are mild vasodilators and result in small, but usually clinically insignificant, drops in blood pressure. When administered to patients already on antihypertensive medicines, they are associated with small additive drops in blood pressure. However, because PDE5 inhibitors prevent the breakdown of cGMP whereas NO donors, such as organic nitrates, increase the production of cGMP, administering PDE5 inhibitors to patients who take organic nitrates is absolutely contraindicated. When PDE5 inhibitors plus organic nitrates are taken together, there may be a large build-up of cGMP with synergistic drops in blood pressure. To date,evidence does not support an increase in MI or cardiac death resulting from the use of PDE5 inhibitors *per se*. Caution is advised in using these agents in the unstable cardiac patients as per guidelines set forth by the ACC/AHA and the Princeton Consensus Guidelines.

REFERENCES

1. Beavo JA. Cyclic nucleotide phosphodiesterases: functional implications of multiple isoforms. Physiol Rev 1995;75:725–748.
2. Polson JB, Strada SJ. Cyclic nucleotide phosphodiesterases and vascular smooth muscle. Annu Rev Pharmacol Toxicol 1996;36:403–427.
3. Jackson G, Benjamen N, Jackson N, et al. Effects of sildenafil citrate on human hemodynamics. Am J Cardiol 1999;83:13C–20C.
4. Wallis RM, Corbin JD, Francis SH, et al. Tissue distribution of phosphodiesterase families and the effects of sildenafil on tissue cyclic nucleotides, platelet function, and the contractile responses of trabeculae carneae and aortic rings in vitro. Am J Cardiol 1999;83:3C–12C.
5. Lue TF. Erectile dysfunction. N Engl J Med 2000;342:1802–1813.
6. Lincoln TM. Cyclic GMP and mechanisms of vasodilation. Pharmacol Ther 1989; 41:479–502.
7. Sáenz de Tejada I. Molecular mechanisms for the regulation of penile smooth muscle contractility. Int J Impot Res 2000;12(Suppl 4):S34–S38.
8. Ückert S, Kuthe A, Stief CG, et al. Phosphodiesterase isoenzyme as pharmacological targets in the treatment of male erectile dysfunction. World J Urol 2001;19: 14–22.
9. Montorsi F, McDermott TED, Morgan R, et al. Efficacy and safety of fixed-dose oral sildenafil in the treatment of erectile dysfunction of various etiologies. Urology 1999;53:1011–1018.
10. Brock GE, McMahon CG, Chen KK, et al. Efficacy and safety of tadalafil in the treatment of erectile dysfunction: results of integrated analyses. J Urol 2002;168: 1332–1336.
11. Porst H, Rosen R, Padma-Nathan H, et al. The efficacy and tolerability of vardenafil, a new, oral selective phosphodiesterase type 5 inhibitor, in patents with erectile dysfunction: the first at-home clinical trial. Int J Impot Res 2001;13: 192–199.
12. Klotz T, Sachse R, Heidrich A, et al. Vardenafil increases penile rigidity and tumescence in ED patients: a Rigi Scan and pharmacokinetic study. World J Urol 2001;19:32–38.
13. Speakman MT, Kloner RA. Viagra™ and cardiovascular disease. J Cardiovasc Pharmacol Ther 1999;4:259–267.
14. Kloner RA. Effect of sildenafil in patients with ED taking antihypertensive medications. Am J Hypertens 2001;14:70–73.

15. Morales A, Gingell C, Collins M, et al. Clinical safety of oral sildenafil citrate (Viagra™) in the treatment of ED. Int J Impot Res 1998;10:69–74.
16. Zusman RM, Morales A, Glasser DB, et al. Overall cardiovascular profile of sildenafil citrate. Am J Cardiol 1999;83:35C–44C.
17. Conti CR, Pepine CJ, Sweeney M. Efficacy and safety of sildenafil citrate in the treatment of ED in patients with ischemic heart disease. Am J Cardiol 1999;83 (Suppl 5A):29C–34C.
18. Hermann HC, Chang G, Klugherz BD, et al. Hemodynamic effects of sildenafil in men with severe coronary artery disease. N Engl J Med 2000;342:1622–1626.
19. Fox KM, Thadani U, Ma PTS, et al. Time to onset of limiting angina during treadmill exercise in men with erectile dysfunction and stable chronic angina: effect of sildenafil citrate. Abstract presented at American Heart Association Scientific Sessions. Circulation 2001;104(17 Suppl II):II.601–II.602.
20. Arruda-Olson AM, Mahoney DW, Nehra A, et al. Cardiovascular effects of sildenafil during exercise in men with known or probable coronary artery disease: a randomized crossover trial. JAMA 2002;287:719–725.
21. Zusman RM, Prisant LM, Brown MJ. Effect of sildenafil citrate on blood pressure and heart rate in men with erectile dysfunction taking concomitant antihypertensive medication. Sildenafil Study Group. J Hypertens 2000;18:1865–1869.
22. Webb DJ, Freestone S, Allen MJ, et al. Sildenafil citrate and blood-pressure-lowering drugs: results of drug interaction studies with an organic nitrate and a calcium antagonist. Am J Cardiol 1999;83:21C–28C.
23. Cheitlin MD, Hutter AM Jr., Brindis RG, et al. ACC/AHA expert consensus document. Use of sildenafil (Viagra) in patients with cardiovascular disease. American College of Cardiology/American Heart Association. J Am Coll Cardiol 1999;33:273–282.
24. Wysowski DK, Farinas E, Swartz L. Comparison of reported and expected deaths in sildenafil (Viagra) users. Am J Cardiol 2002;89:1331–1334.
25. Mittleman MA, Glasser DB, Orazem J, et al. Incidence of myocardial infarction and death in 53 trials of Viagra™ (Sildenafil citrate). J Am Coll Cardiol 2000;35 (Suppl A):302A.
26. Shakir SAW, Wilton LV, Boshier A, et al.Cardiovascular events in users of sildenafil: results from first phase of prescription event monitoring in England. BMJ 2001;322:651–652.
27. Kloner RA. Cardiovascular risk and sildenafil. Am J Cardiol 2000;86(Suppl): 57F–61F.
28. Kloner RA. Sex and the patient with cardiovascular risk factors: focus on sildenafil. Am J Med 2000;109(Suppl 9A):13S–21S.
29. Kloner RA, Jarow JP. Erectile dysfunction and sildenafil citrate and cardiologists. Am J Cardiol 1999;83:576–582.
30. Padma-Nathan H, Eardley I, Kloner RA, et al. A 4-year update on the safety of sildenafil citrate (Viagra). Urology 2002;60:(Suppl 2B):67–90.
31. Webb DJ, Muirhead GJ, Wulff M, et al. Sildenafil citrate potentiates the hypotensive effects of nitric oxide donor drugs in male patients with stable angina. J Am Coll Cardiol 2000;36:25–31.
32. Przyklenk K, Kloner RA. Sildenafil citrate (Viagra) does not exacerbate myocardial ischemia in canine models of coronary artery stenosis. J Am Coll Cardiol 2001;37:286–292.
33. Reffelmann T, Kloner RA. Effect of sildenafil on myocardial infarct size, microvascular function, and acute ischemic ventricular dilation. Cardiovasc Res 2003;59:441–449.

34. Padma-Nathan H, McMurray JG, Pullman WE, et al., for the tadalafil On-Demand Dosing Study Group. On-demand tadalafil (Cialis™) enhances erectile function in patients with erectile dysfunction. Int J Impot Res 2001;13:2–9.
35. Kloner RA, Watkins VS, Costigan TM, et al. Cardiovascular profile of tadalafil, a new PDE5 inhibitor. J Urol 2002;167(Suppl 4):176.
36. Kloner RA, Emmick J, Bedding A, et al. Pharmacodynamic interactions between tadalafil and nitrates [abstract]. J Am Coll Cardiol 2002;39(Suppl A):291A.
37. Emmick JT, Stuewe SR, Mitchell M. Overview of the cardiovascular effects of tadalafil. Eur Heart J 2002;4:(Suppl H):H32–H47.
38. Kloner RA, Mitchell M, Bedding A, et al. Pharmacodynamic interactions between tadalafil and nitrates compared with sildenafil. J Urol 2002;167(Suppl): 176–177.
38a. Kloner RA, Hutter AM, Emmick JT, et al. Time course of the interaction between tadalafil and nitrates. J Am Coll Cardiol 2003;42:1855–1860.
39. Patterson D, MacDonald TM, Effron MB, et al. Tadalafil does not affect time to ischemia during exercise stress testing in patients with coronary artery disease. Circulation 2002;(Suppl II)106:II–330.
40. Kloner RA, Mitchell M, Emmick JT. Cardiovascular effects of tadalafil in patients on commonly used classes of antihypertensive therapy. Am J Cardiol 2003;92(Suppl):47M–57M.
41. Mazzu A, Nicholls A, Zinny M. Vardenafil, a new selective PDE-5 inhibitor, interacts minimally with nitroglycerin in healthy middle-aged male subjects. Int J Impot Res 2001;13(Suppl 5):S64.
42. Kloner RA, Mohan P. Segerson T, et al. Cardiovascular safety of vardenafil in patients receiving antihypertensive medications: a post-hoc analysis of five placebo-controlled clinical trials. J Am Coll Cardiol 2003;41(Suppl A): 276A–277A.
43. Kloner RA, Mohan P, Norenberg C, et al. Cardiovascular safety of vardenafil, a potent, highly selective PDE5 inhibitor in patients with erectile dysfunction: an analysis of five-controlled clinical trials. Pharmacol Ther 2002;22:1371.
44. Padma-Nathan H, Porst H, Eardley I, et al. Efficacy and safety of vardenafil, a selective phosphodiesterase 5 inhibitor, in men with erectile dysfunction on antihypertensive therapy. Presented at the American Society of Hypertension 17th Annual Scientific Meeting. New York, NY, 2002.
45. Thadani U, Smith U, Nash S, et al. The effect of vardenafil, a potent and highly selective phosphodiesterase 5-inhibitor for the treatment of erectile dysfunction, on the cardiovascular response to exercise in patients with coronary artery disease. J Am Coll Cardiol 2002;40:2006–2012.
46. DeBusk R, Drory Y, Goldstein I, et al. Management of sexual dysfunction in patients with cardiovascular disease: recommendation of the Princeton Consensus Panel. Am J Cardiol 2000;86:175–181.
47. Zhao L, Mason NA, Morrell N, et al. Sildenafil inhibits hypoxia-induced pulmonary hypertension. Circulation 2001;104:424–428.
48. Prasad S, Wilkinson J, Gatzoulis MA. Sildenafil in primary pulmonary hypertension. N Engl J Med 2000;343:1342.
49. Wilkens H, Guth A, Konig J, et al. Effect of inhaled iloprost plus oral sildenafil in patients with primary pulmonary hypertension. Circulation 2001;104: 1218–1222.
50. Katz SD, Balideinaj K, Homma S, et al. Acute type 5 phosphodiesterase inhibitor with sildenafil enhances flow-mediated vasodilation in patients with chronic heart failure. J Am Coll Cardiol 2000;36:845–851.

10 Effect of Phosphodiesterase-5 Inhibition on Coronary Blood Flow in Experimental Animals

YingJie Chen, MD, PhD,
Jay H. Traverse, MD,
and Robert J. Bache, MD

CONTENTS

    Coronary Cyclic Guanosine
       Monophosphate-Hydrolyzing Activity
    Effect of PDE5 Inhibition on Coronary Flow
    Effect of PDE5 Inhibition on Coronary
       Reactive Hyperemia
    Effect of PDE5 on Endothelium-Dependent
       Vasodilation
    Effect of PDE5 Inhibition in the Presence
       of a Flow-Limiting Coronary Stenosis
    Congestive Heart Failure
    Acknowledgments
    References

CORONARY CYCLIC GUANOSINE MONOPHOSPHATE-HYDROLYZING ACTIVITY

    Nitric oxide (NO) produced by the endothelium diffuses into the vascular smooth muscle, where it activates soluble guanylyl cyclase (sGC); the resultant increase in cyclic guanosine monophosphate (cGMP)

From: *Contemporary Cardiology: Heart Disease and Erectile Dysfunction*
Edited by: R. A. Kloner © Humana Press Inc., Totowa, NJ

causes vasodilation of the resistance arteries through modulation of calcium channels and by decreasing the calcium sensitivity of the vascular smooth muscle contractile proteins *(1)*. The response to guanylyl cyclase activation is terminated by enzymatic hydrolysis of cGMP. Coronary artery vascular smooth muscle cGMP-hydrolyzing activity is mainly the result of phosphodiesterase-1 (PDE1), a calmodulin-dependent PDE, and PDE5, which is a calcium-calmodulin independent cGMP-specific PDE *(2)*. Of the total cGMP hydrolyzing activity, PDE1 constituted 73% in porcine and approximately 80% in bovine normal epicardial coronary artery *(3)*. Vinpocetin, a selective inhibitor PDE1, has been shown to cause concentration-dependent relaxation of isolated arterial vessel segments *(4)*. Similarly, the PDE5 inhibitors zaprinast, E4021, and sildenafil caused relaxation of isolated porcine or canine normal epicardial coronary artery segments in vitro that was associated with an increase of vascular cGMP concentration *(5–7)*. Comparable results have been obtained in vivo where E4021, 10 µg/kg/min iv, a dose that produced no change in aortic pressure, caused epicardial coronary artery dilation in awake pigs with a 2.9 ± 0.5% increase in coronary diameter *(6)*. The findings indicate that selective inhibition of either PDE1 or PDE5 alone can cause an increase in coronary cGMP content with resultant vasodilation and imply that either PDE pathway alone may be insufficient to maintain normal cGMP levels. It should be noted that these findings apply to epicardial coronary arteries, and that measurements of PDE activity and cGMP content in coronary resistance vessels (where blood flow is regulated) are not available.

EFFECT OF PDE5 INHIBITION ON CORONARY FLOW

PDE5 Inhibition During Basal Conditions

Because inhibition of PDE5 can augment vascular smooth muscle cGMP levels, the effect of PDE5 inhibition might be expected to mimic the effect of NO. Administration of NO donors or intra-arterial infusion of authentic NO can cause dilation of coronary resistance vessels with a modest increase of coronary blood flow *(8,9)*. Nevertheless, inhibition of NO synthesis with competitive inhibitors of arginine did not decrease coronary blood flow in either anesthetized or awake dogs, principally because NO inhibition tended to increase myocardial oxygen consumption *(10)*. Blockade of NO production did cause a slight but significant decrease of coronary venous oxygen tension, indicating that endogenous NO exerts a slight vasodilator effect on the coronary resistance vessels *(10)*. In chronically instrumented normal awake dogs studied during resting conditions, PDE5 inhibition with sildenafil (2 mg/kg) caused a 7 ± 2 mmHg decrease of mean aortic pressure ($p < 0.05$), with no significant change of heart rate, left ventricular (LV) systolic pressure or LVdP/dt$_{max}$ *(11)*. Sildenafil did cause coronary vasodilation with a 19 ± 6% increase in myocardial blood flow ($p < 0.05$) but no change of myocardial oxygen consumption. The finding that inhibition of cGMP degradation caused a modest increase of coronary blood flow implies that some degree of basal guanylyl cyclase activity exists in coronary vessels during resting conditions.

PDE5 Inhibition During Exercise

In the normal heart, coronary blood flow is closely matched to myocardial oxygen requirements so that, even during resting conditions, 75–80% of the oxygen is extracted from the blood traversing the coronary capillaries *(12)*. Because of the limited ability for a further increase in oxygen extraction, increased myocardial oxygen requirements during exercise must be met by essentially parallel increases of coronary blood flow. This increase of blood flow during exercise is mediated by metabolic vasodilation of the coronary resistance vessels. The principal sites of resistance to blood flow are at the level of the small arteries (100–400 µm in diameter) and the coronary arterioles (60–120 µm; refs. *13* and *14*). Metabolic vasoregulation appears to occur principally at the level of the arterioles; increases of myocardial metabolic demands result in opening of ATP-sensitive potassium channels (K_{ATP}) on the coronary arteriolar smooth muscle cell membrane *(15)*. The resultant efflux of potassium causes a decrease in membrane potential that closes voltage-dependent calcium channels in the sarcolemma of the smooth muscle cells. The consequent decrease of cytosolic calcium causes relaxation of the vascular smooth muscle with arteriolar dilation and an increase of coronary flow. The small arteries (100–400 µm in diameter) account for approximately 40% of the total resistance to flow in the coronary circulation *(14)*. These resistance arteries appear to be insensitive to the metabolic state of the myocardium but can undergo endothelium-dependent NO-mediated vasodilation in response to the increased shear forces that result when blood flow is increased by metabolic vasodilation of the arterioles *(16)*. The increased blood flow during exercise would be expected to cause increased endothelial shear forces and an increase in coronary NO production. In agreement with this, direct measurements of the arterial and venous products of NO metabolism (nitrite + nitrate = NOx) have demonstrated that NO production across the coronary cir-

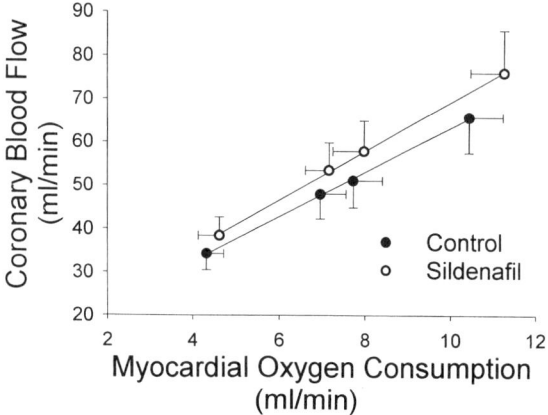

Fig. 1. Effect of PDE5 inhibition with sildenafil on myocardial blood flow in chronically instrumented dogs. Measurements were obtained at rest and during a three-stage graded exercise treadmill protocol. Myocardial blood flow increased in proportion to the increase in oxygen consumption during exercise; sildenafil did not significantly change myocardial oxygen consumption, myocardial blood flow, or the relationship between oxygen consumption and blood flow. Reproduced with permission from ref. *11*.

culation increases during exercise *(17)*. In chronically instrumented dogs, the increase of coronary flow in response to exercise was slightly augmented by PDE5 inhibition with sildenafil; during control conditions, left anterior descending coronary artery blood flow increased from 1.19 ± 0.03 mL/min per g at rest to 2.30 ± 0.18 during treadmill exercise that increased heart rates to approximately 230 beats/min, a 1.11 ± 0.10 mL/min per g increase *(11)*. After sildenafil, coronary flow increased from 1.35 ± 0.09 mL/min per g at rest to 2.69 ± 0.28 during the heaviest level of exercise, an increase of 1.34 ± 0.14 mL/min per g ($p < 0.05$ comparing control with sildenafil; Fig. 1). This difference, although statistically significant, was small and indicates that inhibition of PDE5 does not substantially alter the resistance vessel dilation that occurs during exercise. Furthermore, sildenafil did not significantly change the relationship between oxygen delivery to the heart and myocardial oxygen consumption, indicating that this agent did not interfere with normal physiologic regulation of coronary blood flow during exercise.

The failure of inhibition of PDE5 to increase coronary blood flow relative to myocardial oxygen demands is likely explained by reciprocal vasomotor adjustments at several levels within the coronary microcirculation. In chronically instrumented awake dogs, blockade of NO synthesis caused epicardial coronary artery constriction but had little effect on coronary blood flow *(18)*. Using intravital microscopy to directly visualize coronary microvessels in the beating canine heart, Jones and associates *(19)* observed that inhibition of NO synthesis did cause constriction of the small coronary arteries (>100 μm in diameter) but this was counterbalanced by vasodilation of the arterioles (<100 μm in diameter), demonstrating that compensatory vasomotor adjustments occurred in sequential segments of the coronary microvasculature to maintain blood flow after inhibition of NO production. Thus, in the in vivo heart, the vasodilation produced by cGMP occurs principally at the level of the coronary arteries, including the resistance arteries, whereas regulation of coronary blood flow in response to myocardial metabolic needs is principally a function of the coronary arterioles. The available data indicate that inhibition of PDE5 does not interfere with metabolic coronary vasoregulation at the level of the arterioles.

EXERCISE-INDUCED INCREASES OF HEMOGLOBIN

Exercise normally results in an increase of blood oxygen carrying capacity as the result of an increase in hematocrit. This increase in hematocrit is the result of a decrease in plasma volume secondary to extravasation of fluid from the capillaries, as well as α-adrenergically mediated splenic contraction in animals, such as dogs and horses, in which the spleen has a muscular capsule; during exercise, contraction of the splenic capsule expresses erythrocyte-rich blood into the general circulation, thereby causing an increase of hemoglobin *(20)*. In chronically instrumented dogs, PDE5 inhibition with sildenafil caused an approximately 10% decrease in hemoglobin both at rest and during exercise, although this agent did not interfere with the increase of hemoglobin that occurred during exercise *(11)*. The slight decrease of hematocrit following sildenafil was matched by slightly higher coronary blood flow rates at rest and during exercise so that oxygen delivery to the myocardium was unchanged. Nitroglycerin has been demonstrated to cause splenic dilation in dogs, suggesting cGMP-mediated relaxation of the splenic capsule smooth muscle *(21)*. The decrease in hemoglobin after sildenafil administration in dogs suggests that this agent caused cGMP-dependent relaxation of the splenic capsule with trapping of circulating erythrocytes in the spleen. This effect of sildenafil is likely to be limited to species in which the spleen is surrounded by a muscular capsule (i.e., dog, horse) and likely would not occur in human subjects *(12)*.

EFFECT OF PDE5 INHIBITION ON CORONARY REACTIVE HYPEREMIA

Transient myocardial ischemia results in intense coronary resistance vessel dilation and is followed by a period of increased blood flow termed reactive hyperemia. There is evidence that endogenous NO contributes to coronary reactive hyperemia; thus, in open chest and awake dogs, inhibition of NO synthase decreased total reactive hyperemia blood flow principally by attenuating the late phase of the hyperemic response *(10)*. Because the influence of NO is likely to be mediated by guanylyl cyclase, the effect of PDE5 inhibition with sildenafil on the coronary reactive hyperemia was studied in chronically instrumented awake dogs *(11)*. Sildenafil caused no change in the peak flow rates, the duration of the reactive hyperemic response, or the total volume of excess blood flow during the reactive hyperemia that followed a 10-s coronary occlusion. The failure of sildenafil to augment reactive hyperemia could be the result of an alternate pathway for degradation of cGMP, such as PDE1. Alternatively, it is possible that vasomotor adjustments at the level of the coronary arterioles counter any increase in cGMP-mediated vasodilation of the coronary arteries during the reactive hyperemic response.

EFFECT OF PDE5 ON ENDOTHELIUM-DEPENDENT VASODILATION

Coronary vasodilators, such as acetylcholine, bradykinin, and substance P, are dependent on an intact endothelium to produce vasodilation *(22)*. These agents interact with specific endothelial cell receptors to cause elaboration of NO, endothelium-dependent hyperpolarizing factor, and/or prostacyclin, which diffuses to the smooth muscle to cause vasodilation. In the normal canine heart, PDE5 inhibition with sildenafil significantly augmented the increase in coronary flow produced by intraarterial acetylcholine (Fig. 2; ref. *11*). This is not surprising, inasmuch as NO degradation products (NOx) have been demonstrated to increase during intracoronary infusion of acetylcholine, demonstrating increased coronary NO production *(17)*. Interestingly, sildenafil did not augment the coronary vasodilator response to acetylcholine in dogs with congestive heart failure (CHF) produced by rapid ventricular pacing. This finding is likely explained by reports that NO bioavailability is decreased in the setting of heart failure and suggests that in this situation acetylcholine-induced coronary vasodilation is mediated by factors other than the NO/guanylyl cyclase system, possibly endothelium derived hyperpolarizing factor.

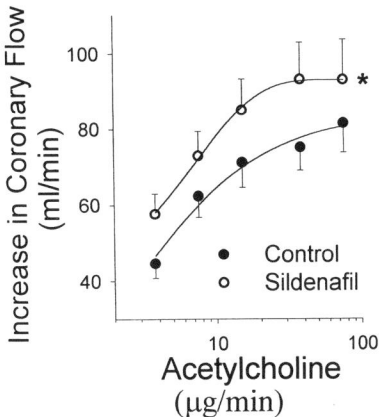

Fig. 2. Effect of sildenafil (2 mg/kg po) on the endothelium-dependent vasodilator response to intracoronary acetylcholine in chronically instrumented awake normal dogs. Acetylcholine caused dose-related coronary vasodilation; sildenafil significantly augmented the response to acetylcholine. Reproduced with permission from ref. *11*.

EFFECT OF PDE5 INHIBITION IN THE PRESENCE OF A FLOW-LIMITING CORONARY STENOSIS

Effect of a Coronary Stenosis With Intact Endothelium

EFFECT OF A CORONARY STENOSIS DURING BASAL CONDITIONS

A coronary stenosis sufficiently severe to limit arterial inflow results in vasodilation of the resistance vessels in the hypoperfused myocardial region. However, even during ischemia, some degree of vasodilator reserve can exist at the level of the coronary resistance vessels *(23)*. When a constrictor on the left anterior descending coronary artery of open-chest dogs was tightened to decrease mean blood flow to 50% of baseline, PDE5 inhibition with sildenafil (total dose 1.5 mg/kg iv) caused no change in blood flow to the ischemic myocardial region during a 2-h observation period *(24)*.

EFFECT OF A CORONARY STENOSIS DURING EXERCISE

In the clinical setting, transient myocardial ischemia and angina pectoris typically occur when a coronary stenosis prevents blood flow from increasing sufficiently to meet the increased myocardial metabolic needs during exercise or other stress. When coronary flow is insufficient to meet myocardial needs, the limited arterial inflow is delivered preferentially to the outer LV layers, whereas hypoperfusion is most severe in the subendocardium *(25)*. This redistribution of blood flow is, in part, a reflection of the transmural gradient of extravascular forces that exists across the wall of the left ventricle. Extravascular forces increase from epicardium to endocardium; the interaction between these compressive forces and the low intracoronary distending pressure that can exist distal to a flow-limiting stenosis acts to collapse the intramural coronary vessels forming vascular waterfalls *(25)*. The resultant impedance to blood flow is most marked in the subendocardium where the extravascular forces are greatest. Factors that increase the extravascular forces, such as an increase in LV diastolic pressure, will exaggerate the redistribution of blood flow away from the subendocardium. An additional factor contributing to the redistribution of blood flow away from the subendocardium relates to the intramural penetrating arteries that deliver blood from the epicardial arteries to the subendocardial vascular plexus *(26)*. In the presence of a coronary stenosis that has caused the arterioles to undergo metabolic vasodilation, the penetrating arteries represent an additional substantial locus of resistance for blood flow to the subendocardium. In this situation, alterations of tone in the penetrating arteries have the potential to influence subendocardial blood flow *(27)*.

The effect of PDE5 inhibition with sildenafil on myocardial blood flow during exercise in the presence of a coronary stenosis has been studied in dogs instrumented with a hydraulic occluder and flowmeter on the left anterior descending coronary artery; a microcatheter allowed measurement of coronary pressure distal to the occluder *(28)*. During normal conditions, treadmill exercise that increased heart rates to approximately 200 beats/min resulted in a near doubling of coronary flow; in these normal hearts, blood flow was distributed preferentially toward the subendocardium so that the subendocardial/epicardial blood flow ratio was 1.34 ± 0.08. When the occluder was partially inflated to produce a stenosis that prevented coronary flow from increasing, exercise caused a redistribution of the limited blood flow away from the subendocardium with a decrease in the subendocardial/subepicardial flow ratio to 0.38 ± 0.07. There was a marked pressure drop across the stenosis; mean aortic pressure during exercise was 124 ± 7 mmHg, whereas pressure distal to the stenosis was 57 ± 2 mmHg. The ischemia resulting from this stenosis caused an increase of LV end-diastolic pressure during exercise from 12 ± 2 to 17 ± 3 mmHg. Sildenafil administered as an oral dose of 2 mg/kg caused no significant change in arterial pressure during exercise but tended to decrease LV end-diastolic pressure in the ischemic ventricle. In the region perfused by the stenotic coronary artery, sildenafil caused a slight but significant increase of myocardial blood flow (mean increase: 11%; $p < 0.05$) at a coronary pressure distal to the stenosis (57 ± 3 mmHg) equal to that during exercise prior to sildenafil (57 ± 2 mmHg). The increase in coronary flow was transmurally uniform, with no change in the subendocardial/subepicardial blood flow ratio. Because the perfusion pressure distal to the stenosis was identical before and after sildenafil, the small increase in blood flow after sildenafil indicated a decrease in small vessel resistance. This decrease in small vessel resistance is unlikely to have occurred at the level of the arterioles, because ischemia would have already caused metabolic vasodilation of these vessels. It is likely that PDE5 inhibition produced vasodilation of the coronary resistance arteries (100–400 µm in diameter), which are unresponsive to the metabolic needs of the myocardium, but where endothelium-dependent cGMP-mediated vasodilation can occur. Previous studies have demonstrated that even during ischemia some degree of vasodilator reserve persists in the coronary resistance vessels, in part because of adrenergic vasoconstriction that competes with metabolic vasodilation during exercise *(29)*. Conversely, sympathetic activation of α_2- and β_2-adrenergic receptors on the coronary endothelium can activate endothelial NOS to increase NO production *(30,31)*. Such an increase of endothelial NO production during exercise might be expected to amplify the effect of PDE5 inhibition, and might explain the lack of effect of sildenafil on blood flow in the presence of a coronary stenosis during resting conditions *(24)*. The finding that PDE5 inhibition increased blood flow in the poststenotic myocardial region during exercise is analogous to reports that nitroglycerin and other NO donors can increase blood flow to a myocardial region that becomes ischemic during exercise in the presence of a coronary stenosis *(9)*. However, the effect of sildenafil was different from that produced by nitroglycerin or the NO donors, because these agents caused a preferential increase of blood flow to the subendocardium, likely as the result of dilation of the penetrating arteries that conduct blood from the epicardial arteries to the subendocardial microvasculature. In contrast, PDE5 inhibition with sildenafil caused no change in the transmural distribution of perfusion *(28)*. An alternate possibility for the increase in poststenotic blood flow is that the tendency toward a lower LV end-diastolic pressure after sildenafil caused a decrease of the extravascular forces compressing the intramural microvasculature.

POTENTIALLY DELETERIOUS EFFECTS OF VASODILATION IN THE PRESENCE OF A CORONARY STENOSIS

In the above studies of single-vessel coronary artery occlusion in experimental animals, PDE5 inhibition had no tendency to worsen myocardial perfusion or to aggravate the subendocardial hypoperfusion that occurs when blood flow was limited by a proximal stenosis. However, this experimental animal model of single vessel coronary artery stenosis does not mimic the complex coronary dynamics that can exist in patients with multivessel coronary disease.

Effects of Resistance Vessel Dilation. Small-vessel dilation has the potential to exert undesirable effects on blood flow in a region of myocardium served by a stenotic coronary artery *(27)*. For example, if a vasodilator causes a substantial decrease of systemic blood pressure, this will reduce the driving pressure across the stenotic segment, thereby causing a decrease in blood flow. Conversely, however, systemic venodilation can cause a decrease of LV diastolic pressure that can enhance blood flow (especially to the subendocardium), because the extravascular forces that act to impede blood flow distal to a coronary stenosis are directly related to the LV filling pressure.

Effect on Stenosis Severity. An agent that causes coronary resistance vessel dilation that results in a decrease of intraarterial pressure distal to a stenosis can worsen stenosis severity. Stenotic arterial segments often demonstrate some degree of compliance and can recoil if the distending pressure is decreased; the distending pressure within the stenotic segment is essentially equal to pressure distal to the stenosis *(32)*. If a pharmacologic agent results in dilation of microvessels distal to the stenosis, the resultant decrease of distal coronary pressure (distending pressure) can cause partial collapse of the stenosis and result in an increase of stenosis severity. The effect of PDE5 inhibition on stenosis severity has not been examined in experimental animal models.

Coronary Steal. In the setting of multivessel coronary artery disease, small-vessel dilators have the potential to cause coronary steal *(27)*. This can occur when two arteries, one having a significant stenosis and the other relatively disease free, are perfused in parallel from a common coronary artery having some resistance to blood flow. In this situation, a resistance vessel dilator will increase flow in the relatively disease-free arterial branch, but this increase in flow will result in an increased pressure drop across the common proximal artery. Because the stenosis in the distal artery has already required vasodilation of the resistance vessels to maintain adequate blood flow, the decreased pressure cannot be countered by additional vasodilation to maintain blood flow. In this situation, the pharmacologic dilator diverts blood to the relatively nondiseased artery at the expense of a decrease in flow in the perfusion bed served by the stenotic artery. This effect can be seen in patients with multivessel coronary disease in which potent coronary resistance vessel dilators, such as adenosine or dipyridamole, can cause an actual decrease of blood flow in myocardial regions perfused by a stenotic coronary artery. Because of the relatively weak vasodilator influence on the coronary resistance vessels, sildenafil is unlikely to exert this deleterious effect.

Epicardial Steal. A decrease of perfusion pressure distal to a stenosis has the potential to divert blood away from the subendocardium as the result of interaction of the decreased intravascular pressure with the extravascular compressive forces *(27)*. Consequently, pharmacologic agents that act to cause vasodilation of coronary resistance vessels could worsen subendocardium hypoperfusion in ischemic myocardial regions by diverting the limited blood flow toward the subepicardium. The weak vasodilator influence of PDE5 inhibition on coronary resistance vessels minimizes the likelihood of redistribution of blood flow from the LV subendocardium toward the outer myocardial layers.

Cyclic Flow Reductions as a Result of Coronary Stenosis With Endothelial Injury

Folts et al. *(33)* observed that when a coronary stenosis that causes a modest reduction of basal blood flow is associated with arterial injury, spontaneous periodic reductions of coronary flow are often observed. These cyclic flow reductions are the result of spontaneous formation of platelet-rich thrombus within the stenotic segment; the formation of thrombus causes the reduction of blood flow, and subsequent dislodgement of the thrombus re-establishes flow. Agents that inhibit platelet aggregation are effective in reducing or eliminating cyclic flow reductions. Platelet cGMP can inhibit agonist-mediated calcium flux and decrease fibrinogen binding to the glycoprotein IIb/IIIa receptor that is essential for aggregation *(33)*. However, in a canine model of coronary artery injury and stenosis, the PDE5 inhibitor zaprinast had no effect on the frequency of cyclic flow reductions *(34)*. Similarly, inhaled NO in a concentration of 20 ppm did not decrease the frequency or duration of flow reductions. However, when inhaled NO was combined with zaprinast coronary flow reductions were decreased from 6.7 ± 0.1 to 1.0 ± 0.5 cycles per hour. An antithrombotic effect of zaprinast is consistent with the finding that PDE5 is present in platelet cytosol *(34)*; the observation that this antithrombotic effect occurred only in the presence of exogenous NO implies that activation of guanylyl cyclase must occur for PDE5 to have an effect. In agreement with this, PDE5 inhibition with sildenafil had no effect on agonist-induced platelet aggregation in vitro but potentiated the antiaggregating effect of sodium nitroprusside against platelet-activating factor, collagen, adenosine diphosphate, and the thromboxane A2 mimetic U46619 *(7)*. Using the coronary stenosis–arterial injury model, Przyklenk and Kloner *(24)* observed that the flow-time area (an index of coronary patency) tended to increase over time in untreated animals, but animals treated with sildenafil did not demonstrate this modest improvement in the flow-time area with time. The investigators subsequently demonstrated that sildenafil prevented the antiaggregatory effect of the adenosine A2 receptor agonist CGS21680 in vitro. The mechanism by which PDE5 inhibition prevented adenosine A2 receptor-mediated inhibition of platelet aggregation (resulting from stimulation of adenylyl cyclase and accumulation of cAMP) is unclear.

CONGESTIVE HEART FAILURE

In the normal heart, the principal mechanism for cGMP production in the coronary vessels involves activation of sGC by NO produced in the vascular endothelium *(1)*. A second parallel system for cGMP production involves activation of particulate guanylyl cyclase by circulating natriuretic peptides that bind to specific receptors (NPR-A) on vascular smooth muscle cells *(35)*. In CHF, NO bioactivity is decreased so that vascular sGC activity would be expected to be reduced *(36)*. However, CHF is associated with increased circulating levels of atrial natriuretic peptide (ANP) and brain natriuretic peptide (BNP) that might be expected to result in increased cGMP production via activation of particulate guanylyl cyclase *(37)*. If vascular cGMP production was increased in CHF, then PDE5 inhibition might have a greater effect in the failing circulation than in the normal heart. We examined the effect of PDE5 inhibition on coronary and systemic hemodynamics in dogs in which heart failure was produced by right ventricular pacing at 240 beats/min for 3–4 wk *(38)*. This protocol results in congestive cardiomyopathy with LV ejection fractions of approximately 30%, elevated LV filling pressures, and marked exercise intolerance *(39)*. In animals with CHF, PDE5 inhibition with sildenafil caused a 4- to 5-mmHg decrease in mean aortic pressure and a slight but significant decrease of LV end-diastolic pressure at rest and during exercise, but did not alter heart rate, LV systolic pressure, or LVdP/dt$_{max}$. Sildenafil had no significant effect on either coronary blood flow or myocardial oxygen consumption in the failing heart. Furthermore, sildenafil did not alter the relationship between coronary flow and myocardial oxygen consumption, indicating that inhibition of PDE5 activity did not alter the coupling between resistance vessel vasomotor activity and myocardial metabolic demands. The finding that sildenafil failed to increase coronary blood flow in animals with CHF but did cause a modest increase in coronary flow in normal animals *(11)* suggests that cGMP is decreased in the coronary microvessels of animals with CHF. Because CHF is associated with increased plasma levels of ANP and BNP *(37)*, both of which can cause coronary vasodilation by activation of particulate guanylate cyclase in vascular smooth muscle, the findings suggest that responsiveness to the natriuretic peptides is decreased in the failing heart. The relaxation of isolated coronary artery segments to ANP and BNP is dramatically decreased in dogs with pacing induced CHF, whereas relaxation to NO or 8-bromo-cGMP is maintained, suggesting that natriuretic peptide receptors are downregulated in response to the persistently elevated circulating levels of natriuretic peptide in the setting of heart failure *(40)*. The finding that PDE5 activity contributes little to regulation of coronary vasomotor activity in animals with CHF implies that the vascular smooth muscle cGMP content is low, likely as the result of endothelial dysfunction with decreased NO bioavailability as well as because of downregulation of vascular smooth muscle natriuretic peptide receptors.

ACKNOWLEDGMENTS

This work was supported by U.S. Public Health Service grants HL20598 and the HL21872 and a grant from the American Heart Association, Northlands Affiliate.

REFERENCES

1. Murad F, Waldman S, Molina C, et al. Regulation and role of guanylate cyclase-cyclic GMP in vascular relaxation. Prog Clin Biol 1987;249:65–76.
2. Polson JB, Strada SJ. Cyclic nucleotide phosphodiesterases and vascular smooth muscle. Annu Rev Pharmacol Toxicol 1996;36:403–427.
3. Ahn HS, Crim W, Pitts B, et al. Calcium-calmodulin-stimulated and cyclic-GMP-specific phosphodiesterases. Tissue distribution, drug sensitivity, and regulation of cyclic GMP levels. Adv Sec Messenger Phosphoprotein Res 1992;25:271–288.
4. Hagiwara M, Endo T, Hidaka H. Effects of vinpocetine on cyclic nucleotide metabolism in vascular smooth muscle. Biochem Pharmacol 1984;33:453–457.
5. Merkel LA, Rivera LM, Perrone MH, et al. In vitro and in vivo interactions of nitrovasodilators and zaprinast, a cGMP-selective phosphodiesterase inhibitor. Eur J Pharmacol 1992;216:29–35.
6. Saeki T, Adachi H, Takase Y, et al. A selective type V phosphodiesterase inhibitor, E4021, dilates porcine large coronary artery. J Pharmacol Exp Ther 1995;272:825–831.

7. Wallis RM, Corbin JD, Francis SH, et al. Tissue distribution of phosphodiesterase families and the effects of sildenafil on tissue cyclic nucleotides, platelet function, and the contractile responses of trabeculae carneae and aortic rings in vitro. Am J Cardiol 1999;83:3C–12C.
8. Chambers JW, Voss GS, Snider JR, et al. Direct in vivo effects of nitric oxide on the coronary circulation. Am J Physiol Heart Circ Physiol 1996;271: H1584–H1598.
9. Duncker DJ, Mizrahi J, Bache RJ. Nitrovasodilators ITF 296 and isosorbide dinitrate exert antiischemic activity by dilating coronary penetrating arteries. J Cardiovasc Pharmacol 1995;25:823–832.
10. Altman JD, Kinn J, Duncker DJ, et al. Effect of inhibition of nitric oxide formation on coronary blood flow during exercise in the dog. Cardiovasc Res 1994; 28:119–124.
11. Chen YJ, Du R, Traverse JH, et al. Effect of sildenafil on coronary activity and reactive hyperemia. Am J Physiol Heart Circ Physiol 2000;279:H2319–H2325.
12. Laughlin MH, Korthuis RJ, Duncker DJ, et al. Control of blood flow to cardiac and skeletal muscle during exercise. In: Rowell LB, Shepherd JT, eds. Regulation and Integration of Multiple Systems: American Physiological Society Handbook Section 12, Oxford Press, New York, 1996, pp. 770–838.
13. Kanatsuka H, Lamping KG, Eastham CL, et al. Heterogeneous changes in epimyocardial microvascular size during graded coronary stenosis. Evidence of the microvascular site for autoregulation. Circ Res 1990;66:389–396.
14. Chilian WM, Eastham CL, Marcus ML. Microvascular distribution of coronary vascular resistance in beating left ventricle. Am J Physiol 1986;251:H779–H788.
15. Komaru T, Lamping KG, Eastham CL, et al. Role of ATP-sensitive potassium channels in coronary microvascular autoregulatory responses. Circ Res 1991;69: 1146–1151.
16. Kuo L, Chilian WM, Davis MJ. Interaction of pressure- and flow-induced responses in porcine coronary resistance vessels. Am J Physiol 1991;261: H1706–H1715.
17. Traverse JH, Wang YL, Du R, et al. Coronary nitric oxide production in response to exercise and endothelium-dependent agonists. Circulation 2000;101:2526–2531.
18. Chu A, Chambers DE, Lin CC, et al. Nitric oxide modulates epicardial coronary basal vasomotor tone in awake dogs. Am J Physiol Heart Circ Physiol 1990; 258:H1250–H1254.
19. Jones CJ, Kuo L, Davis MJ, et al. Regulation of coronary blood flow: coordination of heterogeneous control mechanisms in vascular microdomains. Cardiovasc Res 1995;29;585–596.
20. Sato N, Shen YT, Kiuchi K, et al. Splenic contraction-induced increases in arterial O_2 reduce requirement for CBF in conscious dogs. Am J Physiol Heart Circ Physiol 1995;269:H491–H503.
21. Parameswaran N, Hamlin RL, Nakayama T, et al. Increased splenic capacity in response to transdermal application of nitroglycerine in the dog. J Vet Int Med 1999;13:44–46.
22. Bassenge E, Busse R. Endothelial modulation of coronary tone. Prog Cardiovasc Dis 1988;30:349–380.
23. Laxson DD, Dai XZ, Homans DC, et al. Coronary vasodilator reserve in ischemic myocardium of the exercising dog. Circulation 1992;85:313–322.
24. Przyklenk K, Kloner RA. Sildenafil citrate (Viagra) does not exacerbate myocardial ischemia in canine models of coronary artery stenosis. J Am Coll Cardiol 2001;37:286–292.

25. Ball RM, Bache RJ. Distribution of the myocardial blood flow in the exercising dog with restricted coronary artery inflow. Circ Res 1976;38:60–66.
26. Chilian WM. Microvascular pressures and resistances in the left ventricular subepicardium and subendocardium. Circ Res 1991;69:561–570.
27. Duncker DJ, Bache RJ. Regulation of coronary vasomotor tone under normal conditions and during acute myocardial hypoperfusion. Pharmacol Ther 2000;86: 87–110.
28. Traverse JH, Chen Y-J, Du R, et al. Cyclic nucleotide phosphodiesterase type 5 activity limits blood flow to hypoperfused myocardium during exercise. Circulation 2000;102:2997–3002.
29. Laxson DD, Dai X, Homans DC, et al. The role alpha1- and alpha2-adrenergic receptors in mediating coronary vasoconstriction in hypoperfused ischemic myocardium during exercise. Circ Res 1989;65:1688–1697.
30. Vanhoutte PM. Endothelial adrenoceptors. J Cardiovas Pharmacol 2001;38: 796–808.
31. Kaneko H, Endo T, Kiuchi K, et al. Inhibition of nitric oxide synthesis reduces coronary blood flow response but does not increase cardiac contractile response to beta-adrenergic stimulation in normal dogs. J Cardiovasc Pharmacol 1996;27: 247–254.
32. Schwartz JS, Tockman B, Cohn JN, et al. Exercise-induced fall in flow through stenotic coronary arteries in the dog. Am J Cardiol 1982;50:1409–1413.
33. Folts JD, Schafer AI, Loscalzo J, et al. A perspective on the potential problems with aspirin as an antithrombotic agent: a comparison of studies in an animal model with clinical trials. J Am Coll Cardiol 1999;33:295–303.
34. Schmidt U, Han RO, DiSalvo TG, et al. Cessation of platelet-mediated cyclic canine coronary occlusion after thrombolysis by combining nitric oxide inhalation with phosphodiesterase-5 inhibition. J Am Coll Cardiol 2001;37:1981–1988.
35. Ogawa Y, Itoh H, Nakao K. Molecular biology and biochemistry of natriuretic peptide family. Clin Exp Pharmacol Physiol 1995;22:49–53.
36. Wang J, Seyedi N, Xu XB, et al. Defective endothelium-mediated control of coronary circulation in conscious dogs after heart failure. Am J Physiol 1994;266; H670–H680.
37. Yamamoto K, Burnett JC Jr., Redfield MM. Effect of endogenous natriuretic peptide system on ventricular and coronary function in failing heart. Am J Physiol 1997;273;H2406–H2414.
38. Chen Y, Traverse JH, Hou M, et al. Effect of PPE5 inhibition on coronary hemodynamics in pacing-induced heart failure. Am J Physiol Heart Circ Physiol 2003; 284:1513–1520.
39. Traverse JH, Melchert P, Pierpont GL, et al. Regulation of myocardial blood flow by oxygen consumption is maintained in the failing heart during exercise. Circ Res 1999;5;84:401–408.
40. Matsumoto T, Wada A, Tsutamoto T, et al. Vasorelaxing effects of atrial and brain natriuretic peptides on coronary circulation in heart failure. Am J Physiol 1999;276:H1935–H1942.

11 Safety and Hemodynamic Effects of Sildenafil in Patients With Coronary Artery Disease

Sameer Rohatgi, MD
and Howard C. Herrmann, MD

CONTENTS

INTRODUCTION
SAFETY AND EFFICACY OF SILDENAFIL IN CLINICAL TRIALS
EFFECTS OF SILDENAFIL ON HEMODYNAMICS
EFFECTS OF SILDENAFIL DURING EXERCISE IN PATIENTS WITH CAD
EFFECTS OF SILDENAFIL IN PATIENTS WITH CHF
EFFECTS OF SILDENAFIL ON ARRHYTHMOGENESIS
POTENTIAL CAUSES OF MORTALITY IN MEN TREATED WITH SILDENAFIL
CONCLUSION
REFERENCES

INTRODUCTION

Erectile dysfunction (ED), defined as the persistent inability to attain and/or maintain penile erection sufficient for sexual performance, affects up to 30 million men in the United States *(1)*. Many of these

From: *Contemporary Cardiology: Heart Disease and Erectile Dysfunction*
Edited by: R. A. Kloner © Humana Press Inc., Totowa, NJ

men also suffer from cardiovascular disease because many of the risk factors for ED are also established risk factors for coronary artery disease (CAD). These risk factors include older age, diabetes mellitus, hypertension, smoking, and dyslipidemia. It is also likely, but not proven, that oxidative stress resulting in endothelial dysfunction contributes to the pathogenesis of both diseases. The incidence of ED may also be exacerbated by cardiovascular illness, such as myocardial infarction (MI) and congestive heart failure (CHF), and by the treatment for CAD, including antihypertensive/antianginal medications such as β-blockers.

Sildenafil, a phosphodiesterase inhibitor with vasodilator properties, was originally in development as an antianginal medication. Although more than a dozen isozymes of phosphodiesterases have been identified in mammalian tissue, sildenafil selectively inhibits phosphodiesterase (PDE) type-5, which is found predominantly in the corpus cavernosum of the penis. Sildenafil effectively blocks degradation of cyclic guanosine monophosphate (cGMP) produced in response to nitric oxide (NO), thereby enhancing vasodilatation and erectile function in men with ED.

SAFETY AND EFFICACY OF SILDENAFIL IN CLINICAL TRIALS

The safety and efficacy of sildenafil has been examined in numerous studies in patients with and without CAD. Greater than 3700 patients ages 19–87 yr with ED of various causes received sildenafil therapy in the randomized, placebo-controlled, double-blinded phase II/III clinical studies completed before Food and Drug Administration approval. Importantly, exclusion criteria for these initial randomized trials included recent stroke, MI, or other significant cardiovascular event within 6 months, poorly controlled diabetes, and concomitant nitrate use. In the United States, dose–response and dose–escalation clinical trials *(2)*, sildenafil use resulted in a greater than 80% rate of improved erection with significant increases in the frequency and rigidity of erections compared with placebo. The most common side effects of sildenafil use were headache, flushing, and dyspepsia, which occurred at rates of 6–18%. No serious adverse cardiovascular events were reported.

Concerns regarding the safety of sildenafil use, particularly in patients with cardiac disease, were heightened by postmarketing surveillance data and anecdotal reports revealing numerous serious cardiovascular events, including MI and sudden cardiac death, temporally associated with its use *(3)*. Subsequent analyses suggested that these events did not reflect an increase in expected cardiovascular events in the population with ED *(4–7)*. According to a meta-analysis by Morales et al. *(8)*, serious cardiovascular events occurred at a rate of 4.1 per 100 patient-years of treatment with sildenafil, compared to 5.7 per 100 patient-years of treatment with placebo. The rate of MI was 1.7 per 100 patient-years of treatment with sildenafil compared with 1.4 per 100 patient-years of treatment with placebo. With greater than 6000 patient-years of treatment experience with sildenafil as of December 31, 1998, the incidence of all cause mortality was 0.46 per 100 patient-years with sildenafil compared with 0.84 per 100 patient-years with placebo, and the incidence of MI was 0.84 per 100 patient-years with sildenafil compared with 1.05 per 100 patient-years with placebo. On follow-up of this meta-analysis, the rate of MI remained low, at 0.57 per 100 patient-years of treatment with sildenafil, compared with 0.89 per 100 patient-years of treatment with placebo with greater than 13,000 patient-years of treatment experience as of March 31, 2002 *(9)*. It is important to note that these clinical trials of sildenafil specifically excluded patients with severe CAD, unstable symptoms, or recent MI.

Further evidence for safety in a more general population is shown in the first phase of prescription event monitoring in England, reported by Shakir et al. *(10)*. They reported on 5601 patients with a mean age of 57 yr who were prescribed sildenafil in England and followed for an average of 6 month. Nonfatal adverse cardiac events were angina ($n = 9$), chest pain ($n = 19$), ischemic heart disease ($n = 5$), and MI ($n = 7$). Fatal events included MI ($n = 6$) and ischemic heart disease ($n = 4$). The standardized mortality for this cohort of patients was 20 deaths/yr, and, when compared with the expected mortality of the general population, they found a 30.1% lower mortality in patients using sildenafil, after adjustment for confounding effects of age. The results of this study support that there is no evidence of increased risk of MI or death with sildenafil prescribed to a nonselected diverse population during the first 6 month of use. Further follow-up of this cohort of patients is expected.

Another way to assess safety in clinical trials of sildenafil is to focus specifically on patients with coronary disease. Conti et al. *(7)* reported the results of a retrospective subanalysis of 11 randomized, double-blind, placebo-controlled sildenafil trials involving 357 men with chronic, stable CAD who were not taking nitrates. Sildenafil remained an effective treatment with improved erections noted in 70% of treated men compared with 20% with placebo ($p < 0.0001$). MI rates were comparable at 3% in both the sildenafil and placebo groups, whereas serious cardiovascular events occurred in 7% in the sildenafil group and

10% in the placebo group. The most common adverse effects of sildenafil treatment included headache, flushing, and dyspepsia, and their incidences were comparable with patients with and without CAD. The overall rate of cardiovascular events was low, but there was no suggestion of an increase in events in these men with CAD. Possible reasons for the adverse cardiac events noted by postmarketing surveillance include chance alone with such wide use of sildenafil. In addition, the physical demand of sex may induce the presentation of cardiac events, especially in men who have had decreased sexual activity before using sildenafil. Lastly, although sildenafil is highly selective for PDE5, inhibition of this isozyme, which is present in platelets and vascular smooth muscle, as well as the weak inhibition of other isozymes present in the heart, could potentially cause adverse cardiovascular effects directly *(11)*. Therefore, to determine the effects of sildenafil on the cardiovascular system in patients with CAD, researchers have examined the effect of this drug on systematic, pulmonary, and coronary hemodynamics, as well as its effects on exercise capacity, on CHF, and on arrhythmogenesis.

EFFECTS OF SILDENAFIL ON HEMODYNAMICS

The effects of sildenafil on human systemic and pulmonary hemodynamics was originally studied in healthy volunteers by Jackson et al. *(12)*. They looked at the effects of both intravenous and oral sildenafil on hemodynamics of healthy young men (ages 18–45 yr) and in men with stable CAD (ages 52–70 yr). Sildenafil had a modest effect on blood pressure in normal subjects, producing an average reduction of about 10 mmHg after a single 100-mg oral dose (the maximum recommended dose). The maximum decrease was noted within 1 h after ingestion, and restoration of baseline values occurred within 4–5 h in most subjects. No significant change in heart rate or cardiac index was observed.

In patients with stable CAD, defined by a positive exercise test, nuclear test, or stress echo, or noted on angiography, sildenafil administration resulted in small reductions in right atrial, pulmonary, and systemic pressures. Once again, no significant change in heart rate was observed after sildenafil use. Overall, the authors concluded that sildenafil produced small, transient, well-tolerated decreases in blood pressure, without a significant effect on heart rate or impairment of exercise cardiac function. The overall effect was that of a mixed vasodilator, with resultant hemodynamics resembling those produced by modest nitrate therapy.

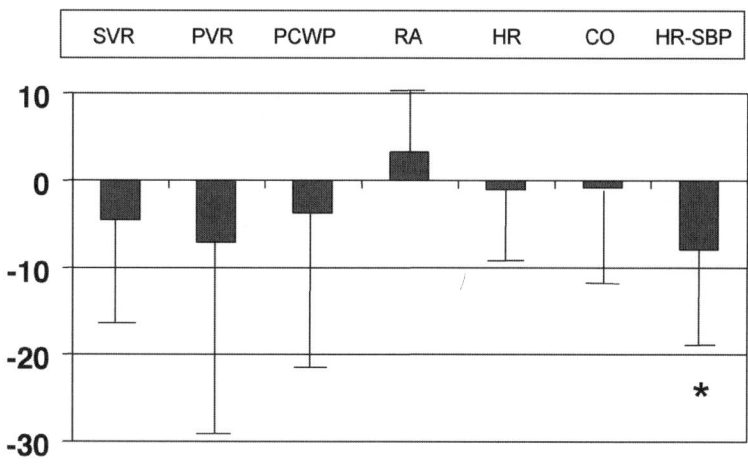

*p-value < 0.05
Adapted from Herrmann et al., (Reference 13)

Fig. 1. Effects of sildenafil (100 mg) on hemodynamics in 14 men with severe coronary artery disease. Percent change (mean ± SD) with sildenafil.

The hemodynamic and coronary effects of sildenafil have been studied in patients with more severe CAD *(13)*. The study population comprised 14 men with a mean age of 61 ± 11 yr who were referred for percutaneous coronary balloon angioplasty and stent placement for severe coronary stenosis (>70% arterial diameter stenosis) in a single coronary artery. Among these men, there was a prevalence of hypertension (57%), diabetes (43%), and smoking (57%). Before percutaneous coronary intervention, all subjects underwent systemic, pulmonary, and coronary artery hemodynamic assessments before and 60 min after a single 100-mg oral dose of sildenafil to allow for peak effect. All subjects had stable angina, which allowed the discontinuation of nitrate therapy 24 h before the study. Coronary hemodynamic assessments were based on results from quantitative coronary angiography and coronary velocity measurements with a doppler steerable guide wire inserted in the stenosed coronary artery and a nonstenosed reference coronary artery.

The systemic and pulmonary hemodynamic effects of oral sildenafil are shown in Figs. 1 and 2. Oral sildenafil produced mild decreases (<10%) in systemic and pulmonary arterial pressures but had no effect on pulmonary capillary wedge pressure, right atrial pressure, or cardiac output. The slightly smaller reductions in calculated systemic vas-

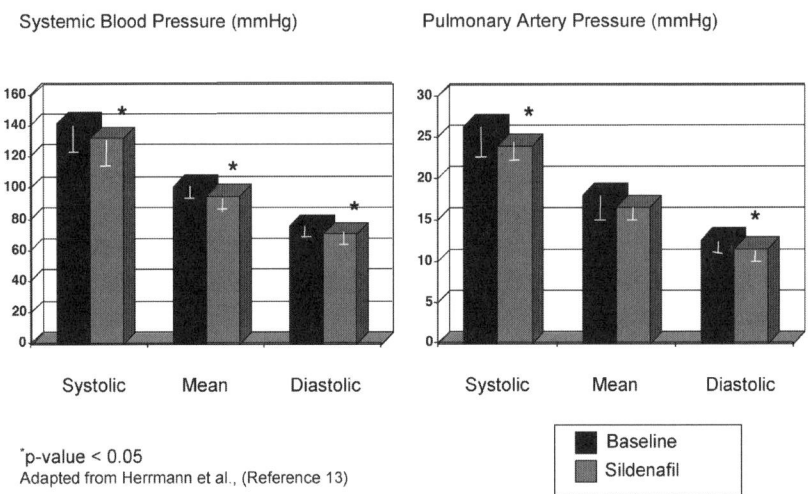

Fig. 2. Effects of sildenafil (100 mg) on systemic and pulmonary hemodynamics in 14 men with severe coronary artery disease.

cular resistance and pulmonary vascular resistance and in the indexes of these measures, which are normalized for body surface area, did not reach statistical significance. The heart rate–systolic blood pressure double product (a surrogate measure of myocardial oxygen demand) was statistically lower in men receiving sildenafil. These findings were similar to those observed by Jackson et al. *(12)* in healthy volunteers.

The coronary hemodynamics are shown in Fig. 3. Hemodynamics are notable for no significant changes in average peak coronary flow velocity, volumetric coronary blood flow, or coronary vascular resistance with the administration of oral sildenafil. On the basis of the decrease in the heart rate–systolic blood pressure double product, one might have expected a parallel decrease in coronary blood flow because of autoregulation. The absence of such a finding in this study may reflect the inaccuracy of the double product as a true measure of myocardial demand, variations in the calculated values for coronary blood flow and resistance, or a vasodilatory effect of sildenafil that blunts the expected reduction in coronary blood flow. Of interest, baseline coronary flow reserve, which was lower in the stenosed than in the nonstenosed arteries (1.26 ± 0.26 vs. 2.19 ± 0.44), increased by about 13% in both groups of arteries (1.70 ± 0.59 to 1.92 ± 0.72; $p = 0.003$) after oral sildenafil administration, as seen in Figure 4.

Coronary flow reserve is the ratio of maximal coronary blood flow (induced by exercise or adenosine-stimulated arteriolar vasodilatation) to resting coronary blood flow. It is this ability of the coronary circu-

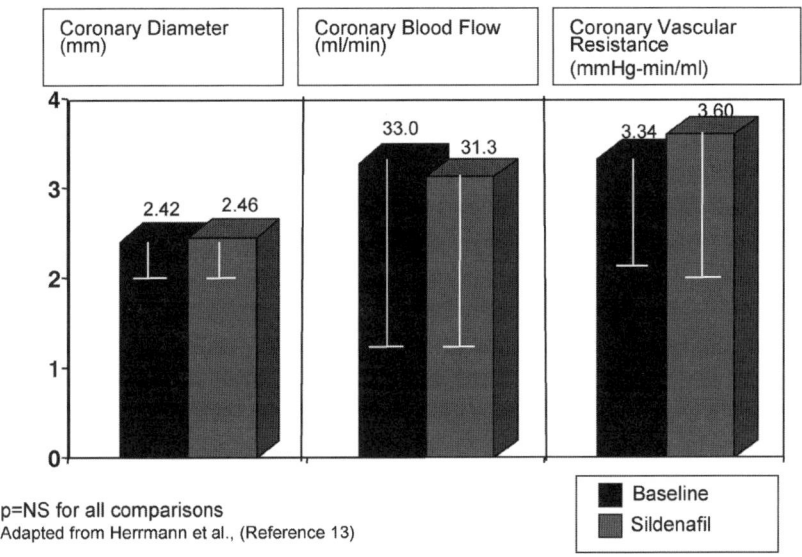

Fig. 3. Effects of sildenafil (100 mg) on coronary hemodynamics in men with severe coronary artery disease for both stenosed and reference vessels.

lation to augment coronary blood flow in response to increased myocardial oxygen demand that allows the left ventricle to increase cardiac output without ischemia. As a coronary artery develops stenosis, autoregulatory vasodilatation occurs to maintain coronary blood flow, limiting the ability to further vasodilate, reducing coronary flow reserve. In this regard, the reduced coronary flow reserve in the stenosed arteries is not unexpected. The augmentation of hyperemic coronary blood flow provided by oral sildenafil in response to intracoronary adenosine occurred to similar degrees in both stenosed and nonstenosed arteries, and the relative coronary flow reserve remained stable before and after sildenafil use at 0.57. The ability of sildenafil to increase hyperemic coronary blood flow suggests a beneficial effect of this agent on the coronary circulation. Although only a small number of men were studied, none had hypotension, chest pain, or any other side effect that could be attributed to sildenafil.

Thus, in this study of men with severe CAD, no adverse cardiovascular effects of oral sildenafil could be detected by measurement of systemic, pulmonary, or coronary hemodynamic variables. Interestingly, hyperemic coronary blood flow after the administration of adenosine, reflected as an increase in coronary flow reserve, increased in all the men treated with sildenafil. Adenosine dilates coronary resistance vessels by stimulating the production of cyclic adenosine monophos-

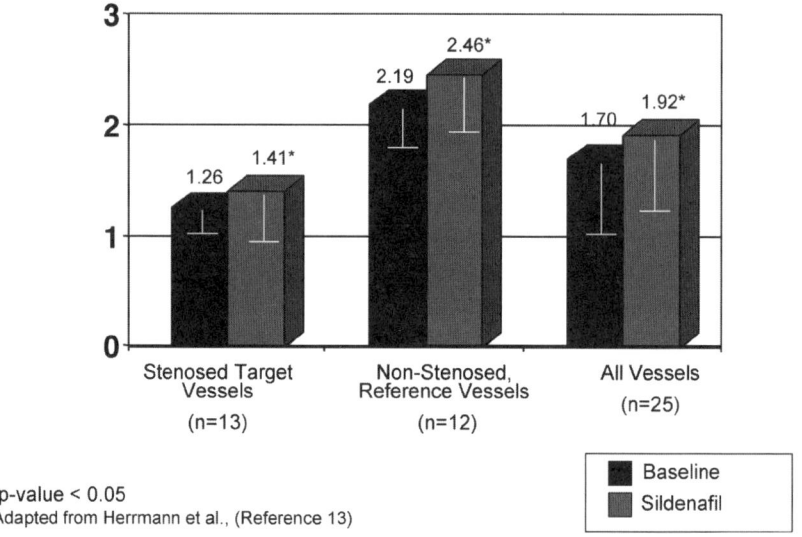

Fig. 4. Effects of sildenafil on coronary flow reserve in men with severe coronary artery disease.

phate. It is possible that adenosine and sildenafil interact and that their interaction potentiates their individual effects on coronary resistance. The doses of adenosine used in our study have been shown to provide maximal coronary vasodilatation, but our data suggest that further vasodilatation is possible. Therefore, PDE5 may play an important role in regulation of coronary blood flow, and sildenafil may have a potential beneficial effect.

The mechanism of action of sildenafil has also suggested the potential for a drug interaction with other agents affecting the NO–cGMP vasodilator pathway. The potential for an adverse reaction with antianginal agents prompted Webb et al. *(14)* to study the interaction between sildenafil and nitroglycerin in healthy men (ages 18–45 yr) and between sildenafil and amlodipine in hypertensive men (ages 26–68 yr). Twelve men received escalating intravenous nitroglycerin (2.5–4.0 µg/min) or a single sublingual nitroglycerin tablet 1 h after receiving sildenafil or placebo in a randomized, double-blind, placebo-controlled, two-way crossover design. A significant synergistic interaction occurred between nitroglycerin and sildenafil, with a larger degree of symptomatic hypotension and a greater than 25 mmHg decrease in blood pressure, compared to nitroglycerin and placebo ($p < 0.01$). Furthermore, a fourfold greater decrease in systolic blood pressure was observed when sublingual nitroglycerin was given with sildenafil than when it was given with placebo. This synergy likely stems from potentiation of sildenafil's effect by donation of NO by nitroglycerin. In the second study, 16 men received sildenafil 100 mg orally or placebo 2 h after their usual morning amlodipine dose, in a double-blind, two-way crossover protocol. Sildenafil plus amlodipine resulted in an additive (not synergistic) 7–8 mmHg reduction in systolic and diastolic blood pressures compared with placebo plus amlodipine ($p < 0.02$).

Additional studies have investigated the effects of sildenafil in patients taking one or more antihypertensive agents (15), such as diuretics, β-blockers, α1-blockers, angiotensin-converting enzyme inhibitor, or a calcium channel blocker. The incidence of treatment-related adverse events was similar to that for sildenafil-treated patients taking antihypertensives and patients taking sildenafil not on antihypertensives. Furthermore, the incidence of adverse events potentially related to blood pressure, such as dizziness, hypotension, and syncope, were similar between the two groups. The study is consistent with the known mechanism of action of sildenafil and suggests that sildenafil is an effective and well-tolerated treatment for ED in patients taking concomitant antihypertensive medication, including those on multidrug regimens, as long as the antihypertensive agent is not a NO donor. There has been a recent precaution regarding the use of sildenafil plus α-blockers (*see* Chapter 9).

EFFECTS OF SILDENAFIL DURING EXERCISE IN PATIENTS WITH CAD

Because sexual intercourse increases myocardial oxygen demand, it is important to examine the cardiovascular effects of sildenafil in patients with CAD during exercise. Arruda-Olson et al. *(16)* studied 105 men (mean age: 66 yr) who had ED and known or highly suspected CAD. Of the study population, 89% had a history of CAD with either greater than 50% stenosis of a major epicardial vessel, history of MI, previous positive stress imaging result, or previous coronary artery bypass surgery. The remaining 11% had a greater than 70% pretest probability of CAD based on the presence of typical anginal symptoms. In a randomized, double-blind, placebo-controlled, crossover design, subjects performed two symptom-limited supine bicycle echocardiograms with oral sildenafil (50 or 100 mg) vs placebo 1 h before exercise. Patients were allowed to continue their cardiac medications, including β-blockers. Baseline resting ejection fraction was 39–68%, with a mean of 56%. Baseline resting wall motion abnormalities were present in 60 patients (57%).

Hemodynamics at peak exercise

	Heart Rate (beats/min)	Systolic BP (mmHg)	Diastolic BP (mmHg)	Double Product (beats-mmHg/min)
Placebo	110 (18)	176 (30)	95 (16)	19503 (5423)
Sildenafil	110 (18)	174 (29)	93 (15)	19294 (5317)

Echocardiography at peak exercise

	WMSI	Ejection Fraction	Ischemic Segments (%)
Placebo	1.4 (0.4)	0.60 (0.09)	20 (17)
Sildenafil	1.4 (0.4)	0.60 (0.10)	19 (17)

All values shown as mean (SD)
p=NS for all comparisons of sildenafil and placebo
WMSI, wall motion score index
Adapted from Arruda-Olson et al., (Reference 16)

Fig. 5. Effects of sildenafil during exercise echo in patients with coronary artery disease.

The hemodynamic effects of sildenafil were assessed by exercise echocardiography. Systolic blood pressure decreased significantly after sildenafil use (from a mean [SD] of 135 [19] mmHg to 128 [17] mmHg with a mean difference of −7 mmHg; (95% CI, −9 to −4 mmHg; $p < 0.001$). Diastolic pressure and heart rate did not change significantly with sildenafil use. Exercise hemodynamic data are summarized in Fig. 5. After exercise, the rate of recovery to baseline was similar between sildenafil and placebo for systolic and diastolic blood pressure, and heart rate.

The resting wall motion severity index and ejection fraction did not change significantly before and after sildenafil use. Reasons for termination of exercise and electrocardiographic interpretation were similar with sildenafil and placebo use with symptoms of dyspnea or angina developing in 69 men taking sildenafil and 70 men taking placebo ($p = 0.89$). There were no deaths, acute MIs, or ventricular fibrillation associated with the exercise studies. In sildenafil and placebo groups, there was no difference in the numbers of subjects with any ischemia or multivessel ischemia, or in wall motion severity index during exercise, ejection fraction, or heart rate at onset of ischemia.

In this study, sildenafil was well tolerated and did not change the onset, extent, or severity of ischemia, as assessed by exercise electrocardiography or echocardiography. There are several limitations to this study, including a low rate of ischemic segments (17%), and the fact that most patients received only 50 mg of sildenafil. Nonetheless, this study supports the safety profile of sildenafil in patients with CAD.

The effects of sildenafil on exercise have also been studied in patients with more significant CAD by Fox et al. *(17)*. In this study, patients with reproducible exercise-induced angina performed exercise treadmill tests in a double-blinded, parallel-group, placebo-controlled, multicenter study. Patients performed a baseline exercise test and then performed a second exercise test after receiving placebo or sildenafil 100 mg 1 h before. In those patients that received placebo, the baseline exercise tolerance was 396 s with an 18 s (4.7%) increase after placebo. In those patients that received sildenafil, the baseline exercise tolerance was 373 s with a 36-s (9.8%) increase after sildenafil. These data further confirm that sildenafil does not adversely affect exercise capacity in patients with CAD. This study supports the use of sildenafil in patients with more severe CAD represented by stable reproducible angina and at a higher dose of sildenafil (100 mg).

EFFECTS OF SILDENAFIL IN PATIENTS WITH CHF

Many patients with CAD will also have left ventricular dysfunction or CHF. In addition, ED may affect up to 60–70% of heart failure patients *(18)*. To retain sexual activity some patients may become noncompliant with medications that they feel exacerbate their ED. Sildenafil is an effective treatment for ED even in patients with CHF. However, concern for the safety of sildenafil in patients with CHF has led to studies of the effects of sildenafil on vascular tone and on exercise capacity.

Katz et al. *(19)* studied 39 men and 9 women between the ages of 21 and 75 yr with New York Heart Association (NYHA) class II or III heart failure. Patients were on a stable heart failure regimen, which was stopped 12 h before study. Flow-mediated, endothelium-dependent vasodilatation was measured by ultrasound of the brachial artery. As a prospective, double-blind study, patients received single oral doses of sildenafil (12.5, 25, and 50 mg) or placebo. After 1 h of ingestion to correspond with peak plasma levels of oral dosing, brachial artery diameter and blood flow velocity were measured at rest and after 1, 3, and 5 min of transient arterial occlusion. Flow-mediated dilatation significantly increased in patients receiving sildenafil 25 mg and sildenafil 50 mg. Mean brachial arterial blood flow velocity did not significantly change. There were no adverse cardiovascular events related to the use of sildenafil in these patients with CHF.

Bocchi et al. *(20)* studied the effects of sildenafil on exercise capacity in 24 men with a history of CHF referred for treatment of ED. The average ejection fraction was 23 ± 7% with predominantly NYHA class II symptoms. In this randomized, double-blind, placebo-controlled, two-way crossover study, patients performed both a 6-min walk test and a maximal exercise test 1 h after receiving sildenafil 50 mg or placebo. As seen in previous studies, sildenafil reduced systolic and diastolic blood pressure at rest; however, at peak exercise both with the 6-min walk test and the exercise test there was a similar increase in systolic and diastolic blood pressure with no difference between placebo and sildenafil (Fig. 6). However, sildenafil attenuated the heart rate increment during the 6-min walk test and during the first 8 min of the exercise test and also reduced the V_E/V_{CO_2} slope during both the 6-min walk test and the exercise test. This resulted in increased maximal exercise capacity with sildenafil. Sildenafil was associated with more nonspecific adverse constitutional symptoms, however none of these resulted in discontinuation from the study. Greater than 80% of patients noted satisfaction with sildenafil for the treatment of ED. The results of this study support the safety of sildenafil in patients with CHF.

EFFECTS OF SILDENAFIL ON ARRHYTHMOGENESIS

Several cases of sudden death have been reported associated with the use of sildenafil, raising the possibility of arrhythmia in addition to ischemia. Studies have shown that, even at twice the recommended dose, sildenafil causes no change in electrocardiogram parameters *(21)*. Recent studies have examined the effects of sildenafil on repolarization at supratherapeutic doses. Geelen et al. *(22)* used a patch clamp technique in isolated hearts to study the electrophysiologic effects of sildenafil. This showed that sildenafil could prolong cardiac repolarization by blocking the rapid component (I_{Kr}) of the delayed rectifier potassium current at supratherapeutic concentrations. Sildenafil is unlikely to reach these concentrations without the presence of an overdose or in the setting of decreased metabolism. Possible causes of decreased metabolism include significant hepatic or renal insufficiency, or coadministration with CYP3A inhibitors such as macrolides or imidazoles. These data would imply that patients with an overdose or decreased metabolism need to be followed for QT prolongation and triggered ventricular tachyarrhythmias. Also, patients with a "drug-revealed" form of silent congenital long QT syndrome would need to be followed carefully.

	Heart Rate (beats/min)	Systolic BP (mmHg)	Diastolic BP (mmHg)	V_E/V_{CO2} Slope
Peak during 6 minute walk test				
Placebo	97 ± 21	126 ± 21	70 ± 13	32 ± 7
Sildenafil	90 ± 19*	120 ± 21	69 ± 13	31 ± 6*
Peak during exercise test				
Placebo	118 ± 23	132 ± 20	74 ± 13	33 ± 8
Sildenafil	118 ± 23	129 ± 26	68 ± 15	31 ± 5*

*p-value < 0.05
Adapted from Bocchi et al., (Reference 20)

Fig. 6. Effects of sildenafil on patients with congestive heart failure.

Piccirillo et al. (23) note that at normal doses sildenafil has no significant effect on QT interval or QT dispersion. Thus, at normal doses sildenafil does not appear to have significant electrophysiologic effects; however, at supratherapeutic doses sildenafil does seem to alter the hearts electrophysiologic properties. Although arrhythmia is a theoretical concern, there have been no reports of torsades de pointes or QT prolongation from the clinical trial database or from postmarketing experience.

POTENTIAL CAUSES OF MORTALITY IN MEN TREATED WITH SILDENAFIL

Other possibilities which have been raised to explain the postmarketing surveillance and anecdotal reports of adverse cardiovascular events temporally associated with the use of sildenafil include coincidence alone, resulting from the high prevalence of both ED and cardiovascular disease in middle-aged men. A second possibility is that sildenafil enables men who may have been previously both sexually and physically inactive to engage in sexual activity. The physical activity of sex is known to be associated with an increased risk of adverse cardiac events. Muller (24) used a case-crossover study design to show that the relative risk of MI after sexual intercourse was 2.5 (95% CI 1.7–3.7) over a 2-h time period after intercourse. Along with this increased risk of sexual activity itself, there is likely an increased reporting bias of adverse cardiovascular events caused by the dramatic nature of MI associated with sexual intercourse. The effects of sexual intercourse on heart rate, blood pressure, and oxygen consumption are similar to moderate exercise. Using 24-h ambulatory electrocardiographic monitoring, Drory et al. *(25)* compared men with CAD having sexual intercourse in their usual settings to a near maximal exercise test. With intercourse, the peak heart rate was 118 ± 21 beats/min, whereas with exercise peak heart rate was 138 ± 19 beats/min. The myocardial oxygen demand of sexual intercourse was estimated to be equivalent to briskly climbing two flights of stairs or the equivalent of five to six metabolic equivalents. Importantly, this study validated the use of stress testing to peak heart rate as a test of the likelihood of sexual activity provoking ischemia.

Lastly, sildenafil itself could have adverse cardiovascular effects. As reviewed earlier, sildenafil can have a significant effect on blood pressure with concomitant nitrate use. However, as described earlier, sildenafil has a safe profile in terms of hemodynamics, exercise capacity, and arrhythmogenesis in patients with both ischemic heart disease and CHF. Based on the available evidence, sildenafil is unlikely to directly cause adverse cardiovascular events.

CONCLUSION

The data presented in this chapter fail to show a direct cardiovascular mechanism for the adverse events reported during postmarketing surveillance. Except for a mild decrease in vascular resistance, sildenafil does not have any adverse effects on systemic, pulmonary, or coronary hemodynamics in normal men and men with severe cardiovascular disease. It is likely that some adverse cardiac events may be the result of interactions with nitrates, which are contraindicated. However, other antihypertensive medications and multiple antihypertensive regimens appear to be safe. The studies of sildenafil with exercise testing show no adverse effects on hemodynamics and no change in exercise capacity, both in patients with coronary disease and in patients with CHF. Lastly, sildenafil at normal doses has been shown to have a benign electrophysiologic profile. From these studies, sildenafil itself is unlikely to be a cause of adverse cardiovascular events and is a safe and effective agent for the treatment of ED in patients with cardiovascular disease.

REFERENCES

1. NIH Consensus Development Panel on Impotence. NIH Consensus Conference: impotence. JAMA. 1993;270:83–90.
2. Goldstein I, Lue TF, Padma-Nathan H, et al. Oral sildenafil in the treatment of erectile dysfunction. N Engl J Med 1998;338:1397–1404.

3. Viagra (sildenafil citrate) [revised package insert]. New York, NY: Pfizer; June, 1999.
4. Zusman RM, Morales A, Glasser DB, et al. Overall cardiovascular profile of sildenafil citrate. Am J Cardiol. 1999;83(Suppl 5A):35C–44C.
5. Kloner RA. Cardiovascular risk and sildenafil. Am J Cardiol 2000;86(Suppl): 57F–61F.
6. Morales A, Gingell C, Collins M, et al. Clinical safety of oral sildenafil citrate (Viagra) in the treatment of erectile dysfunction. Int J Impotence Res 1998;10: 69–74.
7. Conti RC, Pepine C, Sweeney M. Efficacy and safety of sildenafil citrate in the treatment of erectile dysfunction in patients with ischemic heart disease. Am J Cardiol 1999;83(Suppl):29C–34C.
8. Morales A, Gingell C, Collins M, et al. Clinical safety of oral sildenafil citrate (Viagra) in the treatment of erectile dysfunction. Int J Impotence Res 1998; 10:69–74.
9. Pfizer data on file, unpublished.
10. Shakir SA, Wilton LV, Boshier A, et al. Cardiovascular events in users of sildenafil: results from first phase of prescription event monitoring in England. Br Med J 2001;322:651–652.
11. Wallis RM, Corbin JD, Francis SH, et al. Tissue distribution of phosphodiesterase families and the effects of sildenafil on tissue cyclic nucleotides, platelet function, and the contractile responses of trabeculae carneae and aortic rings in vitro. Am J Cardiol 1999;83:3C–12C.
12. Jackson G, Benjamin N, Jackson N, et al. Effects of sildenafil citrate on human hemodynamics. Am J Cardiol 1999;83(Suppl):13C–20C.
13. Herrmann HC, Chang G, Klugherz BD, et al. Hemodynamic effects of sildenafil in men with severe coronary artery disease. N Engl J Med 2000;342: 1622–1626.
14. Webb DJ, Freestone S, Allen MJ, et al. Sildenafil citrate and blood-pressure-lowering drugs: results of drug interaction studies with an organic nitrate and a calcium antagonist. Am J Cardiol 1999;83(Suppl):21C–28C.
15. Kloner RA, Brown M, Prisant LM, et al. Effects of sildenafil in patients with erectile dysfunction taking antihypertensive therapy. Am J Hypertens 2001;14: 70–73.
16. Arruda-Olson AM, Mahoney DW, Nehra A, et al. Cardiovascular effects of sildenafil during exercise in men with known or probable coronary artery disease. JAMA 2002;287:719–725.
17. Fox KM, Thadani U, Ma PTS, et al. Time to onset of limiting angina during treadmill exercise in men with erectile dysfunction and stable chronic angina: effect of sildenafil citrate (abst). Circulation 2001;104:II–601.
18. Jaarsma T, Dracup K, Walden J, et al. Sexual function in patients with advanced heart failure. Heart Lung 1996;25:262–270.
19. Katz SD, Balidemaj K, Homma S, et al. Acute type 5 phosphodiesterase inhibition with sildenafil citrate enhances flow-mediated vasodilatation in patients with chronic heart failure. J Am Coll Cardiol 2000;36:845–851.
20. Bocchi EA, Guimaraes G, Mocelin A, et al. Sildenafil effects on exercise, neurohormonal activation, and erectile dysfunction in congestive heart failure. Circulation 2002;106:1097–1103.
21. Zusman R, Morales A, Glasser D, et al. Overall cardiovascular profile of sildenafil citrate. Am J Cardiol 1999;83:35C–44C.

22. Geelen P, Benoit D, Rail J, et al. Sildenafil (Viagra) prolongs cardiac repolarization by blocking the rapid component of the delayed rectifier potassium current. Circulation 2000;102:275–277.
23. Piccirillo G, Nocco M, Lionetti M, et al. Effects of sildenafil citrate (Viagra) on cardiac repolarization and on autonomic control in subjects with chronic heart failure. Am Heart J 2002;143:703–710.
24. Muller JE. Triggering of cardiac events by sexual activity: findings from a case-crossover analysis. Am J Caridiol 2000;86(Suppl):14F–18F.
25. Drory Y, Shapira I, Fisman EZ, et al. Myocardial ischemia during sexual activity in patients with coronary artery disease. Am J Cardiol 1995;75:835–837.

12 Cardiovascular Effects of Nonphosphodiesterase-5 Inhibitor Erectile Dysfunction Therapies

Harin Padma-Nathan, MD

CONTENTS

BACKGROUND
APOMORPHINE SL
ALPROSTADIL (PROSTAGLANDIN E_1)
PHENTOLAMINE (VASOMAX, Z-MAX)
YOHIMBINE (YOCON)
OTHER AGENTS
CONCLUSION
REFERENCES

BACKGROUND

Worldwide, more than 150 million men experience some degree of erectile dysfunction (ED; refs. *1* and *2*). ED is highly correlated with a range of cardiovascular conditions and risk factors, including ischemic heart disease, hypertension, hypercholesteremia, peripheral vascular disease, and diabetes mellitus *(1–5)*. The presence of these comorbidities has prompted some practitioners and patients to be concerned about the cardiovascular risks associated with resuming sexual activity and about the cardiovascular effects of pharmacologic ED treatments.

From: *Contemporary Cardiology: Heart Disease and Erectile Dysfunction*
Edited by: R. A. Kloner © Humana Press Inc., Totowa, NJ

The belief that sexual activity may increase the likelihood of cardiovascular events such as myocardial infarction (MI) can be traced to the early research of Masters and Johnson, who reported peak coital heart rates of up to 180 beats/min in subjects in the laboratory setting, with increases in systolic and diastolic blood pressure of 80 mmHg and 50 mmHg, respectively *(6)* However, subsequent studies found that peak heart rate and blood pressure during coitus in the home setting are not significantly different from those achieved during normal daily activities *(6,7)*. In a case-crossover study examining the incidence of MI after sexual activity vs MI not temporally related to coitus, Muller and colleagues found the relative risk of MI in the 2 h after sexual activity was 2.5 for patients with no history of MI and 2.9 for those with a previous MI. As this increased risk was transient, the authors concluded that sexual activity is a relatively weak trigger for MI, noting that the absolute risk of postcoital MI in a healthy 50-yr-old man is only 2 in 1 million per hour and only for a 2-h period *(8)*.

Despite the relatively low cardiovascular risk associated with sexual activity, some physicians and patients remain apprehensive about the cardiac risks of pharmacologic ED therapy. At present, numerous agents other than sildenafil are available or in development for the treatment of ED. This chapter examines the cardiac risk profiles of several of these agents, including the dopamine agonist apomorphine, the prostaglandin E_1 analogue alprostadil, the α_{1-2} adrenergic-receptor antagonist phentolamine, and the indole alkaloid yohimbine.

APOMORPHINE SL

Mechanism of Action

Apomorphine (Uprima®; TAP Pharmaceuticals Holdings, Chicago, IL) is a centrally acting, selective dopamine receptor agonist that historically has been used in the treatment of Parkinson's disease. The drug's proerectile effects are caused, in part, by stimulation of the paraventricular nucleus of the hypothalamus, which leads to an increase in parasympathetic outflow and a relaxation of corporal smooth muscle *(9,10)*.

A sublingual preparation of apomorphine has been approved in the European Union for the treatment of ED. The recommended therapeutic dose is 2 or 3 mg, administered approximately 20 min before sexual activity. In clinical trials, 45.6% of 2-mg doses administered produced an erection sufficient for intercourse (placebo: 33.8%), as did 46.9% of 3-mg doses (placebo: 32.3%; ref. *11*). Peak serum levels recorded after treatment at approved doses are significantly lower than those required for direct vascular effects, which should indicate a low risk of systemic vasodilation or interaction with cardiovascular medications *(10,11)*.

Cardiovascular Effects

In clinical trials encompassing more than 5000 patients and 120,000 doses, apomorphine SL was found to have a relatively modest effect on subjects' hemodynamic baseline. Doses as high as 5 mg had little impact on systolic or diastolic blood pressure; overall, apomorphine SL-treated subjects showed a mean maximum reduction of only 2–3 mmHg as compared with placebo-treated subjects *(12)*. The design of one phase III crossover trial included standing and supine blood pressure measurements before dosing and at selected time points after dosing. Data from this trial showed no significant changes in heart rate after the 2- or 4-mg dose, with "a few sporadic statistically significant differences" in blood pressure, none of which were considered clinically significant *(10)*. Holter recordings from a subset of 344 trial participants revealed no significant differences between those who were treated with apomorphine SL and those who received placebo *(11)*.

The most common adverse events reported in apomorphine SL clinical trials were nausea (6.8%), headache (6.7%), dizziness (4.4%), rhinitis (2.8%), and pharyngitis (2.2%; ref. *12)*. A subgroup analysis of subjects with concomitant hypertension or coronary artery disease revealed no "clinically meaningful differences" in adverse event rates in these patients as compared with the general study population *(10,12)*.

The most significant adverse event reported during clinical trials was vasovagal syncope, secondary to hypotension and apparently neurogenic in origin. The majority of syncopal episodes were preceded by prodromal events that included one or more of the following: dizziness, pallor, sweating/hot flashes, moderate-to-severe nausea, and vomiting *(11–13)*. The incidence of syncope was clearly dose-related, occurring in fewer than 0.2% of patients treated at the approved doses of 2 and 3 mg, and rising to 1.1% among patients receiving 6 mg *(11–13)*. Although uncommon, this adverse event was dramatic and potentially life-threatening and is the principle reason for the delay of the drug's approval in the United States. The incidence of syncope has not been significant in field experience after European approval of the lower doses only.

Drug Interaction Data

In phase II and III studies of apomorphine SL, adverse event rates were similar among patients who reported regular alcohol use (63%)

and those who were not alcohol users (37%; ref. *11*). However, alcohol interaction studies in healthy adults revealed more frequent treatment-emergent adverse events in subjects who consumed 0.3 g/kg–0.6 g/kg of alcohol 30 min before a 4-mg dose of apomorphine SL *(11)*.

Approximately 30% of patients in the clinical trial program were being maintained on antihypertensive agents, 21% were taking other cardiac medications, and 9.5% were receiving diuretics. There was no significant difference in the incidence or nature of side effects in patients receiving cardiovascular medications as compared to those who were not on concurrent therapy *(12)*.

More recently, Fagan and colleagues examined the pharmacodynamic interactions between apomorphine SL and commonly used cardiovascular medications in a double-blind, crossover study involving 162 men (mean age: 61 yr) who had been stable on therapeutic doses of angiotensin-converting enzyme inhibitors, β-blockers, α_1 blockers, calcium channel blockers, diuretics, or nitrates for at least 4 wk. Over one-third of the study group was receiving two or more cardiovascular medications, and 75% of patients on nitrates were taking at least three additional cardiovascular medications *(14)*.

Subjects were given 5 mg apomorphine SL 4 h after dosing with antihypertensive medication or long-acting nitrate. (Patients on short-acting nitrates were dosed 30 min prior to nitrate dosing.) Dosing was timed so that peak pharmacologic effects of both medications would occur concurrently *(14)*.

Compared with placebo, no statistically or clinically significant changes from baseline were observed in mean blood pressure or heart rate after apomorphine SL. Symptomatic decreases in blood pressure were recorded in four patients (10%) receiving nitrates and in four patients (3.3%) receiving antihypertensive medications. All eight episodes were associated with a prodrome of dizziness, pallor, diaphoresis, and nausea *(14)*.

Holter monitor readings for eight patients revealed one or more clinically significant abnormalities of cardiac rhythm after apomorphine SL. Five of these subjects showed a similar abnormality following placebo, and one had a predose abnormality. Two clinically relevant sinus pauses (of 11.3 and 7.6 s each) were recorded. Both were associated with nausea, pallor, and diaphoresis, and one was associated with syncope. These pauses appeared to be caused by increased vagal tone, and were consistent with the episodes of vasovagal syncope observed in clinical trials of apomorphine SL *(14)*.

Overall, apomorphine SL at recommended doses produced "only sporadic and clinically insignificant" changes in blood pressure and heart rate in patients on antihypertensives or nitrates. Patients on α_1 blockers and calcium channel blockers showed greater decreases in average systolic blood pressure on standing, which may indicate a potential for orthostatic hypotension after apomorphine treatment in these patients *(14)*. Although syncope occurred in only 1 of the 1028 hypertensive patients involved in the clinical trial program, it is recommended that apomorphine SL "be used with caution in patients receiving antihypertensive medication" *(11)*.

ALPROSTADIL (PROSTAGLANDIN E$_1$)

Mechanism of Action

Alprostadil is a prostaglandin E$_1$ analog derived from free arachidonic acid. When administered via intracavernous injection (Caverject, Edex, Viridal), as transurethral suppository (MUSE™), or as a topical gel (Alprox TD, Topiglan), alprostadil increases levels of cyclic adenosine monophosphate, thereby decreasing intracellular levels of free calcium and promoting corporeal smooth muscle relaxation *(15)*. Because alprostadil is metabolized in local tissue, it is expected to have minimal systemic effects.

Cardiovascular Effects

INTRACAVERNOUS ADMINISTRATION (CAVERJECT, EDEX, VIRIDAL)

Alprostadil has been extensively studied as an intracavernosal agent, both as a monotherapy and in combination with other erectogenic agents. Reported efficacy rates range from 70 to 75% during in-office titration to greater than 90% in the home setting *(15–17)*.

In early studies of intracavernosal alprostadil, Linet and colleagues reported that 1% of subjects experienced side effects that might be attributable to hypotension, including dizziness, diaphoresis, lightheadedness, irregular pulse, vasodilation, and vasovagal reactions *(16)*. When administered to 67 men with ED for up to 12 months, doses of up to 50 µg of alprostadil were "not associated with any clinically relevant changes in laboratory safety variables or vital signs" *(17)*.

Baniel and colleagues evaluated the effects of alprostadil as part of a progressive treatment program for ED. Two hundred and ten subjects received alprostadil ≤ 25 µg as monotherapy or in combination with phentolamine, papaverine, and atropine sulfate. No significant changes in blood pressure were observed at any point during the 3-yr study period *(18)*.

Israilov et al. investigated the efficacy of alprostadil (10–25 µg) as combination therapy in 45 men with known cardiovascular disease who had failed or were ineligible for sildenafil. No significant changes in blood pressure were recorded during the 1-yr study period, and no patient required a change in cardiovascular medications while receiving alprostadil *(19)*.

TRANSURETHRAL ADMINISTRATION (MUSE)

In clinical trials, approximately 50% of administrations of transurethral alprostadil resulted in intercourse *(20)* More recently, Guay and colleagues reported an overall success rate of 56% in 229 men using transurethral alprostadil in the home setting. "Success" was defined as completing intercourse in two-thirds of intercourse attempts *(21)*.

Transurethral alprostadil has been linked to a slightly higher incidence of systemic effects than intracavernous formulations. When administered in the clinic setting during an early double-blind, placebo-controlled study, transurethral alprostadil (125–1000 µg) was associated with hypotension in 3.3% of subjects and with syncope in 0.4%. Hypotension was most frequent among patients in the higher dose groups—occurring in 2.4% of patients receiving 1000 µg of alprostadil. When administered in the home setting, 1.9% of patients reported dizziness, but none reported syncope *(20)*.

Transurethral alprostadil has also been investigated as a combination therapy with the α-adrenergic receptor inhibitor prazosin. Greater than 35% of patients receiving 500 µg alprostadil plus 2000 µg prazosin reported achieving erections sufficient for intercourse. Patients receiving alprostadil plus prazosin also showed a higher incidence of dizziness and hypotension (8.8–13.5%), particularly at the higher dose range for each drug (250–1000 µg alprostadil, 1000–2000 µg prazosin). There was also a higher incidence of syncope in patients receiving high-dose alprostadil *(22)*.

TOPICAL ADMINISTRATION (ALPROX-TD, TOPIGLAN)

Two topical formulations of alprostadil have recently been introduced. Both Alprox-TD cream and Topiglan gel contain varying concentrations of alprostadil combined with a proprietary transdermal permeation enhancer *(23–26)*.

Alprox-TD has been evaluated in two multicenter, placebo-controlled phase II clinical trials involving 303 patients with mild-to-moderate and severe ED. Patients were randomly assigned to receive placebo, 0.05, 0.1, or 0.3 alprostadil cream. Combined analysis of these trials revealed improvement from baseline scores in the Erectile Function domain and questions 3 and 4 of the International Index of Erectile Function (IIEF). These improvements achieved statistical significance in the 0.2-mg and

0.3-mg treatment groups, with a clear dose-related trend in efficacy across all treatment groups *(23,24)*.

More than half of the subjects in each treatment group had a secondary diagnosis of cardiovascular disease. A test dose of study medication was administered in the clinic setting, at which time orthostatic vital signs were measured for up to 2 h postdose. Patients who showed a decrease in systolic blood pressure ≥ 30 mmHg, a decrease of in diastolic blood pressure of ≥ 20 mmHg, or an increase in pulse rate ≥ 30 beats/min were dismissed from the study, regardless of clinical symptoms *(23,24)*.

Eight percent of patients in the highest dose group were dismissed because of postdose hypotension, as were 10.7% of patients in the 0.2-mg group. One patient in the 0.2-mg group experienced a near-syncopal event after the test dose. This event was preceded by tremors and mild weakness and lasted approximately 10 min. During the at-home treatment period, the vast majority of drug-related adverse events were limited to the site of application, and there were no "noteworthy effects" observed in clinical laboratory tests or physical examinations, or electrocardiograms *(23,24)*.

In a single-blind, placebo-controlled trial, McVary and colleagues examined the effects of Topiglan (0.5 mg–2.5 mg alprostadil) in 48 patients with ED. Treatment was associated with "minimal" changes in blood pressure and heart rate, and no clinically significant changes were observed in laboratory values in any patient *(25)*.

Topiglan has also been evaluated in a phase II trial conducted by Goldstein and colleagues. Sixty-two patients were randomly assigned to receive placebo or Topiglan (1% alprostadil) and monitored for 90 min after receiving study medication. One patient (0.02%) reported symptoms of hypotension (diaphoresis and light-headedness) after application of Topiglan. There were no clinically significant changes in vital signs noted in any other patients in either treatment group *(26)*.

PHENTOLAMINE (VASOMAX, Z-MAX)

Mechanism of Action

Phentolamine is an α_1- and α_2-adrenergic antagonist, thereby blocking the action of norepinephrine, a contractile factor that is responsible for maintaining the flaccid state *(27)*. It is a frequent component of combination intracavernous therapies and is currently in development as an oral treatment for ED. At doses of 40 mg or 80 mg, oral phentolamine has been associated with statistically significant improvements in IIEF domain scores. In a recent 13-month trial involving more than 2000 men with mild-to-moderate ED, 87% of men who completed the trial reported improvement in erectile function, with an overall rate of successful vaginal penetration of greater than 90% *(28)*. To date, oral phentolamine has been approved in Mexico and Brazil.

Cardiovascular Effects

Both types of α adrenoceptors are found in other vascular regions other than penile tissue, and intravenous doses of phentolamine have been associated with ischemic cardiac events, tachycardia, arrhythmia, and hypotension *(7)*. Research on oral phentolamine, however, indicates the oral formulation has a more benign side-effect profile than the intravenous form.

In a phase II trial involving 424 patients with ED, Goldstein and colleagues found that oral phentolamine at doses of 40 and 80 mg was not associated with "major cardiovascular hemodynamic changes." Two percent and 7.0% of patients in the 40-mg and 80-mg groups reported dizziness, respectively. Seven percent of patients receiving the 80-mg dose reported tachycardia (vs 1.5% in the 40 mg group and 0.6% in the placebo group). Two percent of patients in the 80-mg group, 0.2% of patients in the 40-mg group, and 0% of patients receiving placebo reported hypotension *(27)*.

In a recent open label study, more than 2000 ED patients received phentolamine 40 mg or 80 mg for up to 13 months. Approximately half of enrolled patients were taking concurrent cardiovascular or diabetes medication. Four patients reported an episode of syncope during treatment, and 40 (2%) discontinued treatment because of tachycardia. There were no serious adverse events or deaths reported *(28)*.

YOHIMBINE (YOCON)

Yohimbine is a centrally and peripherally acting α_2-adrenoceptor antagonist that has been widely promoted as a treatment for psychogenic ED. Inhibition of central α_2-adrenoceptors results in an increase in sympathetic outflow and an increase in blood pressure, theoretically increasing blood flow into erectile tissues while restricting outflow *(29)*. In trials to date, yohimbine has been associated with response rates as high as 86%. In the majority of trials, however, yohimbine was not significantly more effective than placebo *(30)*.

Although there is little evidence that yohimbine has a significant therapeutic effect on erectile function, it continues to be marketed as a "natural" therapy for ED, and there have been reports of hypertensive crisis in patients taking over-the-counter products that contain yohimbine *(31)*. Clinical studies indicate that yohimbine can induce a dose-dependent, transient increase in blood pressure without a concomitant increase in heart rate. At doses of 45.5 mg or higher, yohimbine causes occasional increases in mean arterial blood pressure that peak at 60–90 min postdose and gradually decline over several hours *(30)*. The pressor response to yohimbine seems most pronounced in patients with pre-existing hypertension and tends to become apparent at doses higher than those recommended for therapeutic purposes *(30)*.

Guay and colleagues recently conducted a dose-escalation trial of yohimbine in 18 men with ED who received doses of up to 32.4 mg/d. Nine subjects had hypertension, and seven had atherosclerotic cardiovascular disease. Seven subjects were being maintained on a single cardiovascular medication (primary β-blockers), and five were taking multiple medications. Despite these comorbidities and concomitant medications, side effects were negligible: one subject reported mild hot flashes, another reported mild anxiety. No significant increases in blood pressure or pulse rate were recorded. Fifty percent of subjects reported successful intercourse in at least 75% of attempts *(32)*.

Teloken and colleagues conducted a single-blind study comparing the effects of placebo and yohimbine (100 mg) administered once daily for 30 d. Eight percent of subjects reported adverse effects with yohimbine (vs 20% while receiving placebo), including tachycardia in 27.3% of subjects *(33)*.

OTHER AGENTS

Trazodone (Desyrel)

When administered for the treatment of depression, the selective serotonin reuptake inhibitor trazodone has been associated with priapism, a finding that prompted the investigation of trazodone as a potential treatment for ED *(34,35)*. It is believed that trazodone has α-adrenergic antagonist activity in addition to its serotonergic properties, which may promote both erection and orthostatic hypotension *(34,36)*. To date, randomized, placebo-controlled trials of trazodone in patients with ED have failed to confirm the drug's efficacy as a treatment for ED *(34)*.

As a treatment for ED, trazodone has been administered at doses of 50–200 mg/d, which corresponds to the low end of the recommended dose range for depression *(34,36)*. As the prescribing information for trazodone includes warnings about the possibility of syncope, hypotension, and arrhythmias, the drug should be used with caution in patients with pre-existing cardiac disease or who are being maintained on antihypertensives *(36)*.

PNU-83757

PNU-83757 is a potassium channel blocker under investigation as an intracavernous treatment for ED. It opens ATP-dependent potassium channels and hyperpolarizes the cell membrane. The resulting inhibition of calcium influx through voltage-dependent CA^{2+} channels leads to relaxation of corporeal smooth muscle tissue *(37)*.

In a recent single-dose, single-blind, placebo-controlled study; PNU-83757 (0.25–140 µg) was administered to 55 subjects with vasculogenic ED. Holter monitoring was performed from 1 h before injection through 8 h after dosing, and vital signs were recorded both predose and at selected intervals during the 4 h after injection *(37)*.

Fifteen of the 25 patients who received PNU-83757 at 60–140 µg reported partial erections, and nine reported complete erections. Baseline heart rate and blood pressure were similar across all treatment groups. No significant changes in heart rate or blood pressure were observed in subjects intracavernous PNU-83757, relative to baseline or placebo. There were no acute electrocardiography changes, nor any trend toward hypotension or tachycardia with higher dose levels *(37)*.

CONCLUSION

All pharmacologic ED therapies exert vasoactive effects that may have systemic consequences. Existing research, however, indicates that available therapies pose no significant risk to the majority of ED patients, including those with pre-existing cardiac disease.

Although the relative risk of a cardiovascular event during sexual activity is comparatively low, coitus, like exercise and emotional stress, is a potential trigger for MI *(6)*. It is estimated that a healthy 50-yr-old male has a baseline MI risk of approximately 1% per year, which increases to 1.01% in the 2 h immediately after sexual activity *(38)*. Muller and colleagues reported that regular exercise had a significant protective effect against postcoital MI and may even eradicate the increased risk associated with sexual activity *(8)*. Therefore, a structured exercise program could be an invaluable adjunct to ED therapy, both to reduce the risk of postcoital cardiovascular events and to improve patients' overall cardiac risk profile.

REFERENCES

1. McKinlay JB. The worldwide prevalence and epidemiology of erectile. Int J Impot Res 2000;12(Suppl 4):S6–S11.
2. Aytac IA, McKinlay JB, Krane RJ. The likely worldwide increase in erectile dysfunction between 1995 and 2025 and some possible policy consequences. BJU Int 1999;84:50–56.
3. Chew KK, Earle CM, Stuckey BGA, et al. Erectile dysfunction in general medicine practice: prevalence and clinical correlates. Int J Impot Res 2000;12:41–45.
4. Kloner RS. Cardiovascular risk and sildenafil. Am J Cardiol 2000;86(Suppl):57F–61F.
5. Feldman HA, Goldstein I, Hatzichristou DG, et al. Impotence and its medical and psychological correlates: results of the Massachusetts Male Aging Study. J Urol 1994;151:54–61.
6. Stein RA. Cardiovascular response to sexual activity. Am J Cardiol 2000;86(2A):27F–29F.
7. Andersson K, Stief C. Penile erection and cardiac risk: pathophysiologic and pharmacologic mechanisms. Am J Cardiol 2000;86(2A):23F–26F.
8. Muller JE. Triggering of cardiac events by sexual activity: findings from a case-crossover analysis. Am J Cardiol 2000;86(Suppl):14F–18F.
9. Giuliano F, Allard J. Apomorphine SL (Uprima): preclinical and clinical experiences learned from the first central nervous system-acting ED drug. Int J Impot Res 2002;14(Suppl 1):S53–S56.
10. Heaton JP. Apomorphine: an update of clinical trial results. Int J Impot Res 2000;12(Suppl 4):S67–S73.
11. Abbott Laboratories. Uprima (apomorphine hydrochloride) Product Monograph. Abbott Urology International, 2001.
12. Bukofzer S, Livesey N. Safety and tolerability of apomorphine SL (Uprima). Int J Impot Res 2001;13(Suppl 3):S40–S44.
13. Dula E, Keating W, Siami PF, et al. Efficacy and safety of fixed-dose and dose-optimization regimens of sublingual apomorphine versus placebo in men with erectile dysfunction. The Apomorphine Study Group. Urology 2000;56:130–135.
14. Fagan TC, Buttler S, Marbury T, et al., of the SL APO Study Group. Cardiovascular safety of sublingual apomorphine in patients on stable doses of oral antihypertensive agents and nitrates. Am J Cardiol 2001;88:760–766.
15. Porst H. Current perspectives on intracavernosal pharmacotherapy for erectile dysfunction. Int J Impot Res 2000;12(Suppl 4):S91–S100.
16. Linet OM, Ogrinc FG, Alprostadil Study Group. Efficacy and safety of intracavernosal alprostadil in men with erectile dysfunction. N Engl J Med 1996;334:873–877.
17. Brock G, Tu LM, Linet OI. Return of spontaneous erection during long-term intracavernosal alprostadil (Caverject) treatment. Urology 2001;57:536–541.
18. Baniel J, Israilov S, Engelstein D, et al. Three-year outcome of a progressive treatment program for erectile dysfunction with intracavernous injections of vasoactive drugs. Urology 200;56:647–652.
19. Israilov S, Niv E, Livne PM, et al. Intracavernous injections for erectile dysfunction in patients with cardiovascular diseases and failure or contraindications for sildenafil citrate. Int J Impot Res 2002;14:38–43.
20. Padma-Nathan H, Hellestrom WJG, Hellstrom MD, et al. Treatment of men with erectile dysfunction with transurethral alprostadil. New Engl J Med 1997;336(1):1–7.

21. Guay AT, Perez JB, Velasquez E, et al. Clinical experience with intraurethral alprostadil (MUSE®) in the treatment of men with erectile dysfunction. Eur Urol 2000;38:671–676.
22. Peterson CA, Bennett AH, Hellstrom WG, et al. Erectile response to transurethral alprostadil, prazosin and alprostadil-prazosin combination. J Urol 1998;159:1523–1527.
23. Steidle C, Padma-Nathan H, Salem S, et al. Topical alprostadil cream for the treatment of erectile dysfunction: A combined analysis of the phase 2 program. Urology 2002;60:1077–1082.
24. Padma-Nathan H, Steidel C, Salem S, et al. The efficacy and safety of a topical alprostadil cream, Alprox-TD® for the treatment of erectile dysfunction: two Phase 2 studies in mild-to-moderate and severe ED. Int J Impot Res 2003;15:10–17.
25. McVary KT, Polepalle S, Riggi S, et al. Topical prostaglandin E1 SEPA gel for the treatment of erectile dysfunction. J Urol 1999;162:726–730.
26. Goldstein I, Payton TR, Schechter PJ. A double-blind, placebo-controlled, efficacy and safety study of topical gel formulation of 1% alprostadil (Topiglan) for the in-office treatment of erectile dysfunction. Urology 2001;57:301–305.
27. Goldstein I. Oral phentolamine: an alpha-1, alpha-2 adrenergic antagonist for the treatment of erectile dysfunction. Int J Impot Res 2000;12(Suppl 1):S75–S80.
28. Padma Nathan H, Goldstein I, Klimberg I, et al. Long-term safety and efficacy of oral phentolamine mesylate (Vasomax®) in men with mild to moderate erectile dysfunction. Int J Impot Res 2002;14:266–270.
29. Traish A, Kim NN, Moreland RB, et al. Role of alpha adrenergic receptors in erectile function, Int J Impot Res 2000;12(Suppl 1):S48–S63.
30. Tam SW, Worcel M, Wyllie M. Yohimbine: a clinical review. Pharmacol Ther 2001;91:215–243.
31. Ruck B, Shih RD, Marcus SM. Hypertensive crisis from herbal treatment of impotence. Am J Emerg Med 1999;17:317–318.
32. Guay AT, Spark RF, Jacobson J, et al. Yohimbine treatment of organic erectile dysfunction in a dose-escalation trial. Int J Impot Res 2002;14:25–31.
33. Teloken C, Rhoden EL, Sogari P, et al. Therapeutic effects of high dose yohimbine hydrochloride in organic erectile dysfunction. J Urol 1998;159:122–124.
34. Burnett AL. Oral pharmacotherapy for erectile dysfunction: current perspectives. Urology 1999;54:392–400.
35. Carson CC, Mino RD. Priapism associated with trazodone therapy. J Urol 1988;139:369–370.
36. Mead Johnson Pharmaceuticals. Desyrel® (Trazodone hydrochloride). Princeton, NJ: Bristol Myers Squibb, 1993.
37. Vick RN, Benevides M, Patel M, et al. The efficacy, safety and tolerability of intracavernous PNU-83757 for the treatment of erectile dysfunction. J Urol 2002;167:2618–2623.
38. DeBusk R, Drory Y, Goldstein W, et al. Management of sexual dysfunction in patients with cardiovascular disease: Recommendations of the Princeton Consensus Panel. Am J Cardiol 2000;86:175–181.

13 Potential Cardiac Applications of Phosphodiesterase Type-5 Inhibition

Michael Sweeney, MD
and Richard L. Siegel, MD

CONTENTS

INTRODUCTION
NO/cGMP SIGNALING PATHWAY AND ENDOTHELIAL
 DYSFUNCTION
POTENTIAL CARDIAC APPLICATIONS
CONCLUSION
ACKNOWLEDGMENTS
REFERENCES

INTRODUCTION

The risk factors associated with erectile dysfunction (ED) overlap extensively with risk factors associated with cardiovascular disease and include age, diabetes, hypertension, smoking, and hypercholesterolemia *(1,2)*. This suggests a common pathophysiological basis that is likely to be the vascular endothelium and the nitric oxide (NO)/cyclic guanosine monophosphate (cGMP) signaling pathway. ED is more prevalent and severe in patients with hypertension than in the general population *(3)* and can be a predictor of cardiovascular disease *(1,4)*.

The vascular endothelium is a single layer of cells that lines the luminal surface of the entire vascular system and regulates the transport of macromolecules and blood components. Endothelial cells produce

From: *Contemporary Cardiology: Heart Disease and Erectile Dysfunction*
Edited by: R. A. Kloner © Humana Press Inc., Totowa, NJ

factors that act on (a) vascular smooth muscle cells to maintain vessel tone, (b) both vascular smooth muscle cells and fibroblasts to modify vessel growth and structure, thereby determining vascular architecture, and (c) blood cells to determine platelet aggregation and inflammatory response *(5–7)*. Endothelial dysfunction promotes vasoconstriction, vascular remodeling, and vascular lesion formation—the hallmarks of atherogenic disease processes.

Impaired NO bioactivity is central to the development of endothelial dysfunction and is mediated via several mechanisms, including decreased NO synthesis, increased NO breakdown (e.g., by superoxide anion production and oxidative stress—the redox state), and/or decreased vascular smooth muscle sensitivity to NO *(8)*. Other factors involved in endothelial dysfunction may include (a) alteration in the activity of other vasotonal mediators, such as prostacyclin, endothelium-derived hyperpolarizing factor, and endothelin-1, and (b) the impairment of Gα proteins *(9–11)*. However, decreased bioavailability of NO secondary to superoxide production and oxidative stress may be the major mechanism of endothelial dysfunction *(12)*.

Because endothelial NO promotes vasodilation, inhibits aggregation of platelets and inflammatory cells, and inhibits vascular wall growth *(8,13)*, enhancement of NO activity has generated interest in the treatment of cardiovascular disorders that may have an etiology related to endothelial dysfunction. Organic nitrates, which are NO donors, reduce ventricular filling pressure and increase collateral coronary flow *(14)*. Organic nitrates have a long history of use in the management of coronary artery disease (CAD), but tachyphylaxis limits their utility *(14)*. Inhaled NO is a more recently investigated alternative for the replacement of NO activity. Inhaled NO is approved by the Food and Drug Administration for the treatment of hypoxic respiratory failure associated with persistent pulmonary hypertension of the newborn *(15)* and is used experimentally in the acute management of reversible pulmonary hypertension in cardiac medical and surgical patients *(16)*. However, inhaled NO has a narrow therapeutic index, necessitating therapeutic monitoring to avoid potential toxic effects that include methemoglobinemia secondary to excess NO concentrations and direct pulmonary injury caused by excess levels of nitrogen dioxide *(15)*. Other toxicities include DNA strand breaks and/or base alterations, which may be mutagenic, and the NO/superoxide interaction to form peroxynitrite, which can interfere with surfactant functioning via its cytotoxic activity *(17)*. Additional disadvantages of inhaled NO therapy include difficulties of administration, the possibility of ambient air contamination, and a short duration of pulmonary activity *(16)*. These disadvantages and toxicities have motivated the search for alternative therapies.

Vasodilation, inhibition of platelet aggregation, and many of the other physiological actions of NO are mediated in large part via cGMP generated by the NO/cGMP signaling pathway. NO stimulates guanylate cyclase, which leads to the conversion of guanosine triphosphate to GMP. Thus, the possibility exists to counteract endothelial dysfunction and its cardiovascular consequences at other points in this pathway. Sildenafil is a selective inhibitor of phosphodiesterase type-5 (PDE5), the cGMP-dependent PDE isozyme that specifically metabolizes cGMP *(18)*. Thus, sildenafil has a complementary role to NO in increasing intracellular cGMP activity via the NO/cGMP signaling pathway. However, sildenafil does not appear to be affected by the tolerance that hampers organic nitrates. Tolerance to organic nitrates is mediated via (a) impaired metabolism of organic nitrates to NO and (b) desensitization of soluble guanylyl cyclase (sGC) to the action of NO *(13)*.

The hemodynamic effects of sildenafil, including a possible preferential action on veins as compared with arteries, resemble those of organic nitrates *(19,20)*. Consequently, sildenafil was originally investigated as an antianginal medication *(21)* and is an intriguing alternative to NO to augment the NO/cGMP signaling pathway in various cardiovascular indications. This chapter discusses the relationship between the NO/cGMP signaling pathway and endothelial dysfunction, and reviews data on potential cardiac applications of sildenafil and other PDE5 inhibitors.

NO/CGMP SIGNALING PATHWAY AND ENDOTHELIAL DYSFUNCTION

Vasodilation

NO dilates resistance vessels and amplifies the responses to other endogenous vasodilators, such as prostaglandins, that act by elevating cAMP; the effects of NO are mediated via cGMP, and those of prostaglandins are probably mediated via cGMP-dependent inhibition of the breakdown of cAMP *(22)*. Decreased production of endothelium-derived NO results in vasoconstriction, elevated blood pressure, and bradycardia *(23–26)*. Vasoconstriction probably results both from a decrease of intracellular cGMP-mediated vasodilation and loss of a direct NO effect on smooth muscle potassium channels *(26)*. Renal plasma flow, glomerular filtration rate, and tubular reabsorption of sodium are also decreased *(26)*.

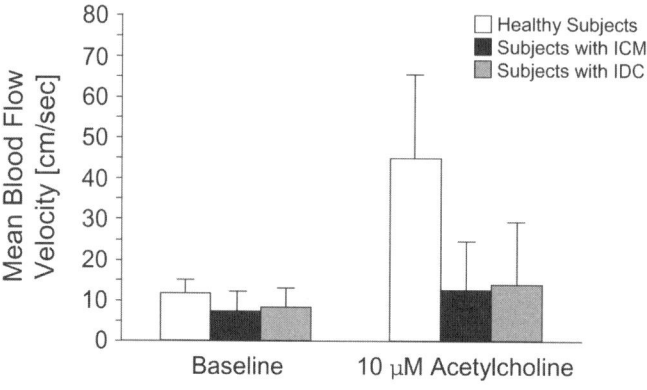

*P<0.05 vs baseline.

Fig. 1. Effects of acetylcholine, an endothelium-dependent vasodilator, on femoral artery blood flow velocity in healthy subjects ($n = 6$), patients with heart failure ($n = 7$) with ischemic cardiomyopathy (ICM), and patients with heart failure ($n = 12$) with idiopathic dilated cardiomyopathy (IDC). Adapted from Katz et al. *(27)*.

Sildenafil improves endothelium-dependent vasodilation in patients with endothelial dysfunction. In patients with normal endothelial function, endothelium-dependent vasodilation of peripheral arteries is induced by blood flow after arterial occlusion and by acetylcholine, a muscarinic endothelium-dependent vasodilator. These endothelium-dependent vasodilatory responses are blunted in the presence of endothelial dysfunction, for example, in patients with congestive heart failure (CHF) (Fig. 1; ref. *27*) or diabetes *(28)*. However, in placebo-controlled comparisons, sildenafil significantly increased the flow-mediated vasodilatory response induced by occlusion of the brachial artery in patients with CHF *(29)* or with diabetes but no overt heart disease *(28)*. In contrast, sildenafil had no statistically significant effect on the maximal NO-mediated vasodilatory response to acetylcholine in the dorsal hand veins or forearm vasculature of healthy men *(30)*. The effect of sildenafil on the endothelium-mediated vasodilatory response in patients with endothelial dysfunction is illustrated by the results of a randomized, double-blind, placebo-controlled study of 48 patients with CHF in whom flow-mediated vasodilation was assessed by ultrasound after release of 1, 3, and 5 min of transient brachial arterial occlusion, at baseline, and 1 h after administration of placebo or increasing doses of sildenafil (12.5, 25, and 50 mg; ref. *29*). Flow-mediated vasodilation was significantly increased by 25 or 50 mg of

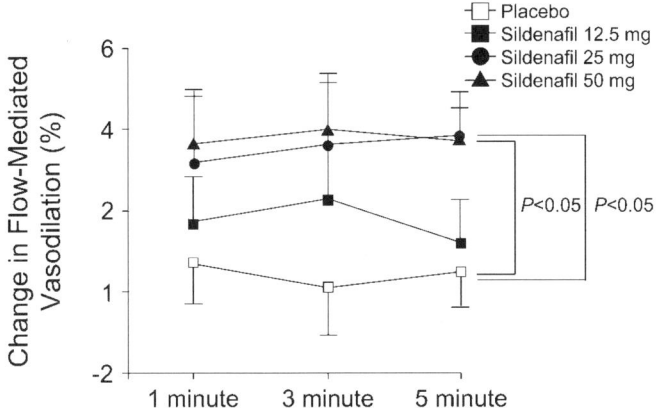

Fig. 2. Change (mean ± SEM) in flow-mediated vasodilation (FMD, %) from pretreatment values after release of 1, 3, and 5 min of brachial arterial occlusion in patients with chronic heart failure treated with placebo (closed squares), sildenafil 12.5 mg (open squares), sildenafil 25 mg (open circles), and sildenafil 50 mg (open triangles). Reprinted with permission from the American College of Cardiology, Journal of the American College of Cardiology *(27)*.

sildenafil, as compared with placebo (Fig. 2), suggesting a potential benefit in patients with heart failure.

Vascular Remodeling and Lesion Formation

Endothelial-derived NO is involved in the control of vascular remodeling and vascular lesion formation (e.g., platelet-thrombus formation and inflammatory cell infiltration) through control of vascular smooth muscle cell growth and migration, the expression of proinflammatory molecules, and endogenous inhibition of endothelial activation and monocyte adhesion *(5,31–33)*. In atherosclerotic cardiovascular diseases, superoxide inactivation of NO leads to oxidation of low-density lipoprotein cholesterol within the vessel wall *(34)*, to decreased vasorelaxation, and to increased adhesiveness of inflammatory cells to the endothelium, predisposing to vascular tissue lesion formation (atherosclerotic plaque; ref. *5*).

The role of NO in the prevention of atherosclerotic cardiovascular diseases is supported by research on the endothelial effects of 3-hydroxy-3-methyl-glutaryl coenzyme A (HMG-CoA) reductase inhibitors (statins). Statins have antiatherosclerotic effects that are independent of their lipid-lowering effects and result in enhanced NO release. For example, endothelial function (flow-mediated vasodilation) in elderly diabetic patients was improved in the absence of any demonstrable effect on lipid profiles within 3 d of initiating cerivastatin treatment *(35)*. Statins activate endothelial cell constitutive NO synthase (NOS), leading to an improved NO/superoxide ratio *(36,37)*. Proposed mechanisms for the effect of statins on NOS expression include attenuation of the upregulation of LOX-1 by its ligand, oxidized low-density lipoprotein cholesterol *(38)*, and inhibition of HMG CoA in endothelial cells stimulated to overexpress HMG-CoA by exposure to homocysteine *(39)*.

Wave reflection along the arterial tree is an important index of arterial stiffening and cardiac afterload and is inversely associated with exercise capacity *(40)*. Carotid-femoral pulse wave velocity is an index of aortic elasticity, which is an important determinant of left ventricular function and coronary blood flow *(41)*. In hypertensive men sildenafil had a beneficial effect on arterial wave reflection *(40,42)* and improved carotid-femoral pulse wave velocity *(41)*. These encouraging improvements in vascular stiffness and elasticity justify speculation that, with prolonged sildenafil use, positive changes in vascular remodeling could occur.

Control of Ischemia/Reperfusion Injury

Ischemia/reperfusion studies in animal models indicate an important role for NO in the prevention of further occlusion and injury. Loss of NO derived from NOS dramatically increased the degree of myocardial reperfusion injury in mice subjected to acute coronary artery ischemia and reperfusion *(43)*. The NO/cGMP signaling pathway in platelets was shown to be essential to the prevention of intravascular adhesion and aggregation of platelets after ischemia, by means of downstream action on cGMP kinase I *(44)*. Exogenous-inhaled NO caused an antithrombotic effect that increased coronary patency in a canine model of platelet-mediated coronary artery reocclusion after thrombolysis *(45)*. Inhaled NO also significantly modified the reduction in perfusion, the increase in leukocyte rolling, adhesion, and emigration, and the endothelial dysfunction caused by ischemia/reperfusion in the peripheral vasculature of cats *(46)*. In a rabbit model, sildenafil offered cardioprotection to ischemia-reperfusion injury *(47)*. Sildenafil reduced infarct size both acutely (68% at 30 min, $p < 0.05$) and delayed (41% at 24 h, $p < 0.05$) compared with vehicle control. The mechanism was suggested to be through opening of mitochondrial K_{ATP} channels.

Cardiac Function

NO influences normal cardiac physiology, both via the actions of cGMP and via independent effects, and it also appears to be important in the pathophysiology of cardiac dysfunction *(48)*. A physiological role has been proposed for NO generated constitutively by endothelial and/or myocyte NOS, but NO generated inducibly by vascular or myocyte NOS is thought to be pathophysiological *(49)*. The pathophysiological effect of NO may be secondary to the interaction of high concentrations of NO (after activation of NOS) with superoxide to form peroxynitrite, which is directly cytotoxic to cardiac myocytes *(50)*.

In heart failure, NO-mediated dysfunction may occur in the cardiac myocyte (negative inotropic effect and induction of apoptosis) and in the vascular endothelium of both the coronary circulation and the peripheral circulation (increased basal vascular tone, impairment of flow-mediated dilation, vascular remodeling, and hyporesponsiveness to vasoactive hormones; refs. *49* and *51*). The pulmonary vascular bed is vulnerable at an early stage of endothelial dysfunction and its resultant pathophysiological changes in compensated heart failure *(52)*.

The impaired endothelium-dependent, flow-mediated vasodilation of heart failure is attributable, at least in part, to hyporesponsiveness of cGMP-mediated vasorelaxation in vascular smooth muscle *(29)*. Reduced NO bioavailability caused by superoxide anion scavenging within the coronary vascular wall appears to be an essential mechanism *(53)*, and the coronary artery vasorelaxant response demonstrated for sildenafil in vitro results from compensation for this defect in the NO/cGMP pathway *(54)*. However, the vasoconstriction that characterizes heart failure does not appear to be solely the result of impaired NO-mediated endothelial vasodilation *(55)*.

POTENTIAL CARDIAC APPLICATIONS

When administered to healthy volunteers, sildenafil is a weak vasodilator that has modest effects on systemic vascular resistance and blood pressure, minimal effects on heart rate and cardiac index, and no consistent or significant dose-related changes in electrocardiogram measurements *(19,20)*. However, sildenafil significantly potentiates the hypotensive effects of glyceryl trinitrate, an organic nitrate *(56)*. Ambulatory blood pressure monitoring revealed that sildenafil causes small, clinically insignificant reductions in blood pressure in normotensive and hypertensive men while awake and asleep *(57)*. Despite these modest effects in healthy volunteers and in hypertensive men, the ability of sildenafil to improve dysfunctional endothelium-dependent vasodilation (*see* "Vasodilation") and of NO to reduce ventricular filling pressure, increase collateral coronary flow, and inhibit platelet aggregation *(13)* suggests a potential role for PDE5 inhibition with sildenafil in the treatment of ischemic heart disease (e.g., angina and the acute coronary syndromes), cardiac failure, and pulmonary hypertension. Thus, sildenafil may have the potential for clinical usefulness independent of the treatment of ED.

PDE5 Inhibition in Ischemic Heart Disease

The hemodynamic and platelet antiaggregation effects of sildenafil have been studied in animal models and in patients with ischemic heart disease. Controlled clinical studies in patients indicate effects on hemodynamic parameters that may be clinically useful, including modestly positive effects at rest and prolonged exercise tolerance.

PLATELET EFFECTS

In studies of human and rabbit platelets, sildenafil potently inhibited PDE5 and potentiated the antiaggregation activity of NO donors such as sodium nitroprusside and glyceryl trinitrate *(58–62)*. Other PDE5 inhibitors (intravenous zaprinast and intravenous dipyridamole) potentiated the antithrombotic properties of inhaled NO in a canine model of platelet-mediated coronary artery thrombosis after thrombolysis, without prolonging the bleeding time or causing systemic hypotension *(63)*.

In a rabbit model, sildenafil demonstrated antithrombotic activity by reducing the cyclical flow reduction and improving blood flow through the damaged vessel *(59)*. However, sildenafil-treated dogs with recurrent thrombosis were apparently unresponsive to the platelet inhibitory effects of an adenosine agonist *(64)*, which was likely because of high dose inhibition of adenosine receptors rather than an inhibitory effect of sildenafil *per se*.

ANIMAL MODELS OF CARDIAC ISCHEMIA

In models of cardiac ischemia in normal dogs, sildenafil has not exacerbated ischemia, and some data indicate that it may improve perfusion during exercise. In a model of stable partial (50%) coronary stenosis, sildenafil did not exacerbate ischemia, resulting in no significant difference from control in coronary blood flow, flow-time area, the overall index of vessel patency, or regional myocardial blood flow *(64)*. Also, sildenafil did not significantly alter debt repayment, the peak blood flow rate during reactive hyperemia, or the duration of reactive hyperemia following 5- to 20-s coronary occlusions *(65)*. However, in dogs with a critical stenosis of the left circumflex artery, sildenafil vasodilated the left anterior descending coronary artery and left circumflex coronary artery, increasing coronary blood flow; not surprisingly, sildenafil potentiated and prolonged the decreases in systemic blood pressure and coronary blood flow induced by isosorbide dinitrate *(66)*. Also, in exercising dogs with a partial stenosis of the left anterior descending artery, sildenafil increased left anterior descending artery flow in the ischemic region distal to the stenosis, from 41 ± 7 mL/min to 50 ± 11 mL/min ($p < 0.05$ vs control), with a small increase in subendocardial blood flow but no change in coronary pressure *(67)*. As discussed previously, in a rabbit model, sildenafil was shown to be highly cardioprotective in both acute and delayed ischemia-induced injury *(47)*. Taken together, these data strongly argue against sildenafil causing any coronary steal phenomenon.

HEMODYNAMIC STUDIES IN PATIENTS WITH ISCHEMIC HEART DISEASE

In a small pilot study of men with ischemic heart disease ($n = 8$), a 40-mg dose of sildenafil was administered intravenously, producing plasma concentrations of two to five times those achievable with a 100-mg oral dose *(19)*. Effects on hemodynamic parameters were comparable with those historically reported for therapeutic doses of nitrates, and the hemodynamic response to exercise was preserved.

In another pilot study, 14 men with severe stable coronary disease (defined as >70% stenosis of at least one coronary artery) who were scheduled for percutaneous coronary revascularization underwent blood-flow velocity and flow reserve assessment with a Doppler guidewire before and after administration of oral sildenafil 100 mg *(68)*. Coronary flow reserve was defined as the ratio of average peak velocity before and after maximal hyperemia was induced with intracoronary administration of adenosine. Sildenafil produced small (<10%) but significant decreases in systemic and pulmonary arterial pressures and a small but nonsignificant reduction in systemic vascular resistance, but it produced no significant change in heart rate or cardiac output. Sildenafil had no adverse effect on coronary blood flow. Indeed, in severely stenosed coronary arteries and in reference coronary arteries, sildenafil produced a small (13%) positive effect on coronary flow reserve ($p < 0.05$). These results prompted several placebo-controlled studies in patients with ischemic heart disease to determine safety and potential therapeutic usefulness.

Hemodynamics at Rest. Given the mechanism of action of PDE5 inhibitors, prevention of the metabolism of cGMP generated via the NO/cGMP pathway, it is not surprising that sildenafil potentiates the hypotensive effects of organic nitrates *(56)*. Double-blind, placebo-controlled, randomized studies have been conducted to determine the additive and comparative effects of sildenafil and organic nitrates on hemodynamics of resting patients with ischemic heart disease.

The magnitude and clinical significance of the additive hypotensive effect of sildenafil and organic nitrates was assessed in two crossover studies in male patients ages 45–78 yr with stable angina *(69)*. In the first study, isosorbide mononitrate 20 mg twice daily was administered for approximately 2 wk to 16 patients. Sitting and standing blood pressure was measured before and for 6 h after administration of a single oral dose of sildenafil 50 mg or placebo, one administered after the first week of isosorbide mononitrate administration, and the alternate administered after the second week. In the second study, 15 patients were challenged with sublingual glyceryl trinitrate 500 µg 1 h after pretreatment with sildenafil 50 mg or placebo; 7 d later, the alternate pretreatment was administered, and the challenge was repeated. Sitting vital signs were measured before and for 6 h after sildenafil or placebo administration. Sildenafil potentiated the hypotensive effects of the organic nitrates, producing significantly greater mean maximum changes from baseline in systolic/diastolic blood pressure as compared with placebo during concomitant administration with isosorbide mononitrate (difference from placebo of –19/–13 mmHg [sitting; $p < 0.01$] and –27/–15 mmHg [standing; $p < 0.001$]) and during concomitant administration with glyceryl trinitrate (difference from placebo of –10/–10 mmHg [sitting; $p > 0.01$]).

The hemodynamics of oral sildenafil 100 mg were compared with those of isosorbide mononitrate 40 mg in a parallel-group study in 31 patients with CAD and ED *(70)*. Hemodynamic parameters were measured at baseline and at 1, 2, 4, and 6 h after administration of sildenafil, isosorbide mononitrate, or placebo; reported values are the mean maximum change. Compared with baseline, sildenafil administration resulted in small increases in cardiac index (0.29 L/min/m^2 at 1 h) and stroke volume index (4.4 mL/m^2 at 2 h, Fig. 3). In contrast, there were small decreases in cardiac index and stroke volume index with isosorbide mononitrate (–0.14 L/min/m^2 and (5.8 mL/m^2, respectively, at 1 h) and placebo (–0.12 L/min/m^2 and –2.8 mL/m^2, respectively, at 4 h). Furthermore, as compared with isosorbide mononitrate, sildenafil caused less reduction in mean arterial pressure (–10 vs –22 mmHg at 2 h), less increase in heart rate (4 vs 7 beats/min at 2 h), and greater reductions in pulmonary vascular resistance. Systemic vascular resistance was reduced similarly by sildenafil and isosorbide mononitrate.

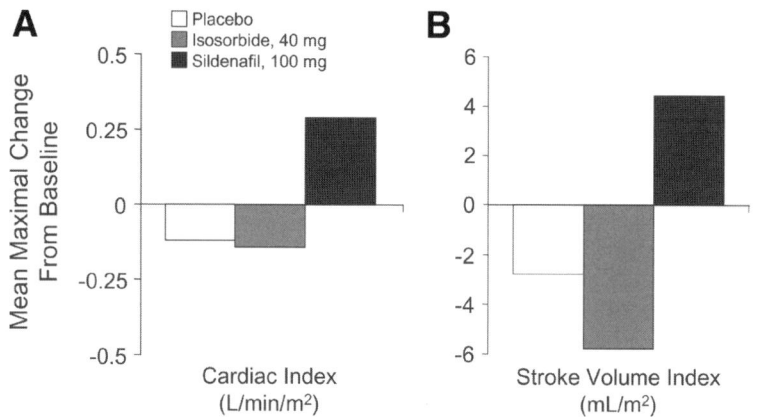

Fig. 3. Mean maximum change from baseline in cardiac index (**A**) and stroke volume index (**B**) within 6 h of administration of oral sildenafil 100 mg ($n = 10$), isosorbide mononitrate 40 mg ($n = 11$), or placebo ($n = 10$) to patients with coronary artery disease and erectile dysfunction. Time to maximal change was 1 h for isosorbide mononitrate, 2 h for sildenafil, and 4 h for placebo. Adapted from Jackson et al. *(70)*.

Halcox et al. also investigated the hemodynamic effects of sildenafil (100 mg) in placebo-controlled studies of patients with CAD *(71)*. Significant epicardial vasodilation (+5.6%) occurred 30 min after sildenafil in patients with CAD (n = 15; $p < 0.001$ compared with baseline). Sildenafil tended to improve myocardial ischemia during exercise testing but not to the level of isosorbide dinitrate: time to ischemic threshold was 538 s after placebo, 563 s after sildenafil, and 598 s after isosorbide ($p < 0.05$ vs placebo). In addition, using quantitative angiography, responses to sildenafil were compared in coronary arteries that were initially constricted with acetylcholine (representing endothelial dysfunction) with those that were dilated (representing normal endothelial function). Interestingly, those vessels with the greatest constriction displayed the most pronounced dilation ($p = 0.02$), suggesting that sildenafil may differentially improve vessels with the greatest endothelial dysfunction. In combination, these data suggest that PDE5 inhibition may be of benefit in treating patients with vascular endothelial dysfunction.

Thus, although most hemodynamic effects of sildenafil and isosorbide were parallel, less hypotension and less reflex tachycardia were observed following sildenafil. Perhaps most importantly, the differential effects on the pulmonary vasculature by sildenafil suggest a potential selective site of action for PDE5 inhibition.

These studies have recently been extended to more closely observe the time frame over which sildenafil-nitrate interactions can take place *(72)*. A double-blind, placebo-controlled trial in 33 healthy male volunteers examined the hemodynamic effects of administering 0.4 mg of glyceryl trinitrate spray from 1 to 48 h after a 100-mg oral dose of sildenafil. The results indicated that significant ($p < 0.01$) decreases in blood pressure (12 mmHg for both systolic and diastolic) occurred only at the 1-h time point. These data suggest that no significant hemodynamic interaction with nitrates occurs after 4 h and that nitrates may be safe to administer 24 h after an oral dose of sildenafil in many patients.

Hemodynamics During Exercise. Double-blind, placebo-controlled, randomized studies in men with ischemic heart disease have demonstrated that sildenafil has no negative effects during exercise when administered alone or concomitantly with a β-adrenergic antagonist and may even prolong exercise tolerance at higher doses.

In a crossover study, 110 male patients (mean age: 66 yr) with known CAD or typical angina were randomized to a single oral dose of sildenafil (median dose 50 mg) or placebo, followed 1 h later by a symptom-limited supine bicycle exercise echocardiogram test. One to 3 d later, the patients crossed over to the alternate treatment and the exercise echocardiogram was repeated *(73)*. Compared with placebo, sildenafil had no significant effect on the extent or severity of exercise-induced regional wall motion abnormalities, symptoms of dyspnea or angina, or arrhythmias. Exercise capacity was similar with sildenafil and placebo.

Sildenafil 50 mg was also assessed in patients with chronic stable angina on chronic treatment with a β-adrenergic antagonist *(74)*. In this crossover study, 14 men (mean age: 51 yr) with documented ED and CAD (a positive exercise test defined as approximately 1 mm ST-segment depression) received atenolol 100 mg once daily. After a week of atenolol therapy, patients were randomized to a single oral dose of sildenafil 50 mg or placebo, with crossover to the alternate treatment after a 2-d washout. Atenolol therapy resulted in a negative exercise test response (eight patients) or a significant prolongation of the time to a positive response (six patients). Sildenafil did not reverse the beneficial effect of atenolol on exercise-induced myocardial ischemia, being similar to placebo in time to 1-mm ST-segment depression (592 ± 35 and 579 ± 52 s, respectively, $p = 0.1$) and exercise time (762 ± 53 and 748 ± 39 s, respectively, $p = 0.1$). The baseline blood pressure and heart rate were not significantly influenced by sildenafil either at rest or during exercise.

In a recently reported controlled clinical trial, the effects of a higher dose of sildenafil were assessed on exercise hemodynamics. In this parallel-group study, 144 men with at least 60% occlusion of a coronary artery and reproducible exercise-induced angina were randomized to receive 100 mg of sildenafil or matching placebo administered 1 h before incremental treadmill exercise, with continuation of their usual antianginal therapy *(75)*. The proportion of patients in the two groups who were using concomitant medications was similar for angiotensin-converting enzyme inhibitors, β-adrenergic blockers, calcium-channel blockers, and HMG CoA reductase inhibitors. For the evaluable population of 108 men, the mean ± SE treatment difference for the time to onset of limiting angina was 19.9 ± 9.6 s (CI, 0.9–38.9; $p = 0.04$) in favor of sildenafil (Table 1). Also statistically significant in favor of sildenafil were treatment differences for time to angina, 31.7 ± 10.7 s (CI 10.5–53.0; $p = 0.004$), and total exercise time, 19.5 ± 9.8 s (CI, 0.04–38.9; $p = 0.049$). Sildenafil was well tolerated, and there were no serious treatment-related adverse events.

Thus, sildenafil has not been associated with negative hemodynamic effects during exercise when administered alone or concomitantly with a β-adrenergic antagonist, and higher doses of sildenafil may prolong exercise tolerance. These results confirm the safety of sildenafil administration to most patients with ischemic heart disease. They also suggest further study of sildenafil in combination with other antianginal therapy for the management of ischemic heart disease, as an alternative to organic nitrates, may be warranted.

PDE5 Inhibition in Heart Failure

Several studies have demonstrated that sildenafil is well tolerated in treating ED in patients with heart failure *(76–78)*. PDE5 inhibition with sildenafil has not been associated with inotropic effects and is not expected to be the cause of the absence of PDE5 in the myocardium *(79)*. However, as discussed previously (*see* "Vasodilation"), the dysfunctional endothelium-dependent vasodilator response of heart failure patients is improved by acute PDE5 inhibition with sildenafil. Furthermore, although comparable data are not available in patients with heart failure, in hypertensive men, sildenafil had a beneficial effect on arterial wave reflection and carotid-femoral pulse wave velocity (*see* "Vascular Remodeling and Lesion Formation"). Arterial wave reflection is an important index of arterial stiffening and cardiac afterload and is inversely associated with exercise capacity *(40)*. Carotid-femoral pulse wave velocity is an index of aortic elasticity, which is an important determinant of left ventricular function and coronary blood flow *(41)*. In patients with CAD, sildenafil (100 mg) produced small increases in cardiac index and stroke volume index, reduced pulmonary vascular resistance, and, as compared with isosorbide mononitrate (40 mg), produced less reduction in mean arterial pressure and less increase in heart rate (*see* "Hemodynamics at Rest"). These data suggest a potential therapeutic role for sildenafil in the treatment of heart failure.

Pulmonary hypertension and elevated pulmonary vascular resistance are common in patients with chronic left heart failure because increased left atrial pressure causes increased pulmonary artery pressure in an effort to maintain forward flow of the pulmonary circulation. Sildenafil has provided therapeutic benefit in a few patients with heart failure and pulmonary hypertension. Three male candidates for heart transplant (mean age: 51 yr) with previously refractory pulmonary hypertension caused by CAD (n = 2) or dilated myocardiopathy (n = 1) were given sildenafil 100 mg sublingually to determine the reversibility of pulmonary hypertension *(80)*. After 30 min, their mean pulmonary artery pressure decreased by one-third and mean transpulmonary gradient decreased by one half ($p < 0.01$). In a study of 22 patients with pulmonary hypertension, 9 of whom had CHF (6 CAD and 3 dilated cardiomyopathy), sildenafil reduced pulmonary vascular resistance and baseline pulmonary artery pressure and augmented the pulmonary vasodilator effect of inhaled NO (Table 2; ref. *81*). Furthermore, sildenafil improved the cardiac index, again augmenting the effect of inhaled NO despite no detectable change in systolic and diastolic myocardial function by sildenafil and/or inhaled NO, as assessed by micromanometer catheterization of the right ventricle (pulmonary vascular disease patients) or left ventricle (CHF patients). It should be kept in mind, however, that because sildenafil potentiates the hypotensive effects of organic nitrates in any form, its coadministration to patients who are using nitrates is contraindicated.

Thus, although there are few data assessing the effects of sildenafil in patients with heart failure, PDE5 inhibition may be a rational basis for treating this condition because it improves endothelium-dependent vasodilation, vessel wall elasticity, and arterial stiffness, resulting in positive hemodynamic effects, particularly on the pulmonary circulation, and an improvement in the cardiac index.

PDE5 Inhibition in Pulmonary Hypertension

Vascular remodeling is a hallmark of pulmonary hypertension, and NO is among the endothelial chemical factors thought to be involved *(82)*. Inhaled NO is approved for the treatment of hypoxic respiratory failure associated with persistent pulmonary hypertension of the newborn *(15)* and is used experimentally in the acute management of reversible pulmonary hypertension in cardiac medical and surgical

Table 1
Endpoints During Incremental Treadmill Exercise After Sildenafil 100 mg Administration to Men With at Least 60% Occlusion of a Coronary Artery and Reproducible Exercise-Induced Angina

	Adjusted mean (SEM)		Time in seconds		
				Treatment difference: sildenafil-placebo[a]	
	Placebo n = 52	Sildenafil n = 56	Mean difference (SEM)	95% CI	p value for superiority
To limiting angina, s[b]	403.7 (8.2)	423.6 (8.3)	19.9 (9.6)	0.92–38.91	0.04
To angina, s	308.6 (9.3)	340.3 (9.3)	31.7 (10.7)	10.46–52.99	0.0039
To 1 mm ST-segment depression, s	327.6 (14.4)	339.2 (14.4)	11.6 (16.6)	−21.27–44.54	0.484
Total exercise, s	405.8 (8.4)	425.3 (8.5)	19.5 (9.8)	0.04–38.94	0.0495

[a]The limit was predefined as a sildenafil minus placebo difference of −50 s, which represents 20% of the mean exercise time in a similar study population. Adapted from Fox et al. (75).
[b]Primary endpoint.

Table 2
Hemodynamic Effects in Patients With Pulmonary Hypertension

Hemodynamic parameter	Mean (± SD)			
	Baseline	Sildenafil 50 mg	Inhaled NO	Sildenafil + Inhaled NO
Pulmonary artery pressure (mmHg)	47 ± 3	44 ± 3[a]	44 ± 3[a]	41 ± 3[a,c]
Pulmonary vascular resistance (dyne·sec/cm^5)	605 ± 88	473 ± 72[a]	490 ± 71[a]	405 ± 69[a–c]
Pulmonary vascular resistance/systemic vascular resistance	0.36 ± 0.04	0.31 ± 0.04[a]	0.35 ± 0.05	0.30 ± 0.05[a]
Cardiac index (L/min/m^2)	2.5 ± 0.2	2.8 ± 0.2[a]	2.8 ± 0.2[a]	3.0 ± 0.2[a–c]

[a]$p < 0.05$ vs baseline (> 90% O_2); [b]$p < 0.05$ vs inhaled NO; [c]$p < 0.05$ vs sildenafil. Adapted from Lepore et al. (118).

patients *(16)*. However, the disadvantages and toxicities of inhaled NO have motivated the search for alternative therapies, such as PDE5 inhibitors *(83,84)*.

EXPERIMENTAL DATA

In vitro studies of bovine-isolated main pulmonary arteries revealed that PDE3, 4, and 5 are the main enzymes involved in the control of vascular tone *(85)*. In isolated perfused rabbit lungs, pulmonary vascular resistance elevated by infusion of U46619, a thromboxane-A2 mimetic, was reduced by dipyridamole and zaprinast, PDE5 inhibitors *(86)*. Sildenafil markedly blunted pulmonary vasoconstriction caused by acute hypoxia of isolated perfused lungs from wild-type and NOS-deficient mice *(87)*.

Short-term studies reveal that PDE5 inhibition reverses U46619-induced or hypoxia-induced pulmonary hypertension in live animal models, usually newborn lambs or rabbits. Efficacy has been reported for dipyridamole either infused intravenously or inhaled, but systemic blood pressure was decreased significantly during infusion *(88,89)*. Sildenafil and zaprinast have also been reported to be effective in animal models and to augment the effect of inhaled NO *(90–93)*. Furthermore, oral sildenafil decreased the pulmonary artery pressure of lambs with U46619-induced pulmonary hypertension *(94)*.

The positive effect of sildenafil has also been demonstrated in several other models of pulmonary hypertension, in animals and in human volunteers. Pulmonary hypertension induced by meconium aspiration in piglets was completely reversed within 2 h of commencing an intravenous infusion of sildenafil 2 mg/kg, and cardiac output was increased by 30%, with no adverse influence on oxygenation or systemic hemodynamics; sildenafil was at least as effective as inhaled NO 20 ppm *(95)*. In a double-blind, randomized comparison, wild-type mice exposed to hypoxia for 3 wk and dosed with oral sildenafil 25 mg/kg daily had right ventricular systolic pressure almost one-third lower, less pulmonary vascular remodeling, and less right ventricular hypertrophy than placebo-dosed animals ($p < 0.05$ for each parameter; ref. *87*). In another double-blind, placebo-controlled, randomized comparison, the 56% increase in pulmonary artery pressure induced in healthy human volunteers challenged with hypoxia (11% O_2 for 30 min) was almost completely absent, and systemic blood pressure was not significantly affected when challenge was preceded by a 100-mg oral dose of sildenafil *(87)*. Thus, experimental data indicate that sildenafil decreases pulmonary artery pressure, improves cardiac index, may be selective for the pulmonary circulation, and, with prolonged use, may decrease vascular remodeling.

TREATMENT OF PULMONARY HYPERTENSION

Most published data on PDE5 inhibition in patients with pulmonary hypertension report acute hemodynamic effects of sildenafil. However, two small uncontrolled case studies assessed acute hemodynamic effects of dipyridamole: 0.2 mg/kg intravenously in 10 consecutive patients with aortic or mitral valvular disease *(96)* and 0.6 mg/kg in 10 consecutive pediatric patients with primary or secondary pulmonary hypertension *(97)*, administered alone and in combination with inhaled NO. Dipyridamole had little or no beneficial effect on pulmonary vasodilation and was not selective for the pulmonary circulation. Thus, the following discussion is limited to sildenafil.

Precapillary Pulmonary Hypertension. Patients with increased pulmonary arteriolar and/or arterial resistance are classified as having precapillary pulmonary hypertension. Examples include primary pulmonary hypertension, hypoxic pulmonary hypertension, pulmonary hypertension secondary to HIV infection, congenital heart disease (e.g., systemic to pulmonary shunt), pulmonary embolism, chronic obstructive pulmonary disease, and scleroderma of the CREST variant (calcinosis, Raynaud's phenomenon, esophageal dysmotility, sclerodactyly, telangiectasias; ref. *98*). Several anecdotal reports have described the acute hemodynamic response to sildenafil in patients with precapillary pulmonary hypertension; there were both no notable effects *(99)* and beneficial effects *(100)* on pulmonary hemodynamics reported in patients with CREST variant scleroderma and beneficial effects reported in patients with pulmonary arterial hypertension secondary to HIV infection *(101)*, severe interstitial pulmonary fibrosis *(102)*, and congenital heart disease *(103)*.

In an uncontrolled case study of 13 consecutive patients (mean age: 44 yr) with severe pulmonary hypertension, mostly precapillary, the acute hemodynamic effects of sildenafil administered alone and in combination with inhaled NO were described *(104)*. Seventy-five mg oral sildenafil and 80 ppm inhaled NO caused similar decreases in pulmonary vascular resistance ($27 \pm 3\%$ and $19 \pm 5\%$, respectively), and the combination was superior to either agent alone ($32 \pm 5\%$). The cardiac index increased with sildenafil and with sildenafil plus NO ($17 \pm 5\%$ and $17 \pm 4\%$, respectively) but not with NO alone ($-0.2 \pm 2.0\%$, $p < 0.003$). Furthermore, NO increased and sildenafil tended to decrease the pulmonary capillary wedge pressure ($+15 \pm 6$ vs

−9 ± 7%, $p < 0.0007$). Systemic arterial pressure did not decrease with treatment. In eight infant children who had congenital heart surgery, acute administration of intravenous sildenafil alone significantly ($p < 0.05$) reduced pulmonary vascular resistance compared with baseline and further reduced resistance when combined with inhaled NO *(105)*. In seven adult patients with pulmonary arterial hypertension, increasing intravenous doses of sildenafil (corresponding to 25, 50, and 100 mg oral) decreased pulmonary arterial pressure from baseline (61 ± 16 to 55 ± 20 mmHg), decreased pulmonary vascular resistance (11.6 ± 4.1 to 8.7 ± 4.2 Wood units), and increased cardiac output (4.6 ± 4.1 to 5.6 ± 4.2 L/min). Importantly, after 3 months of 50 mg oral therapy, the two patients awaiting transplantation were removed from the waiting list *(106)*.

The levels of prostacyclin, a vasodilator and antiaggregant prostaglandin produced by endothelial cells, are reduced in patients with primary pulmonary hypertension *(82)*. Inhaled iloprost, a stable prostacyclin analog, improves exercise capacity and hemodynamic variables, but its use is limited by a short duration of action (30–60 min) and high cost *(107)*. Isolated case reports have established the success of oral sildenafil as an alternative to prostacyclin in primary pulmonary hypertension *(100,108,109)*. A small study of five patients with primary pulmonary hypertension demonstrated that aerosolized iloprost in a cumulative dosage of 8.4–10.5 µg decreased mean pulmonary arterial pressure more than sildenafil 50–100 mg (9.4 ± 1.3 vs 6.4 ± 1.1 mmHg; $p < 0.05$) but less than the combination of sildenafil plus iloprost (9.4 ± 1.3 vs 13.8 ± 1.4 mmHg; $p < 0.009$; *107*). The duration of effect was longer with sildenafil monotherapy (>210 min) than with iloprost monotherapy (60–120 min; Fig. 4). No significant changes in heart rate or systemic arterial pressure were seen during any treatment, and all treatments were well tolerated, without major adverse effects.

Sildenafil administered alone and in combination with inhaled iloprost has also been assessed in a randomized, controlled, open-label study of 30 patients with precapillary pulmonary hypertension, including primary pulmonary hypertension ($n = 10$), the CREST syndrome ($n = 6$), aplasia of the left pulmonary artery ($n = 1$), and chronic thromboembolic pulmonary hypertension ($n = 13$; *110*). Patients were randomized to four treatment groups: sildenafil 12.5 mg ($n = 7$), sildenafil 50 mg ($n = 8$), sildenafil 12.5 mg plus inhaled iloprost 2.8 µg 1 h later ($n = 7$), and sildenafil 50 mg plus inhaled iloprost 2.8 µg 1 h later ($n = 8$). All patients received inhaled NO (20–50 ppm) and aerosolized

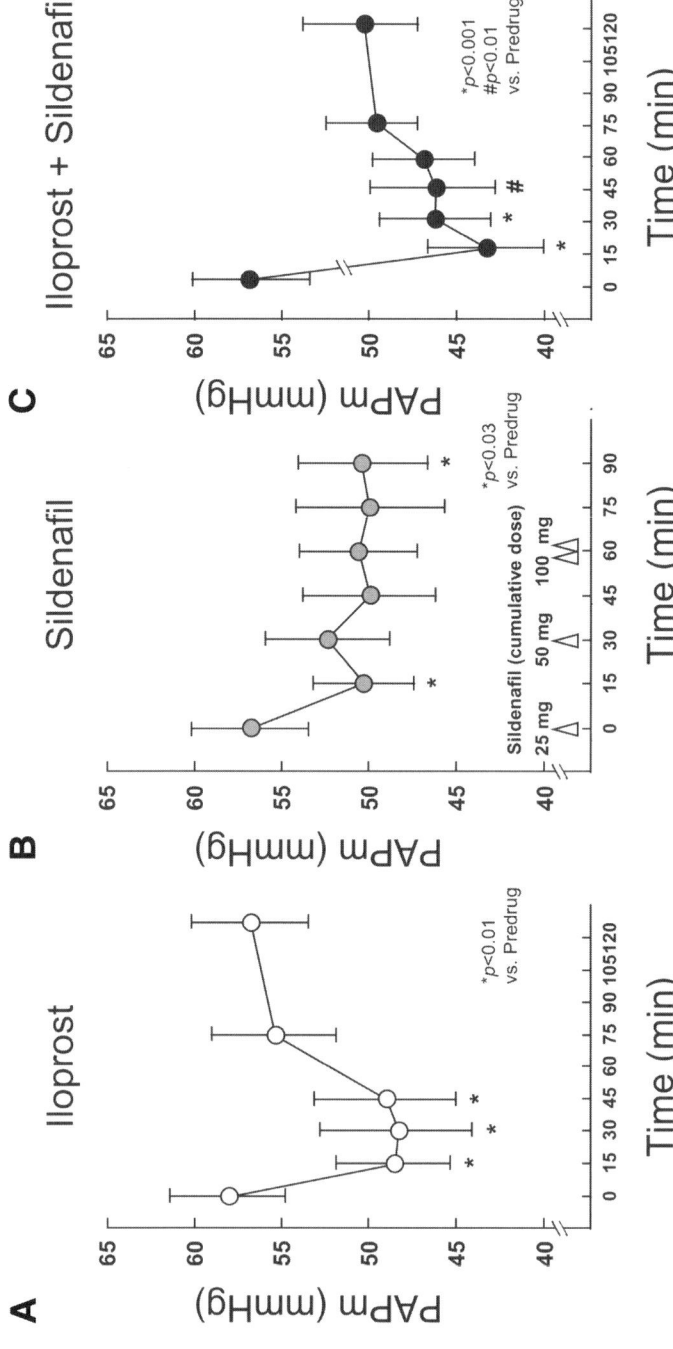

Fig. 4. Time course of mean pulmonary artery pressure in five patients with primary pulmonary hypertension. Iloprost produced a significant reduction, with a return to baseline levels after 120 min (**A**). Sildenafil caused a slightly smaller but significant reduction that was already maximal after ingestion of the first 25 mg dose (**B**). Iloprost plus sildenafil produced a greater maximal reduction than either therapy alone and a more prolonged reduction than that of iloprost alone (**C**). Reprinted from (*107*) with permission.

iloprost (2.8 μg) with hemodynamic parameters measured at 5, 15, 30, 60, 90, 120, and 180 min after dosing. All patients had severe pulmonary hypertension and low cardiac index values at baseline. NO, iloprost alone, sildenafil alone, and sildenafil plus iloprost all decreased mean pulmonary artery pressure, increased the cardiac index, decreased pulmonary vascular resistance, and indicated pulmonary selectivity by a significant reduction in the ratio of pulmonary to systemic vascular resistance (Fig. 5). Pulmonary selectivity was greatest for NO and for the combination of 50 mg of sildenafil plus iloprost. For the other hemodynamic parameters, there was an increasingly beneficial response from NO, to iloprost, to iloprost plus sildenafil (12.5 or 50 mg). The area under the curve for reduction in pulmonary vascular resistance after combination therapy was greater than the sum of the areas under the curve for each single intervention, at either dose of sildenafil plus iloprost ($p < 0.001$, analysis of variance). The effects of NO wore off within 15 min and of iloprost within 60–90 min, but the vasodilatory response to sildenafil was still evident after 120 min when administered alone and after 180 min when administered with iloprost. No significant differences could be detected between subgroups based on diagnosis or in patients with primary pulmonary hypertension as compared with all other patients or with patients with chronic thromboembolic pulmonary hypertension.

Anecdotal reports of chronic therapy with oral sildenafil in a few patients, administered alone or in combination with prostacyclin analog, revealed a persistent 20% decrease in the estimated pulmonary artery pressure over 3 month *(101)*, resolution of cor pulmonale and improved pulmonary artery pressure at 6 month *(100)*, and improved exercise capacity at 12 wk *(111,112)* and 1 yr *(108)*. One recent case report described long-term efficacy in a 39-yr-old man with pulmonary hypertension *(113)*. Substantial improvements were observed in right ventricular systolic pressure (120 mmHg baseline, 85 mmHg at 30 wk) after 50 mg of sildenafil were taken four times daily for 30 wk.

Thus, sildenafil, administered alone or in combination with inhaled NO or inhaled iloprost to patients with precapillary pulmonary hypertension, decreases the pulmonary artery pressure and pulmonary vascular resistance, improves the cardiac index, and shows selectivity for the pulmonary circulation.

Passive Pulmonary Hypertension. Increased pulmonary arterial pressure can occur passively (without active pulmonary arterial vasoconstriction) when the pulmonary venous pressure is elevated, such as in left ventricular failure or mitral stenosis. As discussed in the section "PDE5 Inhibition in Heart Failure," pulmonary hypertension is

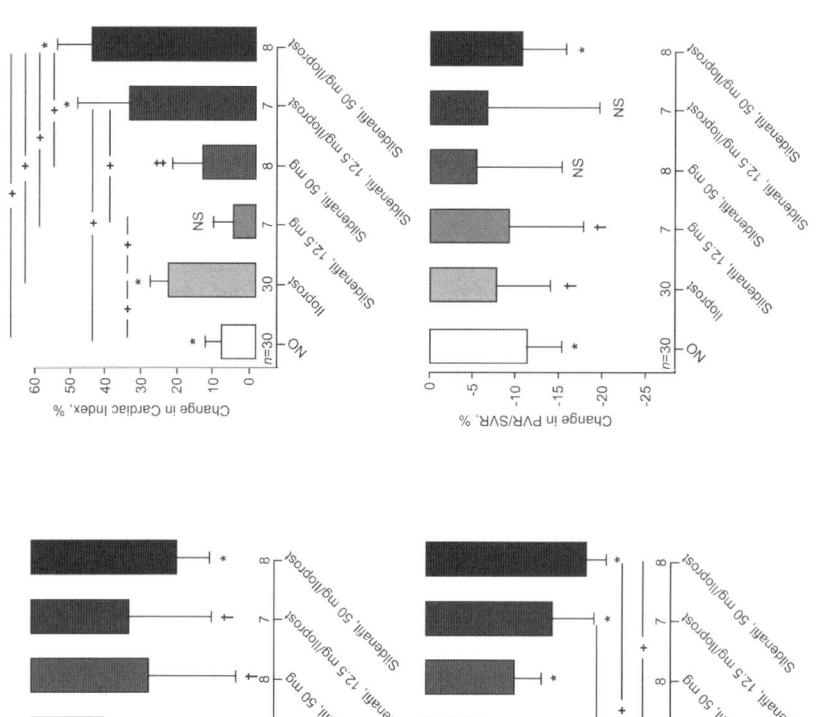
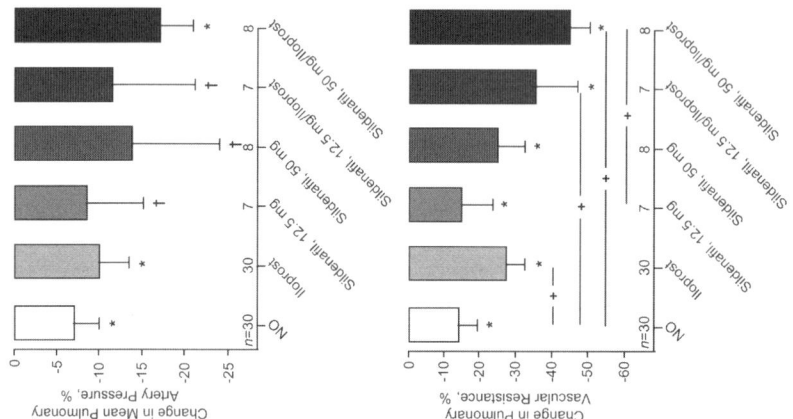

common in patients with chronic left heart failure, and sildenafil has provided therapeutic benefit in a few patients with heart failure and pulmonary hypertension. Also, left ventricular failure and valvular heart disease often culminate in the necessity for surgery, which can be seriously complicated by pre-existing or acute de novo pulmonary hypertension. An anecdotal report describes beneficial effects of sildenafil in two patients who developed acute elevations in pulmonary artery pressure on weaning from cardiopulmonary bypass after cardiac transplantation and redo cardiac bypass, respectively *(114)*.

FACILITATION OF INHALED NO WITHDRAWAL

Discontinuation of inhaled NO can result in rebound pulmonary hypertension for reasons that remain unclear but may include reduced production of endogenous NO and/or reduced ability to rapidly generate cGMP after NO discontinuation *(115)*. Anecdotal reports in a few pediatric patients document the ability of sildenafil *(111,115,116)* and dipyridamole *(117)* to blunt rebound pulmonary hypertension in patients withdrawn from inhaled NO, mostly following cardiac surgery.

CONCLUSION

PDE5 inhibitors appear to be preferentially active in patients with endothelium-mediated disease compared with healthy individuals because of the positive effects on dysfunctional endothelium, mediated via the NO/cGMP signaling pathway. Controlled studies of sildenafil in patients with ischemic heart disease indicate effects on hemodynamic parameters that may be clinically useful include (a) no serious adverse effects; (b) at rest, positive effects on central hemodynamics (e.g., cardiac index and stroke volume index), which are superior to those of isosorbide mononitrate, while causing a similar reduction in systemic vascular resistance, less hypotension and reflex increase in heart rate, and greater reductions in pulmonary vascular resistance; and (c) no

---

Fig. 5. *(opposite)* Maximum change in hemodynamic values from preintervention baseline in patients with precapillary pulmonary hypertension in a randomized, open-label study. Error bars represent confidence intervals. Analysis of variance with the Scheffé posttest for intergroup comparison indicated significant differences ($p < 0.001$); plus signs bracketed by horizontal bars show these relationships. NO, nitric oxide; NS, not significant; PVR/SVR, ratio of pulmonary vascular resistance to systemic vascular resistance. *$p < 0.001$, †$p < 0.05$, ‡$p < 0.001$ for differences between pretreatment and posttreatment values. Reprinted with permission from Annals of Internal Medicine *(110)*.

negative hemodynamic effects during exercise when administered alone or concomitantly with a β-adrenergic antagonist and prolonged exercise tolerance with higher doses (100 mg). Despite limited data assessing the effects of sildenafil in patients with heart failure, PDE5 inhibition may be a rational basis for treating this condition because it improves endothelium-dependent vasodilation, vessel wall elasticity, and arterial stiffness, resulting in positive hemodynamic effects, particularly on the pulmonary circulation, and an improvement in the cardiac index. Results from experimental models and acute hemodynamic studies in patients with precapillary pulmonary hypertension indicate that sildenafil, administered alone or in combination with NO or iloprost, decreases the pulmonary artery pressure and pulmonary vascular resistance, improves the cardiac index, and shows selectivity for the pulmonary circulation.

These results validate the safety of administering sildenafil to patients with cardiac disease. They also suggest further study of sildenafil (a) in combination with other antianginal therapy for the management of ischemic heart disease as an alternative to organic nitrates, (b) in patients with heart failure to further explore the clinical consequences of improved endothelium-dependent vasodilation and vessel wall elasticity and decreased arterial stiffness, and (c) in patients with pulmonary hypertension, both alone and in combination with inhaled NO and inhaled iloprost. If further study confirms the existing data, sildenafil may have broad clinical usefulness independent of the treatment of ED.

ACKNOWLEDGMENTS

We thank Deborah M. Campoli-Richards, RPh, and Peter A. Rittenhouse, PhD, for assistance in the preparation of the manuscript.

REFERENCES

1. Feldman HA, Goldstein I, Hatzichristou DG, et al. Impotence and its medical and psychosocial correlates: results of the Massachusetts Male Aging Study. J Urol 1994;151:54–61.
2. McVary KT, Carrier S, Wessells H. Smoking and erectile dysfunction: evidence based analysis. J Urol 2001;166:1624–1632.
3. Burchardt M, Burchardt T, Baer L, et al. Hypertension is associated with severe erectile dysfunction. J Urol 2000;164:1188–1191.
4. Burchardt M, Burchardt T, Anastasiadis AG, et al. Erectile dysfunction is a marker for cardiovascular complications and psychological functioning in men with hypertension. Int J Impot Res 2001;13:276–281.
5. Dzau VJ, Gibbons GH, Mann M, et al. Future horizons in cardiovascular molecular therapeutics. Am J Cardiol 1997;80(Suppl 9A):331–391.

6. Alberts GF, Peifley KA, Johns A, et al. Constitutive endothelin-1 overexpression promotes smooth muscle cell proliferation via an external autocrine loop. J Biol Chem 1994;269:10,112–10,118.
7. de Nucci G, Thomas R, D'Orleans-Juste P, et al. Pressor effects of circulating endothelin are limited by its removal in the pulmonary circulation and by the release of prostacyclin and endothelium-derived relaxing factor. Proc Natl Acad Sci USA 1988;85:9797–9800.
8. Pudda P, Pudda GM, Zaca F, et al. Endothelial dysfunction in hypertension. Acta Cardiol 2000;55:221–232.
9. Mombouli JV, Vanhoutte PM. Endothelial dysfunction: from physiology to therapy. J Mol Cell Cardiol 1999;31:61–74.
10. Holness W, Santore TA, Brown GP, et al. Expression of Q227L-Galpha(s) inhibits intimal vessel wall hyperplasia after balloon injury. Proc Natl Acad Sci USA 2001;98:1288–1293.
11. Davies MG, Mason DP, Tran PK, et al. G-protein expression and intimal hyperplasia after arterial injury: a role for Galpha(i) proteins. J Vasc Surg 2001;33:408–418.
12. John S, Schmieder RE. Impaired endothelial function in arterial hypertension and hypercholesterolemia: potential mechanisms and differences. J Hypertens 2000;18:363–374.
13. Moncada S, Palmer RM, Higgs EA. Nitric oxide: physiology, pathophysiology, and pharmacology. Pharmacol Rev 1991;43:109–142.
14. Parker JD, Parker JO. Nitrate therapy for stable angina pectoris. N Engl J Med 1998;338:520–531.
15. American Academy of Pediatrics. Committee on Fetus and Newborn. Use of inhaled nitric oxide. Pediatrics 2000;106:344–345.
16. Hayward CS, Macdonald PS, Keogh AM. Inhaled nitric oxide in cardiology. Expert Opin Invest Drugs 2001;10:1947–1956.
17. Weinberger B, Laskin DL, Heck DE, et al. The toxicology of inhaled nitric oxide. Toxicol Sci 2001;59:5–16.
18. Ballard SA, Gingell CJ, Tang K, et al. Effects of sildenafil on the relaxation of human corpus cavernosum tissue in vitro and on the activities of cyclic nucleotide phosphodiesterase isozymes. J Urol 1998;159:2164–2171.
19. Jackson G, Benjamin N, Jackson N, et al. Effects of sildenafil citrate on human hemodynamics. Am J Cardiol 1999;83(Suppl 5A):13C–20C.
20. Zusman RM, Morales A, Glasser DB, et al. Overall cardiovascular profile of sildenafil citrate. Am J Cardiol 1999;83(Suppl 5A):35C–44C.
21. Campbell SF. Science, art and drug discovery: a personal perspective. Clin Sci (Lond) 2000;99:255–260.
22. de Wit C, Bolz SS, Pohl U. Interaction of endothelial autacoids in microvascular control. Z Kardiol 2000;89(Suppl 9):IX/113–116.
23. Vallance P, Collier J, Moncada S. Effects of endothelium-derived nitric oxide on peripheral arteriolar tone in man. Lancet 1989;2:997–1000.
24. Haynes WG, Noon JP, Walker BR, et al. Inhibition of nitric oxide synthesis increases blood pressure in healthy humans. J Hypertens 1993;11:1375–1380.
25. Rees DD, Palmer RMJ, Moncada S. Role of endothelium-derived nitric oxide in the regulation of blood pressure. Proc Natl Acad Sci USA 1989;86:3375–3378.
26. Bech JN, Nielsen CB, Pedersen EB. Effects of systemic NO synthesis inhibition on RPF, GFR, UNa, and vasoactive hormones in healthy humans. Am J Physiol 1996;270:F845–F851.

27. Katz SD, Biasucci L, Sabba C, et al. Impaired endothelium-mediated vasodilation in the peripheral vasculature of patients with congestive heart failure. J Am Coll Cardiol 1992;19:918–925.
28. Desouza C, Parulkar A, Lumpkin D, et al. Acute and prolonged effects of sildenafil on brachial artery flow-mediated dilatation in type 2 diabetes. Diabetes Care 2002;25:1336–1339.
29. Katz SD, Balidemaj K, Homma S, et al. Acute type 5 phosphodiesterase inhibition with sildenafil enhances flow-mediated vasodilation in patients with chronic heart failure. J Am Coll Cardiol 2000;36:845–851.
30. Dishy V, Sofowora G, Harris PA, et al. The effect of sildenafil on nitric oxide-mediated vasodilation in healthy men. Clin Pharmacol Ther 2001;70:270–279.
31. De Caterina R, Libby P, Peng HB, et al. Nitric oxide decreases cytokine-induced endothelial activation. Nitric oxide selectively reduces endothelial expression of adhesion molecules and proinflammatory cytokines. J Clin Invest 1995;96:60–68.
32. Peng HB, Libby P, Liao JK. Induction and stabilization of I kappa B alpha by nitric oxide mediates inhibition of NF-kappa B. J Biol Chem 1995;270:14,214–14,219.
33. Peng HB, Rajavashisth TB, Libby P, et al. Nitric oxide inhibits macrophage-colony stimulating factor gene transcription in vascular endothelial cells. J Biol Chem 1995;270:17,050–17,055.
34. Ohara Y, Peterson TE, Sayegh HS, et al. Dietary correction of hypercholesterolemia in the rabbit normalizes endothelial superoxide anion production. Circulation 1995;92:898–903.
35. Tsunekawa T, Hayashi T, Kano H, et al. Cerivastatin, a hydroxymethylglutaryl coenzyme a reductase inhibitor, improves endothelial function in elderly diabetic patients within 3 days. Circulation 2001;104:376–379.
36. Dobrucki LW, Kalinowski L, Dobrucki IT, et al. Statin-stimulated nitric oxide release from endothelium. Med Sci Monit 2001;7:622–627.
37. Kalinowski L, Dobrucki LW, Brovkovych V, et al. Increased nitric oxide bioavailability in endothelial cells contributes to the pleiotropic effect of cerivastatin. Circulation 2002;105:933–938.
38. Mehta JL, Li DY, Chen HJ, et al. Inhibition of LOX-1 by statins may relate to upregulation of eNOS. Biochem Biophys Res Commun 2001;289:857–861.
39. Li H, Lewis A, Brodsky S, et al. Homocysteine induces 3-hydroxy-3-methylglutaryl coenzyme a reductase in vascular endothelial cells: a mechanism for development of atherosclerosis? Circulation 2002;105:1037–1043.
40. Vlachopoulos C, Hirata K, O'Rourke M. Effects of sildenafil (Viagra®) on wave reflection: a new insight into its cardiovascular effects. J Am Coll Cardiol 2001; 37(Suppl A):260A.
41. Vlachopoulos C, O'Rourke MF, Hirata K. Sildenafil (Viagra®) improves the elastic properties of the aorta. Am J Hypertens 2001;14:6A.
42. Mahmud A, Hennessy M, Feely J. Effect of sildenafil on blood pressure and arterial wave reflection in treated hypertensive men. J Hum Hypertens 2001;15:707–713.
43. Jones SP, Girod WG, Palazzo AJ, et al. Myocardial ischemia-reperfusion injury is exacerbated in absence of endothelial cell nitric oxide synthase. Am J Physiol 1999;276:H1567–H1573.
44. Massberg S, Sausbier M, Klatt P, et al. Increased adhesion and aggregation of platelets lacking cyclic guanosine 3′,5′-monophosphate kinase I. J Exp Med 1999;189:1255–1264.

45. Adrie C, Bloch KD, Moreno PR, et al. Inhaled nitric oxide increases coronary artery patency after thrombolysis. Circulation 1996;94:1919–1926.
46. Fox-Robichaud A, Payne D, Hasan SU, et al. Inhaled NO as a viable antiadhesive therapy for ischemia/reperfusion injury of distal microvascular beds. J Clin Invest 1998;101:2497–2505.
47. Ockaili R, Salloum F, Hawkins J, et al. Sildenafil (Viagra) induces powerful cardioprotective effect via opening of mitochondrial KATP channels in rabbits. Am J Physiol Heart Circ Physiol 2002;283:H1263–H1269.
48. Hare JM, Colucci WS. Role of nitric oxide in the regulation of myocardial function. Prog Cardiovasc Dis 1995;38:155–166.
49. Kelly RA, Balligand JL, Smith TW. Nitric oxide and cardiac function. Circ Res 1996;79:363–380.
50. Ishida H, Ichimori K, Hirota Y, et al. Peroxynitrite-induced cardiac myocyte injury. Free Radic Biol Med 1996;20:343–350.
51. Nakamura M. Peripheral vascular remodeling in chronic heart failure: clinical relevance and new conceptualization of its mechanisms. J Card Fail 1999;5: 127–138.
52. Driss AB, Devaux C, Henrion D, et al. Hemodynamic stresses induce endothelial dysfunction and remodeling of pulmonary artery in experimental compensated heart failure. Circulation 2000;101:2764–2770.
53. Bauersachs J, Bouloumie A, Fraccarollo D, et al. Endothelial dysfunction in chronic myocardial infarction despite increased vascular endothelial nitric oxide synthase and soluble guanylate cyclase expression: role of enhanced vascular superoxide production. Circulation 1999;100:292–298.
54. Sakuma I, Akaishi Y, Tomioka H, et al. Interactions of sildenafil with various coronary vasodilators in isolated porcine coronary artery. Eur J Pharmacol 2002; 437:155–163.
55. Negrao CE, Hamilton MA, Fonarow GC, et al. Impaired endothelium-mediated vasodilation is not the principal cause of vasoconstriction in heart failure. Am J Physiol Heart Circ Physiol 2000;278:H168–H174.
56. Webb DJ, Freestone S, Allen MJ, et al. Sildenafil citrate and blood-pressure-lowering drugs: results of drug interaction studies with an organic nitrate and a calcium antagonist. Am J Cardiol 1999;83(Suppl 5A):21C–28C.
57. Vardi Y, Klein L, Nassar S, et al. Effects of sildenafil citrate (Viagra) on blood pressure in normotensive and hypertensive men. Urology 2002;59:747–752.
58. Wallis RM, Corbin JD, Francis SH, et al. Tissue distribution of phosphodiesterase families and the effects of sildenafil on tissue cyclic nucleotides, platelet function, and the contractile responses of trabeculae carneae and aortic rings in vitro. Am J Cardiol 1999;83(Suppl 5A):3C–12C.
59. Burslem F, Ellis P. Sildenafil enhances the platelet antiaggregatory activity of nitric oxide. Abstract LB11. Presented at: The American Society for Biochemistry and Molecular Biology and The American Society for Pharmacology and Experimental Therapeutics (ASBMB/ASPET) Joint Meeting; June 7, 2000; Boston, MA.
60. Rehse K, Scheffler H, Reitner N. Interaction of Viagra with the NO donors molsidomine and RE 2047 with regard to antithrombotic and blood pressure lowering activities. Arch Pharm (Weinheim) 1999;332:182–184.
61. Berkels R, Klotz T, Sticht G, et al. Modulation of human platelet aggregation by the phosphodiesterase type 5 inhibitor sildenafil. J Cardiovasc Pharmacol 2001; 37:413–421.

62. Hirose R, Okumura H, Yoshimatsu A, et al. KF31327, a new potent and selective inhibitor of cyclic nucleotide phosphodiesterase 5. Eur J Pharmacol 2001;431: 17–24.
63. Schmidt U, Han RO, DiSalvo TG, et al. Cessation of platelet-mediated cyclic canine coronary occlusion after thrombolysis by combining nitric oxide inhalation with phosphodiesterase-5 inhibition. J Am Coll Cardiol 2001;37:1981–1988.
64. Przyklenk K, Kloner RA. Sildenafil citrate (Viagra) does not exacerbate myocardial ischemia in canine models of coronary artery stenosis. J Am Coll Cardiol 2001;37:286–292.
65. Chen Y, Du R, Traverse JH, et al. Effect of sildenafil on coronary active and reactive hyperemia. Am J Physiol Heart Circ Physiol 2000;279:H2319–H2325.
66. Ishikura F, Beppu S, Hamada T, et al. Effects of sildenafil citrate (Viagra) combined with nitrate on the heart. Circulation 2000;102:2516–2521.
67. Traverse JH, Chen YJ, Du R, et al. Cyclic nucleotide phosphodiesterase type 5 activity limits blood flow to hypoperfused myocardium during exercise. Circulation 2000;102:2997–3002.
68. Herrmann HC, Chang G, Klugherz BD, et al. Hemodynamic effects of sildenafil in men with severe coronary artery disease. N Engl J Med 2000;342:1622–1626.
69. Webb DJ, Muirhead GJ, Wulff M, et al. Sildenafil citrate potentiates the hypotensive effects of nitric oxide donor drugs in male patients with stable angina. J Am Coll Cardiol 2000;36:25–31.
70. Jackson G, Keltai M, Csanady M, et al. Sildenafil has mild nitrate-like hemodynamic effects in patients with coronary artery disease and erectile dysfunction (abst). Presented at: American College of Cardiology, Chicago, IL; March 30–April 2 2003;
71. Halcox JPJ, Nour KRA, Zalos G, et al. The effect of sildenafil on human vascular function, platelet activation, and myocardial ischemia. J Am Coll Cardiol 2002;40:1232–1240.
72. Oliver JJ, Bell K, Leckie SM, et al. Interaction between glyceryl trinitrate and sildenafil citrate (Viagra) may last less than four hours. Presented at: 10th World Congress of the International Society for Sexual and Impotence Research; September 22–26, 2002, 2002; Montreal, Canada.
73. Arruda-Olson AM, Mahoney DW, Nehra A, et al. Cardiovascular effects of sildenafil during exercise in men with known or probable coronary artery disease: a randomized crossover trial. JAMA 2002;287:719–725.
74. Patrizi R, Leonardo F, Pelliccia F, et al. Effect of sildenafil citrate upon myocardial ischemia in patients with chronic stable angina in therapy with beta-blockers. Ital Heart J 2001;2:841–844.
75. Fox KM, Thadani U, Ma PTS, et al. Time to onset of limiting angina during treadmill exercise in men with erectile dysfunction and stable chronic angina: effect of sildenafil citrate (abst). Circulation 2001;104(SupplII):601–602.
76. Hebert K, Lee M, Ferguson T. Is sildenafil (Viagra®) safe and effective for the treatment of erectile dysfunction in patients with heart failure? (abst). Circulation 2000;102(Suppl II):413.
77. Hebert KA, Arcement LM, Ewing T, et al. Assessment of erectile dysfunction in a multidisciplinary heart failure program (abst). J Am Coll Cardiol 2001;37 (Suppl A):212A.
78. Bocchi EA, Guimaraes G, Mocelin A, et al. Sildenafil effects on exercise, neurohormonal activation, and erectile dysfunction in congestive heart failure. Circulation 2002;106:1097–1103.

79. Parums DV, Charlton RG, Johnson N, et al. Immunohistochemical (IHC), in situ hybridisation (ISH) and biochemical characterisation of phosphodiesterase type 5 (PDE5) in normal and ischaemic human cardiac tissue (PDE5). Eur Heart J 2000; 21:616.
80. Gomez-Sanchez MA, de la Calzeda CS, Lazaro M, et al. Beneficial acute hemodynamic effects of sublingual sildenafil in refractory pulmonary hypertension due to chronic heart failure. Presented at: Heart Failure Update; June 8–11, 2002; Oslo, Norway.
81. Lepore J, Pereira N, Maroo A, et al. Sildenafil is a pulmonary vasodilator which augments and prolongs vasodilation by inhaled nitric oxide in patients with pulmonary hypertension. Circulation 1999;100:I–240.
82. Veyssier-Belot C, Cacoub P. Role of endothelial and smooth muscle cells in the physiopathology and treatment management of pulmonary hypertension. Cardiovasc Res 1999;44:274–282.
83. Jackson G, Chambers J. Sildenafil for primary pulmonary hypertension: short and long-term symptomatic benefit [case report]. Int J Clin Pract 2002;55:397–398.
84. Hoeper MM, Galie N, Simonneau G, et al. New treatments for pulmonary arterial hypertension. Am J Respir Crit Care Med 2002;165:1209–1216.
85. Pauvert O, Salvail D, Rousseau E, et al. Characterisation of cyclic nucleotide phosphodiesterase isoforms in the media layer of the main pulmonary artery. Biochem Pharmacol 2002;63:1763–1772.
86. Clarke WR, Uezono S, Chambers A, et al. The type III phosphodiesterase inhibitor milrinone and type V PDE inhibitor dipyridamole individually and synergistically reduce elevated pulmonary vascular resistance. Pulm Pharmacol 1994;7:81–89.
87. Zhao L, Mason NA, Morrell NW, et al. Sildenafil inhibits hypoxia-induced pulmonary hypertension. Circulation 2001;104:424–428.
88. Schermuly RT, Weissmann N, Enke B, et al. Urodilatin, a natriuretic peptide stimulating particulate guanylate cyclase, and the phosphodiesterase 5 inhibitor dipyridamole attenuate experimental pulmonary hypertension: synergism upon coapplication. Am J Respir Cell Mol Biol 2001;25:219–225.
89. Dukarm RC, Morin FC 3rd, Russell JA, et al. Pulmonary and systemic effects of the phosphodiesterase inhibitor dipyridamole in newborn lambs with persistent pulmonary hypertension. Pediatr Res 1998;44:831–837.
90. Braner DA, Fineman JR, Chang R, et al. M&B 22948, a cGMP phosphodiesterase inhibitor, is a pulmonary vasodilator in lambs. Am J Physiol 1993;264:H252–H258.
91. Ichinose F, Adrie C, Hurford WE, et al. Selective pulmonary vasodilation induced by aerosolized zaprinast. Anesthesiology 1998;88:410–416.
92. Ichinose F, Erana-Garcia J, Hromi J, et al. Nebulized sildenafil is a selective pulmonary vasodilator in lambs with acute pulmonary hypertension. Crit Care Med 2001;29:1000–1005.
93. Nagamine J, Hill LL, Pearl RG. Combined therapy with zaprinast and inhaled nitric oxide abolishes hypoxic pulmonary hypertension. Crit Care Med 2000;28: 2420–2424.
94. Weimann J, Ullrich R, Hromi J, et al. Sildenafil is a pulmonary vasodilator in awake lambs with acute pulmonary hypertension. Anesthesiology 2000;92: 1702–1712.
95. Shekerdemian LS, Ravn HB, Penny DJ. Intravenous sildenafil lowers pulmonary vascular resistance in a model of neonatal pulmonary hypertension. Am J Respir Crit Care Med 2002;165:1098–1102.

96. Fullerton DA, Jaggers J, Piedalue F, et al. Effective control of refractory pulmonary hypertension after cardiac operations. J Thorac Cardiovasc Surg 1997; 113:363–368; discussion 368–370.
97. Ziegler JW, Ivy DD, Wiggins JW, et al. Effects of dipyridamole and inhaled nitric oxide in pediatric patients with pulmonary hypertension. Am J Respir Crit Care Med 1998;158:1388–1395.
98. Klings ES, Farber HW. Current management of primary pulmonary hypertension. Drugs 2001;61:1945–1956.
99. Patel RV, Karsh J, Jones G. Sildenafil for the treatment of end stage pulmonary hypertension. Presented at: 97th International Conference of the American Thoracic Society; May 18–23, 2001; San Francisco, CA.
100. Pritzker M, Dorman W, Caperton E. The use of sildenafil (Viagra) for the treatment of pulmonary hypertension associated with scleroderma. Arthritis Rheum 2001;44(Suppl 9):S131(abstract 471).
101. Schumacher YO, Zdebik A, Huonker M, et al. Sildenafil in HIV-related pulmonary hypertension. AIDS 2001;15:1747–1748.
102. Bigatello LM, Hess D, Dennehy KC, et al. Sildenafil can increase the response to inhaled nitric oxide. Anesthesiology 2000;92:1827–1829.
103. Li J, Schulze-Neick I, Petros A, et al. Intravenous sildenafil and pulmonary vascular resistance in children with congenital heart disease. Presented at: 3rd World Congress of Pediatric Cardiology and Cardiac Surgery; May 31, 2001; Toronto, Canada.
104. Michelakis E, Tymchak W, Lien D, et al. Oral sildenafil is an effective and specific pulmonary vasodilator in patients with pulmonary arterial hypertension: comparison with inhaled nitric oxide. Circulation 2002;105:2398–2403.
105. Schulze-Neick I, Dietz P, Stiller B, et al. Sildenafil lowers pulmonary vascular resistance in children after heart surgery (abst). Eur Heart J 2002;23:490.
106. Mikhail G, Prasad S, Rogers P, et al. Clinical and haemodynamic effects of sildenafil in pulmonary arterial hypertension [abstract]. Presented at: American Heart Association; November 17–20, 2002, 2002; Chicago, IL.
107. Wilkens H, Guth A, Konig J, et al. Effect of inhaled iloprost plus oral sildenafil in patients with primary pulmonary hypertension. Circulation 2001;104: 1218–1222.
108. Abrams DJR, Gatzoulis MA, Magee AG. Oral sildenafil—a novel therapy for primary pulmonary hypertension. Presented at: 3rd World Congress of Pediatric Cardiology and Cardiac Surgery; May 29, 2001; Toronto, Canada.
109. Prasad S, Wilkinson J, Gatzoulis MA. Sildenafil in primary pulmonary hypertension [Letter]. N Engl J Med 2000;343:1342.
110. Ghofrani HA, Wiedemann R, Rose F, et al. Combination therapy with oral sildenafil and inhaled iloprost for severe pulmonary hypertension. Ann Intern Med 2002;136:515–522.
111. Erickson S, Reyes J, Bohn D, et al. Sildenafil (Viagra) in childhood and neonatal pulmonary hypertension. J Am Coll Cardiol 2002, in press.
112. Siddons TE, Asif M, Armstrong I, et al. Long term effects of oral sildenafil (Viagra®) on haemodynamics and exercise tolerance in patients with pulmonary hypertension. Am J Resp Crit Care 2001;A541.
113. Zimmermann AT, Calvert AF, Veitch EM. Sildenafil improves right-ventricular parameters and quality of life in primary pulmonary hypertension [letter]. Intern Med J 2002;32:424–426.
114. Wheeler EA. Sildenafil-a replacement for inhaled nitric oxide in cardiac surgery? (abst). Anesth Analg 2002;94(Suppl 2):1.

115. Atz AM, Wessel DL. Sildenafil ameliorates effects of inhaled nitric oxide withdrawal. Anesthesiology 1999;91:307–310.
116. Mychaskiw G, Sachdev V, Heath BJ. Sildenafil (Viagra) facilitates weaning of inhaled nitric oxide following placement of a biventricular-assist device. J Clin Anesth 2001;13:218–220.
117. Ivy DD, Kinsella JP, Ziegler JW, et al. Dipyridamole attenuates rebound pulmonary hypertension after inhaled nitric oxide withdrawal in postoperative congenital heart disease. J Thorac Cardiovasc Surg 1998;115:875–882.
118. Lepor JJ, Maroo A, Ginns L. Sildenafil is a pulmonary vasodilator which augments and prolongs vasodilation by inhaled nitric oxide in patients with pulmonary hypertension. Presented at: 7th World Congress on Heart Failure: Mechanisms & Management; July 9–12, 2000; Vancouver, British Columbia.

14 The Physiologic Cost of Sexual Activity

Robert F. DeBusk, MD

CONTENTS

PHYSICAL COMPONENT OF SEXUAL ACTIVITY
EMOTIONAL COMPONENT OF SEXUAL ACTIVITY
   (AROUSAL)
ROLE OF EXERCISE TESTING IN EVALUATING
   THE CARDIOVASCULAR TOLERANCE
   FOR SEXUAL ACTIVITY
EFFECTS OF AGE ON THE CARDIOVASCULAR RESPONSE
   TO SEXUAL ACTIVITY
EFFECTS OF EXERCISE TRAINING
   ON THE CARDIOVASCULAR RESPONSE
   TO SEXUAL ACTIVITY
EFFECTS OF PHOSPHODIESTERASE-5 INHIBITORS
   ON THE EXERCISE TEST RESPONSE
CONCLUSION
REFERENCES

PHYSICAL COMPONENT OF SEXUAL ACTIVITY

Sexual activity is often equated with physical activity, such as walking, running, and lifting and carrying objects *(1)*. However, sexual activity can also be equated with states of arousal such as anger or fear *(2)*. In fact, the model of sex as a state of arousal is in many ways more clinically useful than the model of sex as a form of physical exertion, especially in patients with ischemic heart disease. In most cases

From: *Contemporary Cardiology: Heart Disease and Erectile Dysfunction*
Edited by: R. A. Kloner © Humana Press Inc., Totowa, NJ

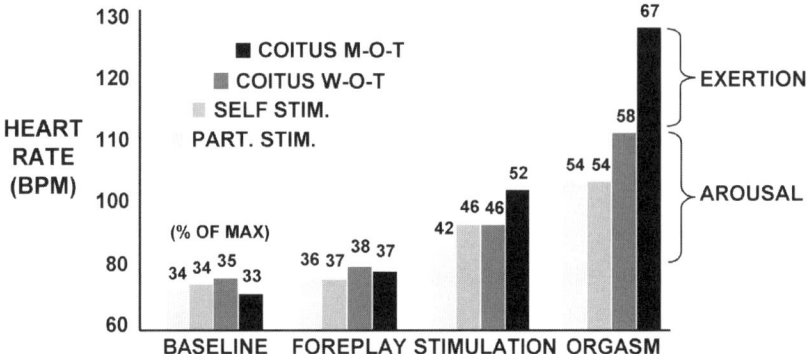

Fig. 1. Hemodynamic response to sexual activity, M-O-T, man on top; W-O-T, woman on top; PART, partner; STIM, stimulation; BPM, beats per minute. Adapted with permission from ref. *4*.

the cardiovascular response to sex is more closely related to sexual arousal than to physical exertion. The distinction between sexual exertion and sexual arousal has important implications when evaluating the cardiovascular tolerance for sexual activity.

Bohlen et al. *(3)* performed an important investigation of hemodynamic and metabolic responses to sexual activity involving 10 healthy, young, married men ages 25–43 yr (mean age: 33 yr) and their wives. Four types of sexual activity, each carried to orgasm, were evaluated in these men: self-stimulation, partner stimulation, coitus with the woman on top, and coitus with the man on top. Oxygen consumption, heart rate, and blood pressure were measured in the men before, during, and after sexual activity. These sexual activities were followed by a symptom-limited treadmill exercise test designed to evaluate peak exercise capacity.

The heart rate response to the four types of sexual activity is shown in Figure 1. The heart rate during sexual activity, expressed as a percentage of the peak treadmill heart rate, varied from 42–53% during the stimulation phase and from 54–67% during the orgasm phase, with little difference between the four types of sexual activity. The peak heart rate during the stimulation/orgasm phase was greater during coitus with the man on top than with the woman on top (heart rate 127 ± 23 beats/min vs 110 ± 24 bpm, $p < 0.02$) compared with a peak heart rate of 102 ± 14 beats/min for the two noncoital sexual activities *(4)*.

As shown in Fig. 2, a similar response to sexual activity was found for oxygen consumption (VO_2) measured as the metabolic equivalent of

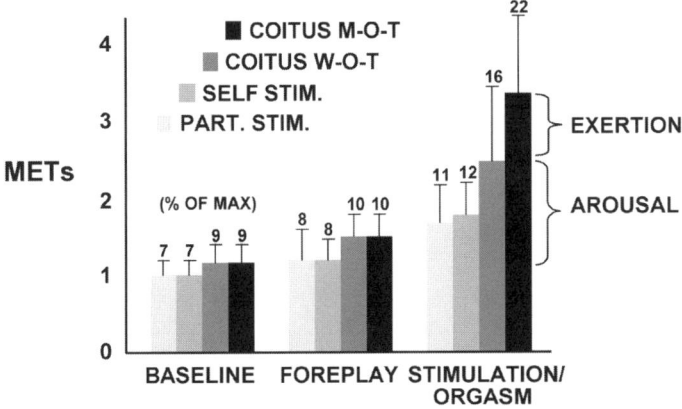

Fig. 2. Metabolic response to sexual activity. M-O-T, man on top; W-O-T, woman on top; PART, partner; STIM, stimulation; METs, multiples of resting energy expenditure; BPM, beats per minute. Adapted with permission from ref *4*.

the task (MET), where one MET is equivalent to 3.5 mL/kg/min. The VO_2 during the two types of coital activities, expressed as a percentage of the peak VO_2 measured during treadmill exercise testing (15.5 METs), was greater than during the two noncoital activities: 22% and 16% for coitus with the man on top and the woman on top, respectively, compared with 11–12% for noncoital activity. The corresponding values of VO_2 during the stimulation/orgasm phase of sexual activity were 3.3 METs for coitus with the man on top, 2.5 METs for coitus with the woman on top, respectively, and 1.7 METs for noncoital sexual activities, differences that were statistically but not clinically significant.

EMOTIONAL COMPONENT OF SEXUAL ACTIVITY (AROUSAL)

The results of this study underscore the distinction between sexual arousal and sexual exertion. Sexual arousal that occurs during self-stimulation, partner stimulation, and coitus with the woman on top is not accompanied by significant physical exertion: the increases in heart rate and VO_2 during these conditions are largely attributable to sexual arousal alone. The greater increase in heart rate and VO_2 noted during coitus with the man on top reflects not only the greater physical exertion associated with this type of sexual activity but perhaps heightened sexual arousal as well *(4)*. A study conducted by Nemec et al. *(1)* in healthy young men showed no significant difference in heart rate and

Table 1
Energy Requirements (METS)
of Selected Physical Activities

Walking 2 MPH, Level	2
Walking 3 MPH, Level	3
"Sexual Activity" Pre-Orgasm	2–3
"Sexual Activity" During Orgasm	3–4
Cycling 10 MPH, Level	6–7
Walking 4.2 MPH, 16% (Bruce Treadmill Stage 4)	13

MET, multiples of resting energy expenditure; MPH, miles per hour. Adapted from ref. *4* with permission.

blood pressure responses between coitus performed in the man-on-top and woman-on-top positions.

The results of studies conducted in healthy young men have been widely extrapolated to older individuals. However, the intensity of sexual arousal and sexual exertion, especially among long-married couples, is almost certainly less than among young couples. In any event, the duration of sexual activity in the study of Bohlen et al. was brief: the stimulation phase involving a sexual partner lasted only 5 min and the orgasm phase during each of the four sexual activities lasted only 10–16 s. Heart rate returned to resting baseline within 30 s for noncoital activities and within 1.5–2.0 min for coitus with the woman on top and man on top, respectively. Other studies also show the brevity of the hemodynamic and metabolic response to sexual activity *(4)*.

ROLE OF EXERCISE TESTING IN EVALUATING THE CARDIOVASCULAR TOLERANCE FOR SEXUAL ACTIVITY

The cardiovascular tolerance for sexual activity can be expressed as the "functional reserve," which represents the difference between peak heart rate and VO_2 measured during treadmill testing and that measured during sexual activity *(4)*. Exercise testing commonly is used to measure the cardiovascular reserve of patients with clinical coronary artery disease (CAD), especially among sedentary individuals. Patients with cardiovascular disease often limit their physical activity, even without being aware of it. Exercise testing enables not only an objective assessment of exercise tolerance in such individuals but also helps

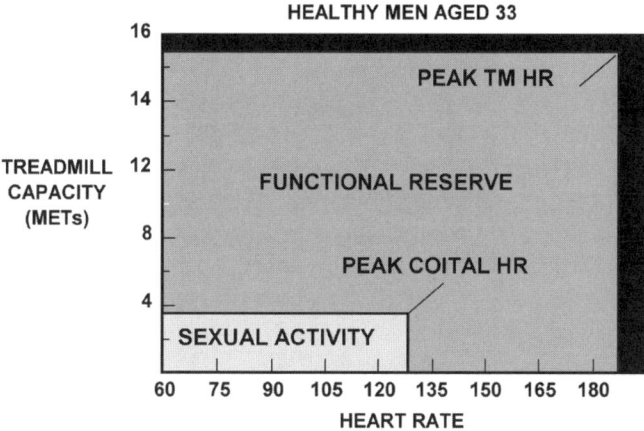

Fig. 3. Workload of sexual activity. TM, treadmill; HR, heart rate; METs, multiples of resting energy expenditure; BPM, beats per minute. In a healthy man aged 33, treadmill exercise elicits a peak functional capacity of 15.5 METs and a peak heart rate of 185 BPM. Sexual activity elicits a peak functional capacity of 3.5 METs and a peak heart rate of 128 BPM. The difference in peak functional capacity during treadmill exercise and sexual activity represents the functional reserve. Adapted with permission from ref. *4*.

to determine the threshold of heart rate, blood pressure, and workload at which symptoms of angina, dyspnea, and fatigue appear *(5)*.

The standard clinical measure of physical exertion is the metabolic equivalent of the task (MET). One MET is equivalent to the resting state. Table 1 shows the energy requirements of selected physical activities. These range from 2 METs for walking at 2 miles per hour (2 METs) to 13 METs for completion of the fourth stage of the Bruce treadmill exercise test. "Sexual activity" is often equated with an exercise workload of 2–3 METs in the preorgasmic phase and 3–4 METs during the orgasmic stage *(3)*. However, the physical exertion associated with sexual activity varies widely among individuals, especially in relation to age.

The functional reserve of the young individuals reported by Bohlen et al. was very great and was not substantially taxed by sexual activity (Fig. 3). Among older individuals, especially those with silent ischemia, the functional reserve is much less (Fig. 4). For patients with coital angina, Drory et al. *(6)* found that the heart rate during sexual activity actually exceeded that noted during treadmill exercise. In this study, cycle ergometry elicited a higher heart rate than coitus in the group as a whole viz. 138 ± 19 vs 108 ± 21 beats/min, respectively ($p < 0.0001$). Moreover, all patients who exhibited myocardial ischemia, with or

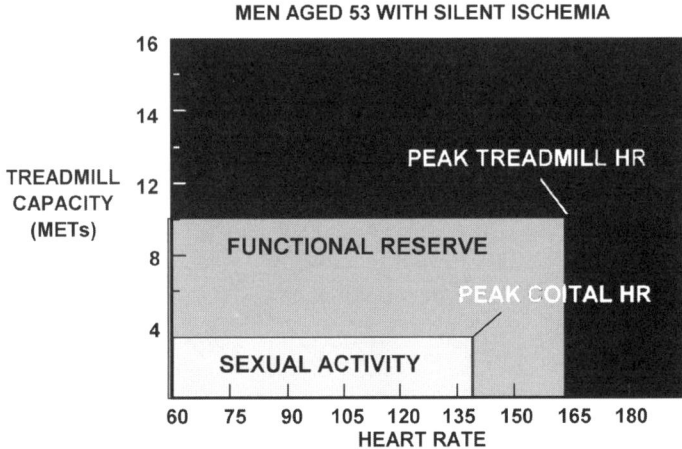

Fig. 4. Workload of sexual activity. TM, treadmill; HR, heart rate; METs, multiples of resting energy expenditure; BPM, beats per minute. In a 53-yr-old man with silent ischemia, treadmill exercise elicits a peak functional capacity of 10.0 METs and a peak heart rate of 165 BPM. Sexual activity elicits a peak functional capacity of 3.5 METs or less and a peak heart rate of 127 BPM. The difference in peak functional capacity for treadmill exercise and sexual activity represents the functional reserve. Adapted with permission from ref. 4.

without angina, during coitus also exhibited myocardial ischemia during exercise testing.

Thus, the exercise test is useful for establishing the functional reserve of patients with and without angina and may elicit angina in a few patients who do not experience angina during other circumstances. However, treadmill testing is not required to evaluate the functional reserve of patients who report no symptoms during vigorous physical activity. For example, the capacity to climb two flights of stairs without limiting symptoms, which is equivalent to 6 METs, is a useful clinical benchmark of exercise tolerance (7). Patients capable of exercising to a 6 MET treadmill workload without cardiovascular symptoms can generally, but not always, engage in sexual activity without experiencing cardiovascular symptoms.

Sexual arousal is an important consideration in patients with ischemic heart disease because it can be equated with the risk of acute coronary events. The influence of arousal on the cardiovascular response to sexual activity can be inferred from observations made during sexual activity with an unfamiliar sexual partner. Cantwell reported on the heart rate during coitus obtained by 24-h ambulatory electrocardiography *(8)*. The patient exhibited a heart rate increase from 96 to 150 beats/min during an extramarital sexual encounter and, later the same day, a heart rate increase from 72 to 92 beats per min during conjugal sexual activity. Reasons for the higher heart rate during sexual activity with a new partner include performance anxiety, an unfamiliar setting, ingestion of alcohol and food, social disapproval, and, especially, a high degree of sexual arousal. Sexual activity with an unfamiliar partner may substantially increase the degree of sexual arousal and thereby the cardiovascular workload and the risk of acute coronary events *(9)*. It is important to recognize that the level of physical exertion associated with coitus may well be less among older individuals than among younger individuals. This is especially true for coitus with the woman on top and for other types of coitus, not reported in previous studies, including the side-by-side position.

Another circumstance in which arousal is the predominant mediator of the cardiovascular response to sexual activity is masturbation. In studies conducted in healthy young men and women, peak heart rates were often substantial, yet the physical exertion associated with masturbation is generally trivial *(10)*. The cardiovascular response to masturbation in men with ischemic heart disease has been little studied. This is an important issue, for masturbation is common among men who engage in coital activity.

EFFECTS OF AGE ON THE CARDIOVASCULAR RESPONSE TO SEXUAL ACTIVITY

The physiologic response to sexual activity among middle-aged and older individuals has been little studied. However, given the tendency for less frequent and less vigorous sexual activity that occurs among even healthy older individuals, it is probably the case that the physiologic demands of sexual activity in older individuals are less than previously had been thought.

In younger men, the hemodynamic and metabolic demands of sexual activity are negligible. Bohlen et al. *(3)* found that oxygen consumption increased to only 23% of the peak oxygen consumption measured during symptom-limited treadmill exercise, even during the most physically taxing forms of sexual activity. Similarly, the heart rate during the most intense sexual activity increased to only 66% of the peak treadmill heart rate in this study. However, the cardiovascular workload of sexual activity has not been extensively studied in older men. Furthermore, the cardiovascular response associated with sexual activity has not been adequately characterized in men with manifest CAD or those at risk for CAD. In particular, data are lacking for patients with CAD who are receiving sildenafil for the management of erectile dysfunction.

The relative cardiovascular workload of sexual activity increases with age, reflecting, in part, a decrease in peak exercise heart rate and workload. This age-dependent decrease in peak heart rate and workload translates to a reduced functional reserve among older individuals. For example, a healthy male aged 63 yr without ischemic heart disease may exhibit a peak treadmill workload of 9 METs, or multiples of resting energy consumption. Sexual activity that elicits a workload of 3.5 METs represents 40% of the peak oxygen consumption for this man. However, it is unknown whether sexual activity in this older man actually elicits the 3.5 MET workload seen in 33-yr-old men. In the setting of chronic deconditioning, or exercise-induced myocardial ischemia, the peak treadmill workload of a 63-yr-old man might be reduced even further to 8 METs. For such an individual, sexual activity that elicited a workload of 3.5 METs would represent 44% of peak oxygen consumption, or roughly twice the relative workload seen in healthy young men.

Therefore, it is important to consider how sexual activity at age 63 yr compares with sexual activity at age 33 yr. In general, the degree of sexual arousal declines over time, even among the most enthusiastic of sexual partners. Moreover, sexual activity tends to be less energetic among middle-aged men than among younger ones. Accordingly, the workload of sexual activity at age 63 yr may well not be 3.5 METs, but only two-thirds this value, or 2.0 METs. This would represent only 26% of the peak oxygen consumption for a well-conditioned man, comparable with the value of 29% for a deconditioned man. The clinical implications of this natural aging phenomenon are important: sexual activity for middle-aged men may be less taxing than previously recognized, and the risks associated with sexual activity may be correspondingly less.

Among a group of 50-yr-old men evaluated 12–15 wk after a heart attack, Stein et al. *(11)* recorded a peak coital heart rate of 127 beats/min, which is equivalent to about 75% of predicted peak heart rate in normal individuals. Hellerstein et al. *(12)* used ambulatory electrocardiography to measure the peak coital heart rate during conjugal sexual activity in middle-aged men. These investigators found that to be even less than that recorded by Stein et al.: 117 beats/min. Both studies demonstrate the modest cardiovascular response to sexual activity in long-established sexual relationships.

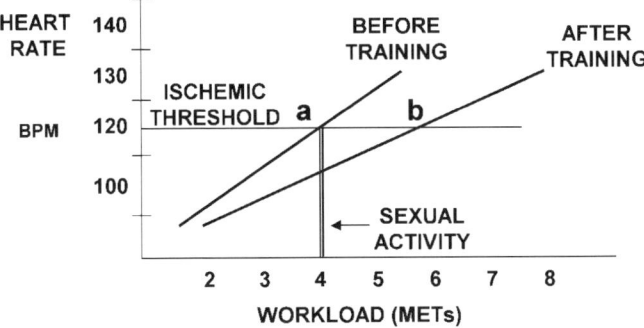

Fig. 5. Effects of exercise training on ischemic threshold during sexual activity. METs, multiples of resting energy expenditure; BPM, beats per minute. In this sedentary individual, exercise training increases the peak exercise capacity increased by 40%, from 6 METs to 8.4 METs. Before training, the patient exhibits ST segment depression and angina pectoris at a heart rate of 120 BPM, which is associated with a workload of 4 METs. After training, the patient still exhibits ischemic ST segment depression and angina pectoris at a heart rate of 120 BPM, but the workload at the onset of ischemia has increased to 6 METs. Adapted with permission from ref. *4*.

EFFECTS OF EXERCISE TRAINING ON THE CARDIOVASCULAR RESPONSE TO SEXUAL ACTIVITY

In men with cardiovascular disease, Stein et al. *(11)* found that the peak heart rate during coitus with the patient's usual sexual partner was less after a 16-wk cycle of training than in an untrained cohort. The peak oxygen consumption after exercise training increased by about 10%, from about 11 METs to 12.2 METs. After exercise training, the peak coital heart rate measured by ambulatory electrocardiography at home decreased by about 5%, from 127 to 120 beats/min. No significant change in peak oxygen consumption or coital heart rate was noted after 16 wk in patients assigned to the control group. No patient in either group exhibited angina during exercise or coitus.

The explanation for the training-induced decrease in coital heart rate is shown in Fig. 5. Exercise training decreases the heart rate response to a given submaximal workload. Accordingly, the workload at which ischemia appears increases from 4 METs (point a) to 6 METs (point b). In this study, the "workload" associated with sexual activity probably remained constant during the 16-wk period, but oxygen consumption was not measured.

Deconditioned patients who exhibit ischemic ST segment depression or angina pectoris on ambulatory electrocardiography during coitus may become ischemia-free after exercise training. This assumes that the workload associated with coitus remains constant. As shown in Fig. 5, exercise training does not significantly increase the heart rate threshold at which ischemia occurs, but it may substantially increase the workload prior to the onset of ischemia. In patients with obstructive CAD, this could reduce the extent of myocardial ischemia, which could reduce the incidence of angina pectoris and the risk of acute coronary events.

The relationship between exercise capacity and prognosis in men with ischemic heart disease is complex. For example, Muller et al. *(13)* noted a substantially lower rate of cardiac events in men who reported a high habitual physical activity score at baseline, soon after acute myocardial infarction. This could reflect the effects of habitual physical exercise, which increases functional capacity. However, an important self-selection process is also at play: physically active individuals generally exhibit less myocardial ischemia and left ventricular dysfunction than those who are less physically active. Self-selection also applies to sexual activity: patients who develop cardiac symptoms of ischemic heart disease are much less likely to continue sexual activity than those who are free of cardiac symptoms.

EFFECTS OF PHOSPHODIESTERASE-5 INHIBITORS ON THE EXERCISE TEST RESPONSE

Studies by Arruda-Olson et al. *(14)* and Thadani et al. *(15)* indicate that phosphodiesterase type 5 (PDE5) inhibitors exert no deleterious effects on the cardiovascular response to exercise among individuals with established heart disease. Whatever the risks of coitus-induced cardiac events, it appears that PDE5 inhibitors do not exert an independent influence on this risk. The risk posed by these events is mediated through the sexual activity that they enable.

CONCLUSION

The physiologic cost of sexual activity reflects arousal and to a lesser extent, exertion. The workload associated with sexual activity is comparatively mild in most individuals and does not represent a significant cardiovascular challenge. However, sexual activity can elicit angina pectoris in individuals with severe CAD. Exercise testing is helpful in evaluating the risk of angina elicited by exercise. Patients who do not experience angina at a treadmill capacity of 6 METs or more rarely experience angina during sexual activity. In patients with angina, exercise training increases the workload, measured in METs, at which ischemic ST segment depression and angina occur.

REFERENCES

1. Nemec ED, Mansfield L, Kennedy JW. Heart rate and blood pressure responses during sexual activity in normal males. Am Heart J 1976;92:274–277.
2. Mittleman MA, Maclure M, Sherwood JB, et al. Triggering of acute myocardial infarction onset by episodes of anger. Determinants of Myocardial Infarction Onset Study Investigators. Circulation 1995;92:1720–1725.
3. Bohlen JG, Held JP, Sanderson MO, et al. Heart rate, rate-pressure product, and oxygen uptake during four sexual activities. Arch Intern Med 1984;144: 1745–1748.
4. DeBusk RF. Evaluating the cardiovascular tolerance for sex. Am J Cardiol 2000;86(Suppl):51F–56F.
5. Froelicher VF. An introduction to the applications, methodology and interpretation of exercise electrocardiography. Cardiology 1980;66:223–235.
6. Drory Y SI, Fisman EZ, Pines A. Myocardial ischemia during sexual activity in patients with coronary artery disease. Am J Cardiol 1995;75:835–837.
7. Jackson G. Sexual intercourse and stable angina pectoris. Am J Cardiol. 2000;86:35F–37F.
8. Cantwell J. Sex and the heart. Med Aspects Human Sexuality 1981;15:14–23.
9. Ueno M. The so-called coition death. Jpn J Leg Med 1963;17:330–340.
10. Sanderson MO, Held JP, Bohlen JG. Heart rate during masturbation. J Cardiac Rehab 1982;2:542–546.
11. Stein RA. The effect of exercise training on heart rate during coitus in the post myocardial infarction patient. Circulation 1977;55:738–740.
12. Hellerstein HK, Friedman EH. Sexual activity and the postcoronary patient. Arch Intern Med 1970;125:987–999.
13. Muller TE, Mittleman MA, Maclure M, et al. Triggering myocardial infarction by sexual activity. JAMA 1996;275:1405–1409.
14. Arruda-Olson AM, Mahoney DW, Nehra A, et al. Cardiovascular effects of sildenafil during exercise in men with known or probable coronary artery disease: a randomized crossover trial. JAMA. 2002;287:719–725.
15. Thadani U, Smith W, Nash S, et al. The effect of vardenafil, a potent and highly selective phosphodiesterase-5 inhibitor for the treatment of erectile dysfunction, on the cardiovascular response to exercise in patients with coronary artery disease. J Am Coll Cardiol 2002;40:2006–2012.

15 Sexual Activity As a Trigger of Myocardial Infarction/Ischemia
Implications for Treating Erectile Dysfunction

Robert A. Kloner, MD, PhD

CONTENTS

PHYSICAL COMPONENT OF SEXUAL ACTIVITY
THE PHYSIOLOGIC COST TO THE SEXUALLY ACTIVE HEART
SEXUAL ACTIVITY AS A TRIGGER FOR ANGINA
IMPLICATIONS FOR THE ED PATIENT
CONCLUSION
REFERENCES

PHYSICAL COMPONENT OF SEXUAL ACTIVITY

Landmark studies by Muller, Mittleman, Tofler and others have suggested that acute myocardial infarctions (MIs) may be triggered by certain phenomena *(1–4)*. It is believed that these triggers, often initiated by an increase in catecholamines and sympathetic nervous system activity, ultimately lead to a disruption of the vulnerable atherosclerotic plaque. Increases in sympathetic vascular tone and sympathetic/catecholamine-related increases in heart rate, blood pressure, ventricular contractility, platelet aggregability, hematocrit, and reductions in fibrinolysis may all contribute *(2)*. For example, an increase in

From: *Contemporary Cardiology: Heart Disease and Erectile Dysfunction*
Edited by: R. A. Kloner © Humana Press Inc., Totowa, NJ

ventricular contractility with changes in dP/dT (change in ventricular pressure over time) and an increase in coronary tone can increase the sheer–stress of blood flowing across a vulnerable atherosclerotic plaque. These mechanical forces may then contribute to rupture of a thin fibrous cap overlying the lipid pool of the plaque. Lipid, foam cells, and tissue factors escape into the lumen of the artery, contributing to platelet aggregation, fibrin deposition, and thrombus, which can then obstruct flow through the coronary artery, causing acute MI and/or sudden death. Reduction in flow also results from an increase in stimulation of alpha sympathomimetic receptors. Increases in heart rate and blood pressure during emotional or physical stress increase oxygen demand, and if O_2 supply is limited by coronary stenosis, coronary artery vasospasm, or flow limiting intra-coronary thrombus, ischemia will be worsened.

Virtually any emotional or physical stress has the potential to trigger acute MI or ischemia—but what are the triggers that actually have been shown to contribute?

Muller and associates showed that one of the most common triggers for acute cardiac events was the time of awakening *(1,5)*. In the multicenter Myocardial Infarction Onset Study, they observed that 19% of over 1700 patients with acute MI woke up in the 2-h period before the infarction. *(6)* Within the first few hours of waking, there is a well-known increase in plasma epinephrine and norepinephrine that is associated with increases in heart rate, blood pressure, ventricular contractility, vasomotor tone, and platelet aggregability. In addition, the morning is associated with increases in hemoglobin and reductions in tissue plasminogen activator coupled with increases in plasminogen activator inhibitor. Such factors result in a relative hypercoagulable state in the morning. These investigators also reported that among patients with acute MI, 11.6% were exposed to psychological stress, 4.9% to heavy exercise, and 2.4% to anger. Of these patients, 1.5% had sexual activity during the 2 h before MI, but following correction for chance occurrence, sexual activity was a contributor to MI in only 0.9% of cases *(3,6,7)*. The use of cocaine increased the risk of MI 23.7 times over baseline *(8)*. Our research group showed that certain major natural disasters such as earthquakes as well as seasonal variations could act as triggers of cardiac events *(9,10)*.

Using a case-crossover study design Muller and associates found that the relative risk of a MI in the 2-h period after sexual activity was increased at 2.5 *(3)*. This relative risk was similar in patients without histories of MI (2.5) vs those with a history of MI (2.9). The relative risk of sexual activity triggering acute MI was 2.1 in those patients with a history of angina vs 2.6 in those patients without angina.

Although the relative risk of having a MI within 2 h of sexual activity was increased at 2.5, the absolute risk was small because the risk of sexually triggered MI occurred only during the 2-h period before acute MI and sexual activity was found to be a contributor to MI in only 0.9% of cases *(7)*.

Using these data and data from the Framingham group, DeBusk et al. *(11)* described another illuminating analysis of this phenomenon. They noted that the baseline annual risk of a MI for a 50-yr-old American man is about 1.0%. As a result of sexual activity this annual risk increases to 1.01%. In a man with a history of MI, the annual risk increases only to 1.10%.

Based on the Framingham Heart Study, Muller pointed out *(7)* that a 50-yr-old healthy man who is physically active has an absolute risk of MI of one chance in a million per hour *(12,13)*. The absolute risk doubles to only two chances in a million per hour with sexual intercourse and, again, only for a 2-h period. The risk of MI is 10 chances per million per hour in a post-MI patient who has been in a rehabilitation program *(14)*. If that patient has sexual intercourse, then the risk is transiently doubled, but, still, the absolute risk is low with the chance of MI at 20 per million per hour *(7)*. Thus, in general, the absolute chance that a person—healthy or with coronary artery disease (CAD)—is going to suffer an acute MI with sexual intercourse is low.

Another important finding from Muller's study was that patients who were physically active and who achieved ≥6 metabolic equivalents of the task (METS) of exertion three or more times a week did not have an increased risk of MI with sexual activity *(3,7)*. Hence, physical activity appears to have an important protective effect, and thus, participation in cardiac rehabilitation programs may reduce the chance of a major cardiac event associated with sexual activity. The research group also observed that patients who were physically active were less likely to have a MI with strenuous physical exertion *(15)*.

THE PHYSIOLOGIC COST TO THE SEXUALLY ACTIVE HEART

Sexual activity has been likened to moderate physical activity *(16)*, and, therefore, there is a physiologic cost to the heart. Studies that have investigated the changes in heart rate and blood pressure that occur during sexual intercourse have shown increases with variability in the increases depending on the setting of the measurements, the age of participants, the health and physical conditioning of the participants, as well as other factors *(11,16,17)*. Although sexual intercourse does increase oxygen demand, in most cases, the duration of the increase in oxygen demand is relatively short.

Early work by Masters and Johnson in which couples engaged in coitus, in laboratories and were attached to electrocardiographic machines, reported increases in heart rate and blood pressure that were impressive (peak heart rates of 140–180 beats/min and increases in systolic blood pressure of 80 mmHg and in diastolic blood pressure of 50 mmHg *(18)*. In 1970, Hellerstein and Friedman *(19)* published an article in which middle-aged men with and without CAD had 24-h ambulatory electrocardiography during coitus in the privacy of their own bedrooms. In men with a mean age of 48 yr with known atherosclerosis, orgasm was associated with an average heart rate of 117 beats/min, and peak coital heart rate usually was lower than heart rates achieved during other normal daily activities (120 beats/min). Also, the peak heart rates associated with sexual intercourse lasted <15 s. They estimated that the myocardial oxygen demands of coitus were about 60% of the subject's maximum achieved oxygen demand and, thus, coitus, in the usual manner in middle-aged men, imposed only a modest physiologic cost to the heart.

Bohlen et al. *(20)* reported that healthy and physically active young men (mean age: 33 yr) in a laboratory setting achieved a mean heart rate of 120 beats/min with woman-on-top coitus and 127 beats/min with man-on-top coitus. Heart rate × systolic blood pressure, or rate-pressure product, peaked at orgasm and was approximately double baseline values. Oxygen consumption expressed as METS (where one MET equals 3.5 mL O_2/kg per min) was 2.5 METS for woman-on-top coitus and 3.3 METS for man-on-top coitus.

In a study by Stein *(21)*, 16 post-MI patients were examined. Heart rate was monitored by 24-h ambulatory monitoring. Mean peak heart rate during sexual intercourse was 127 beats/min before an exercise training period and 120 beats/min after 16 wk of bicycle training.

Jackson et al *(22,23)* studied 14 patients with stable angina using ambulatory electrocardiogram (ECG) monitoring. Sexual intercourse was associated with a mean heart rate of 122 vs 124 beats/min for some other daily ambulatory activity. β-blockers reduced the heart rate response of sexual activity to 82 beats/min. Namec et al. *(24)* made the observation that, in 10 healthy male subjects having coitus with their spouses at home, there was no difference in double product (assessed with ambulatory ECG and automatic blood pressure cuffs) in the "man-on-top" or "woman-on-top" position.

Other analyses have suggested that during sexual intercourse heart rate increases to 120–130 beats/min, systolic blood pressure increases to about 150 mmHg but rarely >170 mmHg, and that diastolic blood pressure increases by about 10 mmHg at orgasm *(25)*. As DeBusk *(16)* notes, the intensity of sexual arousal and exertion will be less among older long-married couples compared with younger couples. Also, duration of increased oxygen demand is usually short. In most studies, the sexual stimulation phase lasted only 5 min, orgasm phase was 10–16 s, and resolution phase <30 min. Thus, the hemodynamic response to sexual activity is brief.

Sexual activity during the preorgasmic phase is associated with 2–3 METS; during orgasm, it is 3–4 METS with a higher range of 5–6 METS *(11,16)*. This can be considered moderate physical exertion.

In the past, the comparison of sexual activity to other activities included the ability to briskly climb two flights of stairs (20 steps in 10 s or about 3 METS; refs. *23* and *26)*, walking 1 mile in 20 min (approximately 3.5 METS), digging in the garden (approximately 5 METS), or 10 min of brisk walking (approximately 5–6 METS) *(23)*. Of course, these comparisons do not take into account the sympathomimetic effect of the arousal phase of sexual activity *(16)*. Of note, a study from Japan suggested that more cases of sudden death during coitus were likely to occur during extramarital coitus *(27)*. As noted by the Princeton Consensus Panel, sexual arousal, through an increase in sympathetic discharge, might contribute to lethal ventricular arrhythmias in some patients *(11)*.

SEXUAL ACTIVITY AS A TRIGGER FOR ANGINA

Drory et al. *(28)* studied men with known CAD with ambulatory ECG monitoring during sexual activity and also monitored them during symptom limited exercise testing. They observed that all patients who experienced myocardial ischemia (associated with angina or silent) during sexual intercourse also experienced myocardial ischemia during exercise stress testing. Therefore, DeBusk has suggested that the exercise test may be useful for determining functional reserve of patients in those who do not experience angina during other circumstances *(16)*. As part of the Princeton Consensus Guidelines, additional cardiovascular testing, including exercise stress testing, was recommended for patients with intermediate cardiac risk *(11)*. An example would be a patient with multiple risk factors for CAD or with moderate stable angina who has been physically and sexually inactive for a long period of time. The patient has erectile dysfunction (ED) and seeks oral pharmacologic therapy. The physician must decide whether a prescription for an oral phosphodiesterase-5 (PDE5) inhibitor, which will enable the patient to have sexual intercourse and achieve the associated increase in oxygen demand, is safe. This is the type of patient in whom an exercise treadmill test may provide valuable information. Suppose the patient exercises long enough and vigorously enough to achieve a heart rate of 130 beats/min, a systolic blood pressure of 140 mmHg, and expends 4–5 METS without chest pain, ST segment depression on the ECG, or other objective evidence of myocardial ischemia. In that case, the patient will be at low risk for developing ischemia during sexual activity. However, if that same patient develops chest pain and objective evidence of ischemia with a low level of physical exertion, then he may need additional intervention, including coronary angiography, percutaneous coronary intervention, coronary artery bypass surgery, and/or additional antianginal/antiatherosclerotic medicines. The same path would be followed if the patient went to see his physician before obtaining a prescription for an exercise or rehabilitation program.

It is important to remember that even if a patient does well on a stress test and does not exhibit signs of ischemia, this cannot absolutely rule out the possibility of a cardiac event with sexual or physical activity. At the present time there is no fool-proof test for identifying who is and who is not going to rupture an atherosclerotic plaque either with sexual activity or any other activity. We have tests that might help determine if any one patient is at high or low risk, but that is about as far as we can go. Determination of biochemical markers of inflammation (high sensitive C reactive protein) and new catheters that can detect a vulnerable plaque (such as thermal catheters and infrared spectroscopy *(29)*) are currently under study.

IMPLICATIONS FOR THE ED PATIENT

ED clearly has been associated with cardiovascular risk factors, such as hypertension, lipid abnormalities, smoking, diabetes, obesity, and lack of physical exertion *(30–32)*. What is the incidence of MI in men with a history of ED who then are successfully treated for ED with oral pharmacologic therapy? Numerous studies have examined this issue in men treated with sildenafil *(33–39)*, vardenafil *(40)*, and tadalafil *(41)*. Obviously, because sildenafil has been available for the longest period of time, more data are available with this agent. Studies have explored the incidence of MI in placebo-controlled randomized trials in which patients received oral therapy vs placebo and in open-label therapy trials, and studies have also compared the incidence of MI in men on these drugs with the expected incidence in the general aged-matched population. The Food and Drug Administration recently released a report from their spontaneous adverse event reporting system examining the number of in deaths in men on sildenafil compared with what is expected *(42)*.

The findings of all these studies *(33–42)* suggest no signal for an increase in either MI rate or death rate in men receiving oral PDE5 inhibitors for ED. In fact, some reports even suggest a lower than expected rate *(39)*. Perhaps healthier men were taking these drugs, or perhaps as some studies suggest PDE5 inhibitors may improve endothelial dysfunction.

A series of recent studies examined the effect of PDE5 inhibitors administered to known coronary artery patients undergoing exercise stress testing. In no cases did these agents exacerbate the threshold for ischemia or angina associated with exercise *(43–46)*. Also, when sildenafil was administered to CAD patients at the time of cardiac catheterization, there was no evidence that it precipitated ischemia *(47)*.

Those patients taking organic nitrates (nitroglycerin, long-acting oral nitrates, others) must not receive the PDE5 inhibitors. That is because organic nitrates are nitric oxide donors that increase the production of the vasodilator cyclic guanosine monophosphate (cGMP), whereas PDE5 inhibitors prevent the breakdown of cGMP *(33,34,48)*. The two agents together result in a synergistic drop in blood pressure in some patients. However, not all CAD patients require nitrates. Nitrates alone have not been shown to improve long-term outcomes. They do relieve angina. Other antianginal and antiatherosclerotic agents, such as β-blockers, calcium blockers, aspirin, and statins, can be used safely with PDE5 inhibitors *(49)*. The optimal CAD patient that may be considered for PDE5 inhibitors has a negative (no ischemia) stress test and perhaps has already been revascularized by either percutaneous coronary intervention or coronary artery bypass surgery.

Both the American College of Cardiology/American Heart Association (ACC/AHA) *(49)* and the Princeton Consensus Panel *(11)* have developed recommendations for the prescription of PDE5 inhibitors (specifically sildenafil at the time of this writing) for the cardiac patient. Although organic nitrate use remains the one contraindication for the use of PDE5 inhibitors, the guidelines caution the use of PDE5 inhibitors or any therapies for sexual dysfunction in the unstable cardiac patient. Details of these guidelines are presented in other chapters of this book. This is, of course, a common sense approach.

CONCLUSION

Although sexual activity is one of the triggers for MI, the absolute hourly risk of having a MI with sexual activity is low. There is a physiologic cost of sexual activity that is likened to moderate physical exertion. Often, the same degree of hemodynamic change occurs during ordinary daily activities. A cardiac stress test, specifically an exercise stress test, may help determine whether a patient is at low risk or high risk for developing myocardial ischemia during sexual activity. However, there is no test that can absolutely predict who is and who is not going to have a cardiac event with sexual activity (or any activity for that matter). As a class, the PDE5 inhibitors have been shown to be safe, without evidence for an increase in MI or cardiac death. In addition, these agents do not appear to worsen the threshold for ischemia during exercise testing in patients with known CAD. The one contraindication to the use of PDE5 inhibitors is concomitant organic nitrate therapy. Other cautions have been recommended by the ACC/AHA and Princeton Consensus Group.

REFERENCES

1. Muller JE, Tofler GH, Stone PH. Circadian variation and triggers of onset of acute cardiovascular disease. Circulation 1989;79:733–743.
2. Muller JE, Abela GS, Nesto RW, et al. Triggers, acute risk factors and vulnerable plaques: the lexicon of a new frontier. J Am Coll Cardiol 1994;23:809–813.
3. Muller JE, Mittleman MA, Maclure M, et al. Triggering myocardial infarction by sexual activity. JAMA 1996;275:1405–1409.
4. Muller JE, Kaufmann PG, Luepker RV, et al. Mechanisms precipitating acute cardiac events: review and recommendations of an NHLBI workshop. Circulation 1997;96:3233–3239.
5. Muller JE. Circadian variation in cardiovascular events. Am J Hypertens 1999; 12:35S–42S.
6. Muller JE. Sexual activity as a trigger for cardiovascular events: what is the risk? Am J Cardiol 1999;84 (Suppl 5B):2N–5N.
7. Muller JE. Triggering of cardiac events by sexual activity: findings from a case-crossover analysis. Am J Cardiol 2000;86 (Suppl):14F–18F.
8. Mittleman MA, Mintzer D, Maclure M, et al. Triggering of myocardial infarction by cocaine. Circulation 1999;99:2737–2741.
9. Leor J, Poole WK, Kloner RA. Sudden cardiac death triggered by an earthquake. N Engl J Med 1996;334:413–419.
10. Kloner RA, Poole WK, Perritt RL. When throughout the year is coronary death most likely to occur? A twelve-year population based analysis of over 220,000 cases. Circulation 1999;100:1630–1634.

11. DeBusk R, Drory Y, Goldstein J, et al. Management of sexual dysfunction in patients with cardiovascular disease: recommendations of the Princeton Consensus Panel. Am J Cardiol 2000;86:175–181.
12. Anderson KM, Wilson PW, Odell PM, et al. An updated coronary risk profile: a statement for health professionals. Circulation 1991;83:356–362.
13. Anderson KM, Odell PM, Wilson PW, et al. Cardiovascular disease risk profiles. Am Heart J 1993;121:293–298.
14. Moss AJ, Benhorin J. Prognosis and management after a first myocardial infarction. N Engl J Med 1990;322:743–753.
15. Mittleman MA, Maclure M, Tofler GH, et al. Triggering of acute myocardial infarction by heavy physical exertion. N Engl J Med 1993;329:1677–1683.
16. DeBusk RF. Evaluating the cardiovascular tolerance for sex. Am J Cardiol 2000; 86(Suppl):51F–56F.
17. Stein RA. Cardiovascular response to sexual activity. Am J Cardiol 2000;86 (Suppl):27F–29F.
18. Masters WH, Johnson VE. Human Sexual Response. Little, Brown and Co., Boston, 1966.
19. Hellerstein HK, Friedman EH. Sexual activity in the postcoronary patient. Arch Intern Med 1970;125:987–999.
20. Bohlen JG, Hel JP, Sanderson MO, et al. Heart rate, rate-pressure product, and oxygen uptake during four sexual activities. Arch Intern Med 1984;144: 1745–1748.
21. Stein RA. The effect of exercise training on heart rate during coitus in the post myocardial infarction patient. Circulation 1977;738–740.
22. Jackson G. Sexual intercourse and angina pectoris. Int. Rehab Med 1981;3:35–37.
23. Jackson G. Sexual intercourse and stable angina pectoris. Am J Cardiol 2000; 86(Suppl):35F–37F.
24. Namec ED, Mansfield L, Kennedy JW. Heart rate and blood pressure responses during sexual activity in normal males. Am Heart J 1976;92:274–277.
25. Pollock M, Schmidt DH. Heart Disease and Rehabilitation, 3rd ed. Human Kinetics, Champaign, IL, 1995, p. 372.
26. Larson JL, McNaughton MW, Kennedy JW, et al. Heart rate and blood pressure responses to sexual activity and stair-climbing test. Heart Lung 1980;9: 1025–1030.
27. Ueno M. The so-called coition death. Jpn J Legal Med 1969;17:333–340.
28. Drory Y, Shapira I, Fisman EZ, et al. Myocardial ischaemia during sexual activity in patients with coronary artery disease. Am J Cardiol 1995;75: 835–837.
29. Moreno PR, Lodder RA, O'Connor WN, et al. Characterization of vulnerable plaques by near infrared spectroscopy in an atherosclerotic rabbit model (abst.). J Am Coll Cardiol 1999;33(Suppl A):66A.
30. Feldman HA, Goldstein I, Hatzichristou DG, et al. Impotence and its medical and psychosocial correlates; results of the Massachusetts Male Aging Study. J Urol 1994;151:54–61.
31. Feldman HA, Johannes CB, Derby CA, et al. Erectile dysfunction and coronary risk factors: prospective results from the Massachusetts Male Aging Study. Preventive Med 2000;30:328–338.
32. Virag R, Bouilly P, Frydman D. Is impotence an arterial disorder? A study of arterial risk factors in 400 impotent men. Lancet 1985;322:181–184.
33. Kloner RA, Jarow J. Erectile dysfunction and sildenafil citrate and cardiologists. Am J Cardiol 1999;83:576–582.

34. Kloner RA. Cardiovascular risk and sildenafil. Am J Cardiol 2000;86(Suppl): 57F–61F.
35. Morales A, Gingell C, Collins M, et al. Clinical safety of oral sildenafil citrate (VIAGRA) in the treatment of erectile dysfunction. Int J Impot Res 1998; 10:69–74.
36. Kloner RA, Brown M, Prisant LM, et al., for the Sildenafil Study Group. Efficacy and safety of Viagra® (sildenafil citrate) in patients with erectile dysfunction taking concomitant antihypertensive agents. Am J Hypertens 2001;14:70–73.
37. Conti CR, Pepine CJ, Sweeney M. Efficacy and safety of sildenafil citrate in the treatment of erectile dysfunction in patients with ischemic heart disease. Am J Cardiol 1999;83(Suppl):29C–34C.
38. Zusman RM, Morales A, Glasser DB, et al. Overall cardiovascular profile of sildenafil citrate. Am J Cardiol 1999;83(Suppl):35C–44C.
39. Padma-Nathan H, Eardley I, Kloner RA, et al. A 4-year update on the safety of sildenafil citrate. Urology 2002;60(Suppl 213):67–90.
40. Kloner RA, Mohan P, Norenberg C, et al. Cardiovascular safety of vardenafil, a potent, highly selective PDE5 inhibitor in patients with erectile dysfunction: an analysis of five-controlled clinical trials. Pharmacotherapy 2002;22:1371.
41. Emmick JT, Stuewe SR, Mitchell M. Overview of the cardiovascular effects of tadalafil. Eur Heart J Suppl 2002;4(Suppl 14):H32–H47.
42. Wysowski DK, Farinas E, Swartz L. Comparison of reported and expected deaths in sildenafil (Viagra) users. Am J Cardiol 2002;89:1331–1334.
43. Arruda-Olson AM, Mahoney DW, Nehra A, et al. Cardiovascular effects of sildenafil during exercise in men with known or probable coronary artery disease. A randomized crossover trial. JAMA 2002;287:719–725.
44. Fox KM, Thadani U, Ma PT, et al. Time to onset of limiting angina during treadmill exercise in men with erectile dysfunction and stable chronic angina: effect of sildenafil citrate (abst). Circulation 2001;107:II601.
45. Thadani U, Smith W, Nash S, et al. The effect of vardenafil, a potent and highly selective phosphodiesterase-5 inhibitor for the treatment of erectile dysfunction, on the cardiovascular response to exercise in patients with coronary artery disease. J Am Coll Cardiol 2002;40:2006–2012.
46. Patterson D, MacDonald TM, Effron MB, et al. Tadalafil dose not affect time to ischemia during exercise stress testing in patients with coronary artery disease. Circulation 2002;106(Suppl II):II–330.
47. Hermann HC, Chang G, Klugherz BD, et al. Hemodynamic effects of sildenafil in men with severe coronary artery disease. N Engl J Med 2000;342:1662–1666.
48. Webb DJ, Freestone S, Allen MJ, et al. Sildenafil citrate and blood-pressure lowering drugs: results of drug interaction studies with an organic nitrate and a calcium antagonist. Am J Cardiol 1999;83(Suppl 5A):21C–28C.
49. Cheitlin MD, Hutter AM, Brindis RG, et al. ACC/AHA Expert Consensus Document. Use of sildenafil (Viagra) in patients with cardiovascular disease. J Am Coll Cardiol 1999;33:273–282.

16 Sex After Cardiac Events and Procedures

Counseling From the Cardiovascular Specialist's Perspective

Herman A. Taylor, Jr., MD, FACC, FAHA

CONTENTS

INTRODUCTION
WHAT YOUR PATIENTS ARE ACTUALLY DOING
IMPORTANCE OF RAISING THE ISSUE
ED, DEPRESSION, AND CVD
REASSURANCE AND PERSPECTIVE: PLACING SEXUALITY IN CONTEXT
AGE-SPECIFIC NORMS
COUNSELING AFTER THE EVENT
"SEXUAL REHABILITATION" AFTER CARDIAC EVENTS
ED POST-MI-SPECIFIC THERAPY
CONCLUSION
REFERENCES

INTRODUCTION

The current era of cardiovascular medicine has been referred to as a "golden age" because of the impressive array of technological and pharmaceutical tools at the disposal of the cardiologist and other cardiovascular (CV) specialists. However, most cardiologists and their col-

From: *Contemporary Cardiology: Heart Disease and Erectile Dysfunction*
Edited by: R. A. Kloner © Humana Press Inc., Totowa, NJ

leagues in CV health are more than technicians—we generally ascribe to ideals of medicine that seek to remove suffering and to do so in a more general sense than the merely biological. We certainly aim primarily to add years to life for our patients; however, increasingly we see a need to facilitate "adding life to their years." The cardiovascular literature is replete with publications on quality of life, consistent with the more "holistic" look at outcomes of our interventions.

Sexual intimacy is an important aspect of life for the vast majority of adults; impediments to sexual intercourse are barriers for expression of that intimacy and may result in a significant loss in quality of life. Perhaps the most common physical barrier to successful intercourse among patients with manifest cardiovascular disease (CVD) is male erectile dysfunction (ED). Studies cited earlier in this volume suggest that approximately half of the men with CVD also suffer from significant ED *(1)*. ED, therefore, represents a significant issue for our patients, although often they do not openly mention it. Furthermore, given data demonstrating that ED can play a role in the development of depression, ED can be an especially relevant concern of the cardiologist. Depression is lethal for cardiac patients *(2)*. Avoiding depression is helped by maintaining quality of life, which for many people implies a satisfactory sex life.

WHAT YOUR PATIENTS ARE ACTUALLY DOING

Current data (reviewed in preceding chapters) suggest that the prevalence of impaired sexual relationships is high among couples in which one of the partners has manifest heart disease. After myocardial infarction (MI), approximately one-fourth of patients report total cessation of sexual activity. About half describe their level of activity as reduced. Only about a quarter of patients claim that their level of activity did not change at all after the MI. This suggests that approximately 75% of post-MI patients have a significant lessening in their level of sexual activity. The vast majority of these patients do not have reduced left ventricular function or persistent coronary insufficiency as the underlying cause for this change *(3–5)*.

Coronary artery bypass surgery patients also report significant reduced sexual activity after the procedure, although the statistics appear to be substantially better than among the MI patients *(6)*. In a study of 134 surgery patients, 84 of the 92 previously sexually active and 2 of the inactive patients resumed sexual activity. Thirty-nine percent of patients decreased the frequency of intercourse. Fear was a significant factor for many couples: 17% of patients and 35% of their partners expressed fear of resumption of sexual activity. The couples who resumed sexual activity had a closer emotional relationship ($p < 0.02$). This study concluded that bypass surgery does not provide a net gain in sexual functioning compared with preoperative rates. However, much more optimistic (though still limited) data are reported from other groups. For instance, one Austrian study reported that rates of sexual activity rose substantially after surgery, from over 90% abstinence (often because of physician advice or fear) to 47% sexually active *(7)*.

Little is published regarding sexual habits after other procedures. Percutaneous coronary intervention appears to have less impact on sexual behavior than bypass surgery in the short term; however, by 15 month, there are no discernible differences in sexual activity between the two patient groups *(8)*. At a glance, automatic internal cardiac defibrillator (AICD) placement appears to have little impact on sexual behavior. However, the 59% "no change" status reported for AICD may include good and bad news: the usual AICD patient has severe coronary artery disease or congestive heart failure (CHF) and may start from a baseline of very low activity *(9)*. Similarly, transplantation appears to produce no change or a worsening in function in the large majority (71%) of transplant recipients *(10)*. Only approximately 8% of pacemaker recipients report improvement in frequency of sexual activity after the procedure is performed *(11)*.

Data on CHF are few. The available literature suggests that the diagnosis of CHF has dramatic impact on both libido and the actual activity of intercourse. A small study of 62 patients in Los Angeles with class III or IV CHF revealed that approximately 70% of them showed no interest or a marked loss of interest in sex after diagnosis. Only 25% reported no change in libido. Three-fourths of the group reported a marked decrease in sexual activity; nearly half of these had ceased intercourse altogether *(12)*.

These data suggest that the nature of the disease, or procedures a cardiovascular disease patient experiences, is a prominent factor in the level of sexual activity they assume. However, in each category of cardiac disease, a substantial fraction suffers significant impairment. For most, this is a source of concern.

IMPORTANCE OF RAISING THE ISSUE

Although the issues of survival and return to useful function are paramount after a CVD event or procedure, the impact of the event on the patient's relationship with his/her partner is usually a source of significant anxiety *(13)*. For the majority of patients, such worry includes concern over whether sexual intercourse can be safely resumed. However, this concern may frequently go unstated. Patients may feel a bit intimidated by the specialist, or that discussions about sex would distract from a focus on the heart disease. (S)he may fear that sex is an inappropriate, perhaps "trivial," concern given the seriousness of cardiovascular disease. Silence about sexual function may be particularly common among older patients who grew up at a time when societal norms were generally less permissive of frank discussions of sexuality. Also, the older patient may assume that sexual interest is inappropriate for the elderly or embarrassing evidence of misplaced priorities.

Such reticence appears to be waning. An increased willingness to discuss such issues (on survey questionnaires and with providers) has revealed that older men retain interest in sex into advanced ages *(14)*. Elderly women are also likely to be interested in sexual relationships if spouses or loving partners are available (the gender difference in longevity produces many more widows than widowers). Younger patients tend to be less inhibited in addressing this issue, and most expect an active sex life. Given this high prevalence of interest, the physician can feel reasonably certain that a discussion of the issue of sexual activity would be welcomed by most patients. The provider should, therefore, specifically raise the issue if the patient does not, after more urgent issues of prognosis and survival have been adequately discussed. The timing of such a discussion is highly individual, but most patients will signal readiness for such a talk with questions like, "Doctor, what can I do?" that is, how much physical exertion is safe. The best answer to this question may be readily apparent or may need to await exercise stress test results (see below). In either case, questions about physical limitations or return to work open the door for the important discussion about sex after MI, bypass, percutaneous coronary intervention, or other event. This is a juncture in the patient's recuperation that must be handled with sensitivity and confidence by the provider. Even if the patient is initially silent with regard to sex, the approbation implied by the physician's raising the topic may open the door for frank discussions when the patient is ready. For CVD patients, cardiovascular specialists may be among the most trusted to counsel on sexual activity, given their specialized knowledge of the potential risks of physical exertion and/or the specific therapies for ED.

Currently, most physicians do not elect to discuss sexual questions with their CVD patients *(15,16)* and thereby miss an important opportunity to impact their patients' overall well-being. Allowing sexual issues to surface and be faced directly will help avoid incorrect assumptions about the risk of an active sex life. Such assumptions, if left silent and uncorrected, may do significant harm to the patient's most important human relationship. As stated earlier, fear and/or ED (secondary to fear or physiology) are often twin challenges to sexual intimacy after CVD is manifest.

ED, DEPRESSION, AND CVD

There is a well-documented association between depression, ischemic heart disease, and cardiovascular mortality. The pioneering work of Frasure-Smith and subsequent studies by many others have shown that depression after MI is associated with increased cardiac mortality, that depressed patients have a higher than expected rate of sudden cardiovascular death, and also that patients with depression are at greater risk for developing fatal coronary disease than their nondepressed counterparts *(2,17)*.

As there is a clear association between depression and heart disease, there is also a well-documented association between sexual dysfunction (mainly ED) and depression. Depression may precede the ED, or, alternatively, sexual dysfunction may contribute to the development of depression. This latter pathway suggests another reason why sexual issues warrant discussion during consultation with cardiac patients *(18)*.

REASSURANCE AND PERSPECTIVE: PLACING SEXUALITY IN CONTEXT

After the subject is broached by doctor or patient, the physician must provide facts. The patient may be consumed with uncertainties: "Is having sex too risky? Will sexual activity damage my stent/pacemaker/AICD (or other device), or hurt my surgical site? When can I resume sexual activity? Will I be able to perform?" The patient's sexual partner may be stressed to at least the same degree: "Can (s)he really have sex now? Will it overtax his/her heart? What should I do if (s)he develops chest pain/shortness of breath? Am I being too selfish?" and so on. Such fears can cloud the couple's view of physical intimacy and may precipitate or aggravate various negative emotions such as anxiety, frustration, anger, denial, and even (as noted above) depression. A couple already coping with the stress of the illness and recuperation may suffer even more if such negative emotions develop in either partner. It is imperative that the physician/counselor be prepared and willing to provide perspective in this area.

AGE-SPECIFIC NORMS

First, it is helpful for the patient to have an understanding of some key aspects of sexuality and sexual responses in his/her age group.

Sexual function issues in CVD can be complicated by the fact that patients with manifest major CVD are usually middle-aged or older. This stage of life is visited by physiological changes in various organ systems. Most physicians (and many laypeople) are acquainted with normative changes associated with healthy aging, such as changes in muscle and bone mass, metabolic and endocrine changes associated with the menopause (for women), and other developments of mid-life. However, there is less general awareness of normal changes in the human sexual response.

The best data available suggest that the human sexual response undergoes a significant evolution over the lifespan. According to the Kinsey report of 1990 *(14)*, healthy older men experience fewer spontaneous erections, require more stimulation to achieve erections, and report that erections tend to be slightly less firm than in their youth. Once satisfactory erections are achieved, however, older men can generally sustain the act of intercourse for a longer time than their younger counterparts. Ejaculations tend to be less forceful in older men, and refractory time is longer.

Older women are the usual partners of older men. They experience less lubrication and, after menopause, greater sensitivity and fragility of vaginal tissues. Orgasms are physically less intense. Taken together with male changes listed above, sexual intercourse could be naturally more challenging in the advanced years, whether CVD is superimposed or not. Furthermore, these normative changes may be accelerated or aggravated in the CVD patient because of abnormal vascular function related to the atherosclerotic process, or to medications commonly used in these patients *(3–5)*.

The potential for these challenges to produce significant frustration is particularly high in the postevent/diagnosis patient. The CVD event may suddenly focus attention on changes in sexual response (and other physical capabilities) that may have been developing gradually prior to the event. Attribution of these changes to the cardiac event or disease or interpretation of them as further evidence of a decline in health status can be disheartening. Less lubrication and less intense orgasm in the female partner may cause additional worry about a loss of virility in the male partner. A psychologically mediated worsening of erectile function may occur. Erectile failure can initiate a vicious cycle of failure, increasing anxiety and frustration followed by more failure and worry. Ultimately, avoidance of sexual intimacy may become preferable to the negative emotions produced by attempting intercourse *(19)*.

However, awareness of age-related changes in physical responses in intercourse suggests specific actions couples can take to enhance their sexual relationships. With additional caveats specifically aimed at the cardiac patient and his partner, many couples can return to a high level of enjoyment of sex.

COUNSELING AFTER THE EVENT

The challenge before the couple seeking to resume sexual activity after a major CVD event involves re-establishing intimacy in the broadest sense. A major disruption has occurred in the life of the couple. To re-establish the connection between partners, it is essential that the partners be encouraged to relax, go slow, and focus on nonphysical dimensions of intimacy first *(20)*. This can be summarized as "dating behavior" or "romancing" one another. "Making love" should be thought of as a long series of interactions (many of which are non-physical and occur outside the bedroom) that create warm feelings between the partners. Deep communication, nongenital touching, caressing, and kissing are important parts of this phase of reconnection. This behavior can intensify sexual desire and arousal as well as produce many emotional rewards besides enhancing sex.

When actual intercourse is desired by the couple, the guiding principle again is to relax and go slow. One to 3 wk after MI is safe for most postevent patients without significant ischemia at 3–5 metabolic equivalents of the task . This level of activity is roughly equivalent to walking 2–4 mph on a level surface *(21)* or to the old "two flights of stairs" rule of thumb but is best tested formally by a graded exercise test *(22)*. Successful completion of stage 2 of a standard Bruce protocol (or equivalent) is good assurance that the exertion of sexual intercourse is safe.

Little data exist on the question of optimal timing after bypass surgery or angioplasty. Data from the 1980s suggest that the average time before resumption of sexual activity after bypass was greater than 7 wk *(7)*. Contemporary bypass procedures and rehabilitation practices may allow for a comfortable return to sexual intercourse sooner. Certainly, if substantial revascularization was successfully achieved, no cardiac reason exists for such a lengthy delay *(23)*. The degree of healing of the sternotomy wound is probably the key variable in well-revascularized postbypass patients. The Princeton Consensus Panel guidelines are useful for counseling the patient on his readiness to resume coitus.

Physical acts of sex should be timed to allow thorough relaxation, well after any large meal (2–3 h). A familiar, relaxed setting free of distraction should be chosen. The focus should be on a relaxed pace, romantic sensuality, and erotic foreplay. (Foreplay has low metabolic demands, allows intimate communication and functions as an effective "warm-up" period for any more strenuous activity to follow.) "Goal-oriented sex,"that is, the approach to sex that considers penetration and orgasm the measures of success/fulfillment, should be discouraged. After adequate "warm-up," if the couple wishes to progress to intercourse, they should be prepared to use lubricants to ease penetration. Also, even after prolonged foreplay, the male may require direct tactile stimulation of the penis to achieve adequate stiffness. Familiar, comfortable positions are best in most cases. Female-on-top may be the preferred position if the male is a recent postcoronary artery bypass grafting patient. If discomfort occurs during coitus, a rest should be taken. Intercourse should stop if symptoms of severe shortness of breath, dizziness, or angina occur. Such an occurrence should be reported to the physician. Sublingual nitroglycerin should be taken if prescribed for angina but avoided if the male patient has taken sildenafil *(24)*.

"SEXUAL REHABILITATION" AFTER CARDIAC EVENTS

Sexual intercourse brings a special level of closeness that most couples desire to resume. The good news is that for the large majority this is achievable. Cardiac rehabilitation programs may be especially helpful in this regard *(5,25)*. Monitored exercise is the core activity; however, modern cardiac rehabilitation is not exclusively focused on exercise training. Many programs integrate smoking cessation, diet and weight modification, information on lipid management, stress-coping techniques and other interventions into their protocol. Furthermore, abnormal developments in the patient's recuperation (e.g., uncontrolled blood pressure, blood sugar, or other risks; worrisome symptoms) can be detected by skilled nursing staff readily reported to the managing physician.

All of these features of cardiac rehabilitation programs have advantages for both the overall health and the sexual health of the postevent/ diagnosis patient. Because most ischemia during sexual activity occurs at elevated heart rates, exercise programs, which eventually lower the heart rate and blunt the tachycardic response to exertion, are specifically cardioprotective with regard to sex *(26)*. Smoking is associated with ischemia, MI, and sudden death; cessation substantially lowers that risk. Smoking is also directly associated with ED; cessation may improve penile blood flow and reduce the incidence of ED *(27)*. In addition to reducing measurable risk factor levels in the cardiac patient, rehabilitation builds confidence, as the patient demonstrates to himself and his partner an ability to tolerate significant exertion as the program progresses. The rebounding self-esteem this provides is of incalculable benefit to the patient's overall outlook and his sex life.

Rehabilitation programs also make educational tapes and literature available on a wide variety of topics, including sexuality for couples affected by CVD.

ED POST-MI-SPECIFIC THERAPY

Of the available therapies for ED, none are inherently dangerous for CVD patients if used within guidelines. Please see the other chapters of this book for detailed discussions of therapeutic approaches, potential drug interactions, and related topics. It is perhaps important to restate that the combination of nitrates and sildenafil can produce precipitous, and potentially dangerous, drops in blood pressure.

CONCLUSION

The advances in revascularization techniques, cardiac transplantation, cardiac devices, and other therapies have all improved the longevity and vigor of our patients. Along with these improving outcomes, patients also want a return to normal living. Indeed, the dream of reclaiming a normal life (or nearly so) is often the reason the patient consents to interventions. The vast majority of CVD patients are not sexually incapacitated by their disease. With modern therapeutic approaches and physician sensitivity and insight, a resumption of normal sexual relations can be accomplished in most cases.

REFERENCES

1. Dhabuwala CB, Kumar A, Pierce JM. Myocardial infarction and its influence on male sexual function. Arch Sex Behav 1986;15:499.
2. Lesperance F, Frasure-Smith N, Talajic M, et al. Five-year risk of cardiac mortality in relation to initial severity and one-year changes in depression symptoms after myocardial infarction. Circulation 2002;105:1049–1053.
3. Jackson G. Erectile dysfunction and cardiovascular disease. Int J Clin Pract 1999;53:363.
4. Drory Y, Kravetz S, Florian V, et al. Sexual activity after first acute myocardial infarction in middle-aged men: demographic, psychological, and medical predictors. Cardiology 1998;90:207.
5. Rosal MC, Downing J, Littman AB, et al. Sexual functioning post-myocardial infarction: effects of beta-blockers, psychological status and safety information. J Psychosom Res 1994;38:655.
6. Papadopoulos C, Shelley SI, Piccolo M, et al. Sexual activity after coronary bypass surgery. Chest 1986;90:681.

7. Penckofer SH, Holm K. Early appraisal of coronary revascularization on quality of life. Nurs Res. 1984;33:60–63.
8. Raft D, McKee DC, Popio KA, et al. Life adaptation after percutaneous transluminal coronary angioplasty and coronary artery bypass grafting. Am J Cardiol 1985;56:395–398.
9. Clinical Progress in Electrophysiology and Pacing. Futura Pub. Co., Mount Kisco, NY, 1985, p. 306.
10. Bunzel B, Wollenek G, Grundbock A, et al. Heart transplantation and sexuality. A study of 62 male patients [in German]. Herz 1994;19:294–302.
11. Mickley H, Petersen J, Nielsen BL. Subjective consequences of permanent pacemaker therapy in patients under the age of retirement. PACE Pacing Clin Electrohysiol 1989;12:401–405.
12. Jaarsma T, Dracup K, Walden J, et al. Sexual function in patients with advanced heart failure. Heart Lung 1996;25:262–270.
13. Egger J. "[Psychological adaptation in coronary patients]." Wien Med Wochenschr 1984;134361–367.
14. The Kinsey Institute new report on sex: what you must know to be sexually literate c1990. Reinisch, June Machover.
15. Papadopoulos C, Beaumont C, Shelley SI, et al. Myocardial infarction and sexual activity of the female patient. Arch Intern Med 1983;143:1528.
16. Papadopoulos C, Larrimore P, Cardin S, et al. Sexual concerns and needs of the postcoronary patient's wife. Arch Intern Med 1980;140:38.
17. Lesperance F, Frasure-Smith N. Depression in patients with cardiac disease: a practical review. J Psychosom Res 2000;48:379–391.
18. Goldstein I. The mutually reinforcing triad of depressive symptoms, cardiovascular disease, and erectile dysfunction. Am J Cardiol 2000;86:41F–45F.
19. Renshaw DC, Karstaedt A. Is there (sex) life after coronary bypasss? Comprehen Ther 1988;14:61–66.
20. Taylor HA Jr. Sexual activity and the cardiovascular patient: guidelines. Am J Cardiol 1999;84:6N–10N.
21. Bohlen JG, Geld JP, Sanderson MO, et al. Heart rate, rate-pressure product, and oxygen uptake during four sexual activities. Arch Intern Med 1984;144:1745.
22. DeBusk RF. Evaluating the cardiovascular tolerance for sex. Am J Cardiol 2000; 86:27F.
23. DeBusk R, Drory Y, Goldstein I, et al. Management of sexual dysfunction in patients with cardiovascular disease: recommendations of the Princeton Consensus Panel. Am J Cardiol 2000;86:62F.
24. Kloner RA. Cardiovascular risk and sildenafil. Am J Cardiol 2000;86:57F.
25. Papadopoulos C, Beaumont C, Shelley SI, et al. Myocardial infarction and sexual activity of the female patient. Arch Intern Med 1983;143:1528.
26. Stein RA. The effect of exercise training on heart rate during coitus in the post myocardial infarction patient. Circulation 1977;55:738–740.
27. Jeremy JY, Mikhailidis DP. Cigarette smoking and erectile dysfunction. J R Soc Health 1998;118:151–155.

17 American College of Cardiology/American Heart Association Guidelines on the Use of Sildenafil in Patients With Cardiovascular Disease

Adolph M. Hutter, Jr., MD, MACC

CONTENTS

INTRODUCTION
INFORMATION ON CARDIAC EFFECTS OF SILDENAFIL
  IN 1998
ACC/AHA RECOMMENDATIONS
NEW INFORMATION ON THE USE OF SILDENAFIL
  IN PATIENTS WITH CARDIOVASCULAR DISEASE
CURRENT PERSPECTIVE OF THE ACC/AHA
  GUIDELINES
REFERENCES

INTRODUCTION

The American College of Cardiology (ACC) and the American Heart Association (AHA) developed an Expert Consensus Document in 1999 on the use of sildenafil in patients with cardiovascular disease *(1)*. This type of document is intended to inform practitioners, payers, and other interested parties of the opinion of the ACC concerning evolving areas of clinical practice and/or technologies that are widely available or are

From: *Contemporary Cardiology: Heart Disease and Erectile Dysfunction*
Edited by: R. A. Kloner © Humana Press Inc., Totowa, NJ

new to the practice community. Topics chosen for coverage by the Expert Consensus document are so designated because the evidence base and experience with the technology or clinical practice are not sufficiently well developed to be evaluated by the formal ACC/AHA Practice Guidelines process. This is an attempt to inform and guide clinical practice in areas in which vigorous evidence is not yet available. Sildenafil, a selective inhibitor of phosphodiesterase-5 (PDE5), became widely available in 1998 for the treatment of erectile dysfunction (ED). In response to inquiries from various parties about the safety of using sildenafil in patients with cardiovascular disease, the ACC leadership decided to develop an Expert Consensus Document on this topic. The writing committee members were selected for specific expertise in clinical cardiology, managed care, vascular reactivity, nitric oxide donors and pharmacology of antihypertensive agents. The AHA was invited to jointly author the document. After the document was developed, 10 external referees reviewed the text. The final document was approved by the ACC Board of Trustees and the AHA Scientific Advisory Committee and published in January 1999 *(1)*.

INFORMATION ON CARDIAC EFFECTS OF SILDENAFIL IN 1998

The information available about the cardiovascular effects of sildenafil at the time of the recommendations indicated it was not present in cardiac myocytes and had no direct inotropic effects on isolated dog trabeculae muscle. Sildenafil is highly selective for PDE5 over human PDE3 (>4000-fold). This is important because cyclic adenosine monophosphate-specific PDE3 inhibitors (milrinone, vesnarinone, and enoximone) have been shown to increase long-term mortality in patients with heart failure *(2,3)*. At the time of the recommendations, however, little information was available about the use of sildenafil in patients with congestive heart failure (CHF).

Sildenafil causes a transient modest reduction in systolic (8–10 mmHg) and diastolic (5–6 mmHg) blood pressure, with a peak effect occurring about 1 h after the dose. The hypotensive effects of sildenafil were neither age dependent nor dose related. No significant effects were observed on heart rate. In normal volunteers, oral sildenafil caused no significant changes in cardiac index. The drug has both arteriodilator and venodilator effects on the peripheral vasculature.

Nitrates were known to markedly amplify the hypotensive effects of sildenafil leading to dangerous drops in blood pressure and clinical events. The effect was assumed to occur for up to 24 h after a dose of sildenafil based on the pharmacokinetics of sildenafil (five half lives). Similarly, there was concern about patients taking sildenafil in the 24 h period after taking a nitrate, because the presence of even trace amounts of nitrates may have unknown effects on the action of sildenafil.

Limited information was available about the use of sildenafil in conjunction with single antihypertensive drugs, and there was virtually none available about using the drug in patients on multiple antihypertensive agents.

ACC/AHA RECOMMENDATIONS

Based on information available in 1998, the ACC/AHA recommendations are summarized as follows (1):

1. Sildenafil is absolutely contraindicated in patients taking any nitrate drug therapy because of the risk of developing potentially life-threatening hypotension.
2. Nitrates should not be taken for 24 h after use of sildenafil, and sildenafil should not be used for 24 h after taking nitrates.
3. The use of an exercise test before taking sildenafil is recommended in patients with coronary artery disease (CAD) to assess the risk of cardiac ischemia during sexual intercourse. "If the patient can achieve >5–6 METS on an exercise test without ischemia, the risk of ischemia during coitus with a familiar partner, in familiar settings, without the added stress of a heavy meal or alcohol ingestion, is probably low. We wish to stress that the physical and emotional stresses of sexual intercourse can be excessive in some people, particularly those who have not performed this activity in some time and who are not in good condition. These stresses themselves may produce acute ischemia or precipitate myocardial infarction. Such patients should be advised to use common sense and to moderate their physical exertion and their emotional expectations" as they resume sex.
4. Caution was raised about the use of sildenafil in patients on antihypertensive medications because of the "possibility of sildenafil-induced hypotension." "Initial monitoring of the blood pressure with the institution of sildenafil" would "identify patients with an undesired hypotensive blood pressure response. This is an area of particular concern for the patient with congestive heart failure who has a borderline low blood volume and a low blood pressure status as well as for the patient who is following a complicated, multidrug antihypertensive therapy regimen."

NEW INFORMATION ON THE USE OF SILDENAFIL IN PATIENTS WITH CARDIOVASCULAR DISEASE

Since these recommendations were published in 1999 the safety of using this drug has been reported in a large number of patients including those with CAD, those on multiple antihypertensive agents, and those with CHF.

Angina

Sildenafil has no deleterious effects during exercise in patients with CAD and stable angina. In one study of 105 such men, sildenafil lowered resting systolic blood pressure (4.3 mmHg) and diastolic blood pressure (3.7 mmHg) more than placebo *(4)*. There was no difference in the resting or exercise heart rate, exercise capacity, or exercise blood pressure. There was also no difference between sildenafil and placebo in symptoms with exercise, in exercise-induced electrocardiographic changes, or exercise-induced wall motion abnormalities. The resting and exercise ejection fraction were also not affected by sildenafil compared with placebo. In another study of 118 evaluable patients randomized to sildenafil or placebo, there was no difference in time to 1-mm ST depression or total exercise. Sildenafil actually prolonged the time to angina compared with placebo ($p = 0.04$) *(5)*.

Congestive Heart Failure

Bocchi et al. *(6)* studied the effects of sildenafil on the exercise performance in patients with CHF. They found that sildenafil reduced resting heart rate, systolic blood pressure, and diastolic blood pressure. It actually increased exercise time and oxygen consumption while not changing the duration of exercise, the exercise systolic blood pressure, exercise diastolic blood pressure, or peak heart rate. It had no effect on norepinephrine levels and actually reduced renin activity. Thus, sildenafil was beneficial to the exercise performance in patients with CHF.

Safety in CAD

Sildenafil has now been used by millions of men throughout the world and has no associated increase in risk of serious cardiovascular events or myocardial infarction (MI) in placebo-controlled studies or in open label studies *(7)*. A review of 53 clinical trials, including 30 double-blind, placebo-controlled and 23 open-label trials, showed no difference between placebo and sildenafil in the incidence of MI or death *(7)*. Furthermore, the rate of MI or ischemic heart death as tested by prescription event monitoring in 5000 English men was similar to those of the general population of men *(8)*.

Safety With Antihypertensive Agents

Sildenafil has also been used in thousands of men receiving antihypertensive agents. Zussman *(9)* found that the mild reduction in blood pressure was similar for sildenafil doses of 50, 100, and 200 mg. Kloner et al. assessed the safety of sildenafil in men with ED taking multiple antihypertensive agents *(10)*. The investigators performed a subanalysis of patients in 18 double-blind, placebo-controlled studies. The studies included 4274 men, 1393 of whom were taking antihypertensive medications, of which 704 were in the sildenafil group. Of the 2881 patients not taking any antihypertensive agents, 1827 were randomized to sildenafil. There was no increase incidence of angina, coronary artery disorder, or MI in the patients taking one, two, three, or more antihypertensive agents compared to the patients taking no antihypertensive agents. Hypotension occurred in less than 1% of patients taking two antihypertensive drugs and less than 1% of patients on no antihypertensive drugs. It did not occur in patients on one, three, or more antihypertensive drugs. Thus, the incidences of treatment-related adverse cardiovascular events were negligible and similar to those observed in patients not taking antihypertensive drugs.

CURRENT PERSPECTIVE OF THE ACC/AHA GUIDELINES

In my opinion, the ACC/AHA guidelines are clearly still valid concerning the absolute contraindication of using nitrates and sildenafil together. Nitrates should not be used within 24 h of sildenafil (about five half-lives for sildenafil). The duration between nitrates and other PDE5 inhibitors should be increased for PDE5 inhibitors with a longer half life. Similarly, sildenafil should not be used while nitrates are still in the body even in trace amounts. Thus, 24 h seems to be a reasonable interval after the duration of action of the last nitrate use.

A screening exercise test looking for active ischemia before resuming sex is still a rational recommendation for patients with stable ischemic heart disease who are not taking nitrates.

It makes sense to monitor the blood pressure of patients with borderline low blood pressure after taking sildenafil. This can be performed by the patient himself with a home blood pressure cuff. I usually advise patients to check their blood pressure 30 min after taking 25 mg of sildenafil and then, at another time, to check it after 50 mg and then 100 mg if that dose is needed. If no untoward drop in blood pressure occurs, the patient can then use sildenafil for the purpose of having intercourse without worrying about his blood pressure.

I think there is now no concern about using sildenafil in patients with CHF as long as the congestion is controlled and the blood pressure is in normal range. There are now extensive data indicating that sildenafil is perfectly safe in patients on multiple antihypertensive agents as long as their blood pressure is not too low. If it is, the antihypertensive agents can be reduced. Thus, the caution expressed in the original guidelines in these two groups of patients is probably no longer warranted.

The vast majority of patients with cardiovascular disease can safely use sildenafil. Because of effective preventive and therapeutic therapy, cardiovascular disease, especially CAD, has become a chronic disease that people can live with rather than die of. Therefore, quality of life is important to these people and sexual activity is important for a good quality of life for most people. We, as physicians, should inquire about sexual activity when we evaluate our patients and should point out to both men and women that there are now effective agents which can safely help ease ED in men with cardiovascular disease.

REFERENCES

1. Cheitlin MD, Hutter AM Jr., Brindis RG, et al. Use of sildenafil (Viagra) in patients with cardiovascular diseases. Circulation 1999;99:168–177; J Am Coll Cardiol 1999;33:273–282.
2. Packer M, Carver JR, Rodenheffer RJ, et al. Effect of oral milrinone on mortality in severe chronic heart failure: the PROMISE Study Research Group. N Engl J Med 1991;325:1468–1475.
3. Nony P, Boissel JP, Lievre M, et al. Evaluation of the effect of phosphodiesterase inhibitors on mortality in chronic heart failure patients: a meta-analysis. Eur J Clin Pharmacol 1994;46:191–196.
4. Arruda-Olson AM, Mahoney DW, Nehra A, et al. Cardiovascular effects of sildenafil during exercise in men with known or probable coronary artery disease: a randomized crossover trial. JAMA 2002;287:719–725.
5. Jackson G, Keltai M, Gillies H, et al. Viagra is well-tolerated by subjects with stable angina and erectile dysfunction during incremental treadmill exercise. Eur Urol 2002;1(Suppl 1):151.
6. Bocci EA, Guimaraes G, Mocelin A, et al. Sildenafil effects on exercise, neurohormonal activation, and erectile dysfunction in congestive heart failure: a double-blind, placebo-controlled, randomized study followed by a prospective treatment for erectile dysfunction. Circulation 2002;106:1097–1103.
7. Mittleman MA, Glasser D, Orazem J, et al. Incidence of myocardial infarction and death in 53 clinical trials of viagra (abst). J Am Coll Cardiol 2000;35 (Suppl 1):302A.

8. Shakir SAW, Wilton CV, Heeley E, et al. Sildenafil prescription-event monitoring study. No evidence of an increase in cardiovascular outcomes among 5000 men prescribed sildenafil in general practice in England. J Am Coll Cardiol 2001;37 (Suppl A):1302–162.
9. Zusman RA, Morales A, Glasser DB, et al. Overall cardiovascular profile of sildenafil citrate. Am J Cardiol 1999;83:35C–44C.
10. Kloner RA, Brown M, Prisant LM, et al. Efficacy and safety of Viagra (sildenafil citrate) in patients with erectile dysfunction taking concomitant antihypertensive therapy. Am J Hypertens 2001;14:70–73.

18 Risk of Heart Attack After Sexual Activity
The Princeton Guidelines and Their Rationale

Robert F. DeBusk, MD

CONTENTS

BACKGROUND
DETERMINANTS OF SEXUAL FUNCTIONING
CARDIOLOGIC ASPECTS OF SEXUAL FUNCTIONING
ASSESSMENT OF PATIENTS WITH ESTABLISHED
 CORONARY ARTERY DISEASE
DIAGNOSTIC TESTING
THERAPEUTIC INTERVENTIONS FOR CAD
ASSESSMENT OF PATIENTS AT HIGH RISK FOR CAD
CLINICAL MANAGEMENT OF CAD
CONCLUSION
REFERENCES

BACKGROUND

Erectile dysfunction (ED) is a clinical condition affecting nearly one-third of men ages 40–70 yr *(1)*. Since the release of sildenafil in 1998, more than 10 million men with ED have received this agent *(2)*. Double-blind and postmarketing studies have demonstrated the safety of sildenafil in men with ED *(3)*. However, there is concern among the public and the medical profession that patients undergoing treatment with sildenafil may experience acute myocardial infarction (MI) and

From: *Contemporary Cardiology: Heart Disease and Erectile Dysfunction*
Edited by: R. A. Kloner © Humana Press Inc., Totowa, NJ

death related to sexual activity. This concern prompted a multidisciplinary conference in 1999 at Princeton, New Jersey, that considered the risks associated with sexual activity and developed guidelines for evaluating the risk of heart attack after sexual activity *(4)*.

DETERMINANTS OF SEXUAL FUNCTIONING

Determinants of lifelong sexual functioning include sociocultural as well as biological factors. Among the former are sexual desire, arousal, and satisfaction, which are culturally determined. Among the latter are aging and vascular disease involving the penile and coronary circulation. Complex interactions exist among these factors: even healthy young men may experience psychogenic ED. Among older individuals with or without cardiovascular symptoms, ED may result from occult vascular disease, medication used to treat vascular disease and its antecedents (diabetes, hypertension), and the psychological sequelae of acute vascular events such as acute MI—or from various combinations of all of these *(5,6)*. Thus, in evaluating the cardiovascular tolerance for sexual activity in older individuals, it is important to explore the expectations for sexual activity of patients and their partners. Many patients elect to discontinue sexual activity after the onset of clinical coronary artery disease, even in the absence of limiting cardiac symptoms or an unfavorable prognosis. For them and for their partners, sexual activity may have been unsatisfying before the onset of coronary artery disease. Such patients may be reluctant to broach the subject of sexual activity with their physicians. Likewise, physicians are often reluctant to initiate the discussion of an aspect of their patients' lives about which they know little *(7)*.

CARDIOLOGIC ASPECTS OF SEXUAL FUNCTIONING

Physicians' reluctance may result also from their uncertainty about how to address patients' concern over the safety of sexual activity. The concern of the physician is at two levels: What is the cardiovascular tolerance of the individuals for sexual activity? Also, what is the physiologic demand of sexual activity for the individual patient? The former can be addressed by techniques familiar to the physicians such as exercise testing *(8)*, but the latter requires discussion with the patient that many physicians are reluctant to initiate. In general, patients who can climb two flights of stairs without cardiovascular symptoms will be free of such symptoms during sexual activity *(9)*. Among sedentary patients, an exercise test can provide insights into the threshold at which cardiovascular symptoms, if any, occur.

Reassuring patients about the risk of heart attack and sudden cardiac death associated with sexual activity is more problematic. This is because most acute coronary events result from rupture of vulnerable but nonobstructive coronary artery plaques *(10)*. Therefore, the absence of exercise-induced ST segment depression or angina does not exclude the possibility of an acute coronary event such as MI or death. However, only 1% of heart attacks are associated with sexual activity *(11)*.

ASSESSMENT OF PATIENTS WITH ESTABLISHED CORONARY ARTERY DISEASE

The Princeton Conference addressed two important methodologic issues in evaluating the diagnosis and prognosis of patients with documented or suspected coronary artery disease (CAD). The first issue is diagnostic: the coronary lesions responsible for acute coronary events are heterogeneous. The thin-walled, nonobstructive coronary plaques that account for most coronary events generally do not cause myocardial ischemia that can be detected by noninvasive testing *(12)*. Even coronary angiography does not resolve the issue, for there are presently no techniques that reliably distinguish vulnerable plaques from stable ones. The second issue is prognostic: currently available diagnostic techniques cannot reliably identify the individual patients who are destined to experience acute coronary events.

These are not new issues, and they are not likely to be resolved soon. The challenge to the clinician is to advise patients with ED on how to decrease their risk of future cardiac events, including those related to sexual activity. Patients with ED exhibit a greater number of coronary risk factors and experience a greater frequency of acute coronary events than patients without ED *(13)*. Likewise, patients who have experienced acute coronary events exhibit a higher prevalence of ED than patients who have not experienced acute coronary events such as unstable angina pectoris, acute MI, and sudden coronary death *(14)*.

The management approach adopted by the Princeton conference is one of stepwise risk stratification based on evaluation of coronary risk factors, historical features, and the results of specialized cardiac testing (Fig. 1). The clinical evaluation is designed to distinguish the great majority of patients (60–70%) who are at low risk from the minority of patients (10–15%) who are high risk, based largely on clinical and standard laboratory measurements. This leaves approximately 15–30%

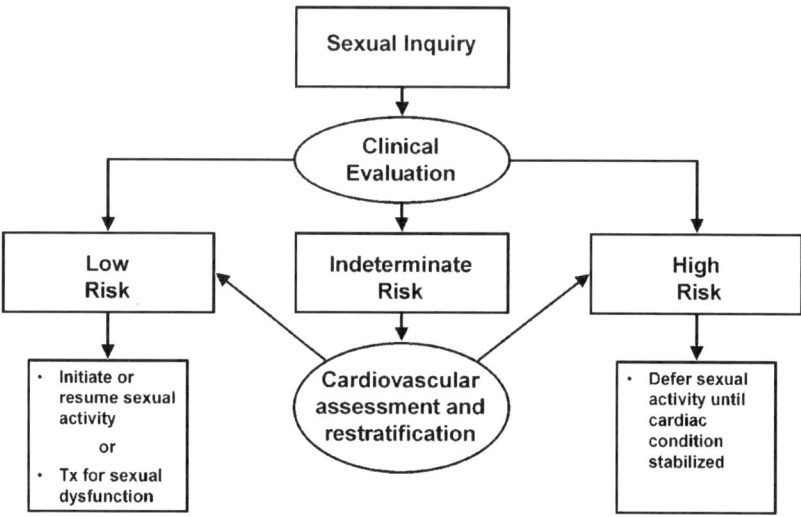

Fig. 1. Stepwise risk stratification and patient management. Tx, treatment.

of patients whose risks lie between the low- and high-risk groups. Specialized cardiac testing is often useful in reclassifying these intermediate-risk patients into low- or high-risk categories. Accordingly, many moderate- to high-risk patients will be referred to cardiologists for further assessment. In general, the low-risk patients described below do not require cardiologic evaluation.

Low-risk patients are described in Table 1. These patients experience a relatively low-risk for acute coronary events, including those associated with sexual activity. Coronary risk factors used in this classification include age, male sex, postmenopausal female, hypertension, diabetes, cigarette smoking, dyslipidemia, obesity, and sedentary lifestyle. Low-risk patients are asymptomatic. They can be advised to initiate pharmacotherapy for ED without the need for further diagnostic evaluation.

High-risk patients are described in Table 2. They are often symptomatic as a result of angina pectoris or heart failure. Patients who experience ongoing cardiac symptoms after an acute cardiac event often discontinue sexual activity, especially if their concerns are reinforced by their sexual partner. Even asymptomatic patients with a good prognosis based on clinical information may elect to discontinue sexual activity. The patient's decision to forego sexual activity often forecloses the opportunity for a medical evaluation that could dissipate unwarranted concerns about prognosis in general and the risks of sexual activity in particular. Before these patients are considered for pharmacotherapy for ED, they should receive treatments designed to reduce

Table 1
Low-Risk Features

Asymptomatic, <3 major risk factors for CAD
Controlled hypertension
Mild, stable angina
Post-successful coronary revascularization
Uncomplicated post-MI (>6–8 wk)
Mild valvular disease
Mild heart failure

CAD, coronary artery disease; wk, week; Post-MI, post-myocardial infarction.

Table 2
High-Risk Features

Unstable or refractory angina
Uncontrolled hypertension
Moderate/severe heart failure
Recent MI (<2 wk), CVA
High-risk arrhythmias
Cardiomyopathies
Moderate/severe valvular disease

Wk, week; MI, myocardial infarction; CVA, cerebrovascular accident.

Table 3
Intermediate-Risk Features

≥3 major risk factors for CAD, other than gender
Moderate, stable angina
Recent MI (> 2, < 6 wk)
Moderate heart failure
Cerebrovascular or peripheral vascular disease

CAD, coronary artery disease; Wk, week; MI, myocardial infarction.

their risk of subsequent cardiac events. This may entail anti-ischemic pharmacotherapy such as β-blockers, angiotensin-converting enzyme inhibitors, statins, and antiplatelet agents, or percutaneous coronary interventions, such as percutaneous transluminal coronary angioplasty or coronary artery bypass grafting surgery.

Intermediate-risk patients are described in Table 3. These patients exhibit a pattern of coronary risk factors and historical features that falls between low- and high-risk groups. Specialized cardiovascular testing is of particular value in stratifying the risk of this group of patients. The chief determinants of risk in these patients are the extent of myocardial ischemia, the extent of left ventricular dysfunction, and the risk factor profile.

DIAGNOSTIC TESTING

Treadmill exercise testing has been used for many years to stratify prognosis in patients with coronary artery disease, including those who are recovering from acute cardiac events *(15)*. Adverse prognostic features on the exercise test include a low peak workload (less than 5 metabolic equivalents of the task [METS]), low heart rate and blood pressure, and marked ischemic ST segment depression >0.2 mV that occurs at a low heart rate and workload, especially if it persists for greater than 3 min after the cessation of exercise. Angina that limits exercise to a workload less than 5 or 6 METS or persists for more than 3 min after the cessation of exercise is likewise an adverse prognostic feature. Standardized exercise testing is appropriate for patients with an interpretable baseline electrocardiogram (ECG), that is, no evidence of left bundle branch block or resting ST segment depression. In the presence of these confounding ECG features, the sensitivity and specificity of exercise testing may be augmented by techniques for evaluating myocardial perfusion and left ventricular wall motion. Patients who are unable to exercise because of musculoskeletal limitations, extreme debility, or other noncardiac limitations may undergo pharmacologic stress testing performed at rest *(16)*. Patients with evidence of marked myocardial ischemia on exercise or pharmacologic stress testing, especially at a low heart rate and workload, should be considered for coronary angiography and revascularization. However, even marked ischemic ST segment depression at a high heart rate and workload generally are associated with a good prognosis.

THERAPEUTIC INTERVENTIONS FOR CAD

Coronary revascularization should be based on symptoms that are significantly limiting or the demonstration of one or more of the adverse prognostic features described previously. The urgency to proceed to coronary revascularization after acute coronary events has been muted in recent years by the dramatic improvements in prognosis resulting from the use of aggressive combination pharmacotherapy, including angiotensin-converting enzyme inhibitors, β-blockers, statins, and antiplatelet agents *(17,18)*. The effects of these agents may be evident within weeks or months. Because CAD is increasingly being understood as a diffuse condition, mediated in large part by an inflammatory process involving the coronary plaque, it is appropriate to consider pharmacotherapy as the mainstay of treatment in most patients recovering from acute cardiac events.

Exercise testing is often valuable in assessing patients' capacity for sexual activity, especially in habitually sedentary individuals. Angina that occurs exclusively with sexual activity is rare, except in habitually sedentary individuals for whom sexual activity may be the most strenuous of their customary activities. Patients capable of completing a treadmill exercise workload equivalent to 6 or more METS or multiples of resting oxygen consumption without cardiovascular symptoms generally are asymptomatic during sexual activity. Exercise testing is especially recommended for patients who report coital angina. Such testing helps to establish the threshold at which angina occurs and the magnitude of ischemic ST segment depression that is associated with coital angina.

ASSESSMENT OF PATIENTS AT HIGH RISK FOR CAD

The stepwise approach to risk factor modification adopted by the Princeton conference is of particular value to patients who have clinically manifest coronary artery disease. Patients with subclinical coronary artery disease, who exhibit only coronary risk factors, present a more difficult challenge. For example, patients with one or more coronary risk factors number approximately 100 million, of whom 50 million are at high risk for CAD based on the presence of two or more coronary risk factors (19). These patients are classified as high-risk for CAD. Likewise, among the 18 million patients with clinically manifest CAD (angina, MI, history of coronary revascularization) approximately 9 million are at high risk for subsequent cardiac events based on two or more cardiovascular risk factors (20). These patients are classified as high-risk CAD.

Among the 50 million patients at high risk for CAD, approximately 10% exhibit exercise-induced myocardial ischemia (21). Among the 9 million high-risk CAD patients, approximately 33% will exhibit exercise-induced myocardial ischemia (Fig. 2). Based on epidemiologic studies, as many as 40% of the 50 million patients at high risk for CAD harbor vulnerable but nonobstructive coronary plaques (Fig. 3). Thus, noninvasive exercise testing fails to detect the great majority of the 20 million patients with vulnerable but clinically silent plaques (Fig. 3). Likewise, up to 4 million (40%) of the 9 million high-risk CAD patients harbor vulnerable plaques. As noted previously, about half of the ischemic treadmill responses in these individuals reflect obstruc-

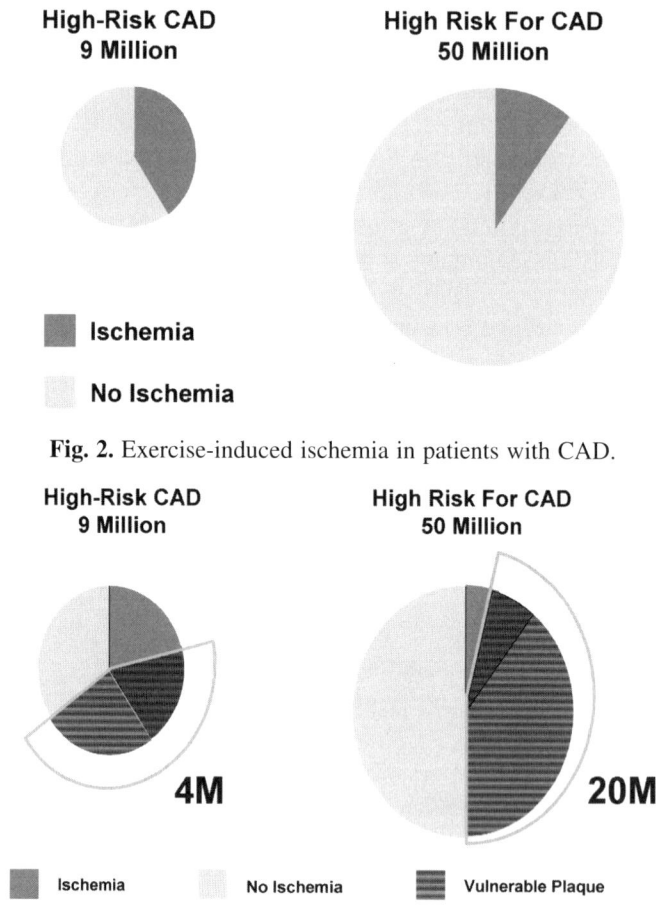

Fig. 2. Exercise-induced ischemia in patients with CAD.

Fig 3. Prevalence of vulnerable plaque in patients with CAD. M, million

tive but stable plaques. Nonobstructive plaques generally do not cause myocardial ischemia. However, patients with nonobstructive plaques may also harbor obstructive plaques that do cause myocardial ischemia. Indeed, nonobstructive coronary plaques are more numerous than obstructive ones: For every obstructive plaque, there may be as many as three nonobstructive plaques (Fig. 4).

CLINICAL MANAGEMENT OF CAD

The inability to identify patients with vulnerable plaques based on noninvasive testing has important clinical consequences. Among the 20 million patients at high risk for CAD based on the presence of vulnerable coronary artery plaques, the incidence of acute MI and

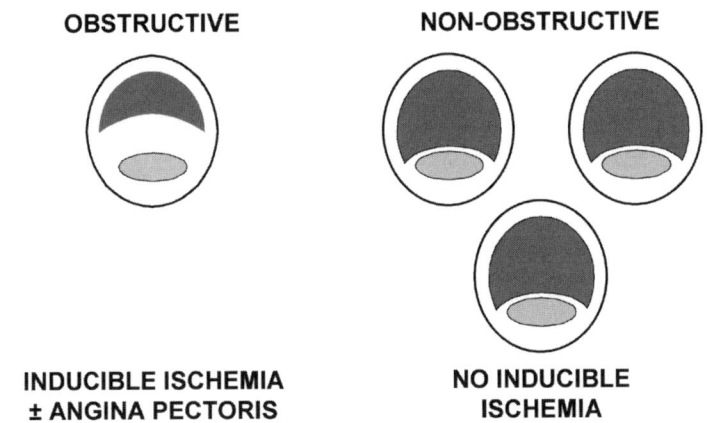

Fig. 4. Pattern of coronary plaques.

death is about 2% per year, accounting for a total of 400,000 new events annually. Among the 4 million high-risk patients with CAD, the annual incidence of acute MI and death is about 4%, accounting for a total of 160,000 new events annually. Thus, the number of new cases of acute MI and death occurring annually is more than twice as great in patients at high risk for CAD as in high-risk patients with CAD. This is a compelling indication for a broad-based preventive approach based on risk factor modification and the use of aggressive pharmacotherapy to stabilize the widespread vulnerable coronary artery plaques that are responsible for the great majority of acute coronary events. Considering that only 1% of all acute MIs are related to sexual activity, it is clear that the appropriate evaluation and management of patients with ED must incorporate the principles of comprehensive care.

CONCLUSION

A stepwise approach to risk stratification combined with an individualized approach to treatment of clinical or subclinical coronary artery disease will enable most patients with ED to continue or resume sexual activity with safety.

REFERENCES

1. Feldman HA, Goldstein I, Hatzichristou DG, et al. Impotence and its medical and psychosocial correlates: results of the Massachusetts Male Aging Study. J Urol 1994;151:54–61.
2. Padma-Nathan H, Eardley I, Kloner RA, et al. A 4-year update on the safety of sildenafil citrate (Viagra). Urology 2002;60(2 Suppl 2):67–90.

3. Osterloh I, Gillies H, Siegel R, et al. Efficacy and safety of VIAGRA™ (sildenafil citrate). Presented at the 4th Congress of the European Society for Sexual and Impotence Research; September 30–October 3, 2001, Rome, Italy.
4. DeBusk R, Drory Y, Goldstein I, et al. Management of sexual dysfunction in patients with cardiovascular disease: recommendations of the Princeton Consensus Panel. Am J Cardiol 2000;86:62F–68F.
5. Jackson G, Betteridge J, Dean J, et al. A systematic approach to erectile dysfunction in the cardiovascular patient: a consensus statement. Int J Clin Pract 1999;53:445–451.
6. Grimm RH Jr, Grandits GA, Prineas RJ, et al. Long-term effects on sexual function of five antihypertensive drugs and nutritional hygienic treatment in hypertensive men and women. Treatment of Mild Hypertension Study (TOMHS). Hypertension 1997;29:8–14.
7. Levine LA, Kloner RA. Importance of asking questions about erectile dysfunction. Am J Cardiol 2000;86:1210–1213,A1215.
8. DeBusk RF. Evaluating the cardiovascular tolerance for sex. Am J Cardiol 2000; 86:51F–56F.
9. Muller JE, Mittleman A, Maclure M, et al. Triggering myocardial infarction by sexual activity. Low absolute risk and prevention by regular physical exertion. Determinants of Myocardial Infarction Onset Study Investigators. JAMA 1996; 275:1405–1409.
10. Kullo IJ, Edwards WD, Schwartz RS. Vulnerable plaque: pathobiology and clinical implications. Ann Intern Med 1998;129:1050–1060.
11. Muller TE, Mittleman MA, Maclure M, et al. Triggering Myocardial Infarction by Sexual Activity. JAMA 1996;275:1405–1409.
12. Prakash M, Myers J, Froelicher VF, et al. Clinical and exercise test predictors of all-cause mortality: results from > 6,000 consecutive referred male patients. Chest 2001;120:1003–1013.
13. Kloner RA. Cardiovascular risk and sildenafil. Am J Cardiol 2000;86:57F–61F.
14. Jackson G. Erectile dysfunction and cardiovascular disease. Int J Clin Pract 1999;53:363–368.
15. Pryor DB, Bruce RA, Chaitman BR, et al. Task Force I: Determination of prognosis in patients with ischemic heart disease. J Am Coll Cardiol 1989;14: 1016–1025.
16. Kim C, Kwok YS, Heagerty P, et al. Pharmacologic stress testing for coronary disease diagnosis: a meta-analysis. Am Heart J 2001;142:934–944.
17. Gibbons RJ, Abrams J, Chatterjee K, et al. ACC/AHA 2002 guideline update for the management of patients with chronic stable angina—summary article: a report of the American College of Cardiology/American Heart Association Task Force on Practice Guidelines (Committee on the Management of Patients With Chronic Stable Angina). Circulation 2003;107:149–158.
18. Klungel OH, Heckbert SR, de Boer A, et al. Lipid-lowering drug use and cardiovascular events after myocardial infarction. Ann Pharmacother 2002;36:751–757.
19. Lloyd-Jones DM, Larson MG, Beiser A, et al. Lifetime risk of developing coronary heart disease. Lancet 1999;353:89–92.
20. Gotto AM Jr. High-density lipoprotein cholesterol and triglycerides as therapeutic targets for preventing and treating coronary artery disease. Am Heart J 2002; 144:S33–S42.
21. Ghayoumi A, Raxwal V, Cho S, et al. Prognostic value of exercise tests in male veterans with chronic coronary artery disease. J Cardiopulm Rehabil 2002; 399–440.

INDEX

A

Acetylcholine
  endothelium-dependent
    vasodilation, 210
Adenosine
  sildenafil citrate (Viagra), 185
Adrenergic antagonists, 30
Adverse effects
  sildenafil citrate (Viagra), 77–81
Aging process
  erectile response, 7, 9
  sexual activity, 265–267
    cardiovascular response,
      245–246
    specific norms, 265–267
AICD
  sexual activity, 263
Alcohol use, 29
  apomorphine SL (Uprima),
    197–198
Alprostadil (prostaglandin E1), 20,
  66, 199–201
  cardiovascular effects, 199–201
  intracavernous administration,
    199–200
  mechanism, 199
  topical administration, 200–201
  transurethral administration, 200
Alprox-TD, 200–201
American College of Cardiology
  nitrates and sildenafil, 148
  phosphodiesterase type-5 (PDE5)
    inhibitors, 257–258
  sildenafil prescribing practices, 145
  cardiovascular disease
    patients, 271–276
American Heart Association
  nitrates and sildenafil, 148
  phosphodiesterase type-5 (PDE5)
    inhibitors, 257–258
  sildenafil prescribing practices, 145
  cardiovascular disease
    patients, 271–276
Amitriptyline, 10, 30
Amoxapine, 10
Angina
  sexual activity triggering, 248,
    255–256
  sildenafil citrate (Viagra), 218, 274
  tadalafil with, 151
Angioplasty
  sexual activity resumption, 267
Angiotensin-converting enzyme
  inhibitors, 10
Angiotensin receptor blockers
  tadalafil with, 154
Anorgasmia, 58
Antiandrogen hormones, 30
Antidepressants, 10, 22, 29, 30, 54
Antihypertensives, 10, 22, 28–29
  apomorphine SL (Uprima)
    with, 198
  sildenafil citrate (Viagra) with,
    145, 275
Antipsychotics, 10
Anxiety, 50, 55–56
  performance, 56–57
Apomorphine SL (Uprima), 196–199
  alcohol use, 197–198
  with antihypertensives, 198
  cardiovascular effects, 197
  drug interactions, 197–198
Arginase, 4–5
Arousal. *see* Sexual activity
Arrhythmogenesis
  sildenafil citrate (Viagra), 190–191
Arteriogenic
  erectile dysfunction, 32

Atenolol
  sildenafil citrate (Viagra), 218
Atherosclerosis, 23
Automatic internal cardiac
    defibrillator (AICD)
  sexual activity, 263
Autonomic nerves
  erectile dysfunction, 32
Awakening
  time of, 252

B

β-adrenergic antagonists, 30
Binuclear manganese
    metalloenzyme, 4–5
Brief Male Sexual Function
    Inventory for Urology, 26
Bruce treadmill exercise test, 243

C

cAMP. *see* Cyclic adenosine
    monophosphate (cAMP)
Carbamazepine, 10
Cardiac applications
  phosphodiesterase type-5 (PDE5)
      inhibitors, 207–230
  vasodilation, 213–229
Cardiac function
  nitric oxide cyclic guanosine
      monophosphate
      (NO-cGMP), 212–213
Cardiologic aspects
  sexual functioning, 280–281
Cardiovascular disease
  aging process specific norms,
      266–267
  depression, 265
Cardiovascular effects
  phosphodiesterase type-5 (PDE5)
      inhibitors, 195–204
  sexual activity, 242–245, 261–269
  sexual rehabilitation, 268–269
Cardiovascular response
  sexual activity
    age, 245–246
    exercise training, 247–248

Cardiovascular risk factors
  erectile dysfunction, 37–45, 50–51
Cardiovascular safety
  phosphodiesterase type-5 (PDE5)
      inhibitors, 139–158
Central antiadrenergic agents, 10
cGMP. *see* Cyclic guanosine
    monophosphate (cGMP)
Chlorpromazine, 10
Chlorthalidone, 10
Cholesterol, 38
Chronic illnesses
  erectile dysfunction, 24
Cimetidine, 30
Clofibrate, 10, 30
Clomipramine, 10
Clonidine, 10
Cocaine, 29, 30
  myocardial infarction, 252
Comorbid depression, 11–12
Congestive heart failure
  endothelium-dependent
      vasodilation, 210
  phosphodiesterase type-5 (PDE5)
      inhibitors for, 157–158,
      174–175, 219–220
  sexual activity, 263
  sildenafil citrate (Viagra),
      189–190, 219–220, 274
Coronary artery bypass surgery
  sexual activity, 262, 267
Coronary artery disease
  assessment, 281–284
    high risk, 285–286
  clinical management, 286–287
  sildenafil citrate (Viagra),
      274–275
    exercise, 187–189
  tadalafil with, 150–151, 153
  therapeutic interventions, 284–285
  vardenafil, 156
  vardenafil with, 156
Coronary blood flow
  phosphodiesterase type-5 (PDE5)
      inhibitors
    basal conditions, 164–167

exercise, 165–167
experimental animals, 163–175
Coronary cyclic guanosine monophosphate
  hydrolyzing activity, 163–164
Coronary flow reserve, 184
  sildenafil citrate (Viagra), 186
Coronary heart disease
  erectile dysfunction, 43–45
  sildenafil citrate (Viagra)
    hemodynamic studies, 132–134
Coronary plaques, 287
Coronary reactive hyperemia
  phosphodiesterase type-5 (PDE5) inhibitors, 168
Coronary steal, 172–173
Coronary stenosis
  phosphodiesterase type-5 (PDE5) inhibitors, 169–174
    basal conditions, 169
    cyclic flow reduction, 173–174
    exercise, 169–171
    vasodilation, 172–173
Corpora cavernosa, 3
Corpus spongiosum, 3
Counseling
  sexual activity
    after cardiac events and procedures, 267–268
Cross-talk, 124–125, 149
  phosphodiesterase type-5 (PDE5) inhibitors, 124–125
Crura, 3
Cyclic adenosine monophosphate (cAMP), 96
  and PDE families, 96–101
    cross-talk, 149
    domain structure models, 118
    inhibition, 149
Cyclic guanosine monophosphate (cGMP), 94–96
  hydrolyzing activity, 103, 163–164
  nitrate and sildenafil, 148–150
  pathway
    phosphodiesterase type-5 (PDE5), 125–126

and PDE families, 96–101
  domain structure models, 118
  penile erection mechanism, 140
  structure comparison, 102
  vascular smooth muscles, 120–122
Cyclic nucleotide phosphodiesterase. *see* Phosphodiesterase (PDE)
Cytotoxic agents, 10

D

Dehydroepiandrosterone (DHEA), 31
Delayed ejaculation, 58
Depression, 11–12, 23, 50–51
  cardiovascular disease, 52–55, 265
  heart disease, 52–55
Derby's study, 42
Desipramine, 10
Desire
  sexual, 28, 59
Desyrel, 203–204
Detumescence
  biochemistry, 4–6
  hemodynamics, 4–6
DHEA, 31
Diabetes, 23, 29, 38, 42–43, 50–51
  sildenafil citrate (Viagra), 76–77
    adverse effects, 79
  type 2, 50–51
Diagnostic testing, 284
Diagnostic tests
  erectile dysfunction, 32
Digital rectal examination, 29
Digoxin, 10, 30
Dipyridamole
  phosphodiesterase type-5 (PDE5) inhibitor cardiac application, 223
Disulfiram, 10
Doppler flow studies
  duplex ultrasound color, 32–33
Dorsal penile nerves, 3
Drugs
  recreational, 29
Duplex ultrasound color Doppler flow studies, 32–33
Dyspareunia, 58

E

Ejaculation
  delayed, 58
Elderly. *see* Aging process
Emotional component
  sexual activity, 241–242
Endothelial dysfunction
  erectile dysfunction, 7, 39, 41
  nitric oxide cyclic guanosine
      monophosphate (NO-cGMP)
      signaling pathway, 209–213
Endothelial nitric oxide synthase
    (eNOS), 41, 93
Endothelin-1, 5
Endothelium-dependent vasodilation.
    see also Vasodilation
  acetylcholine, 210
  cardiac applications, 213–229
  congestive heart failure, 210
  mechanism, 141
  phosphodiesterase type-5 (PDE5)
      inhibitors, 168
  sildenafil citrate (Viagra), 168, 210
eNOS, 41, 93
Epicardial steal, 173
Erectile dysfunction, 17–33
  aging process, 7
  cardiovascular risk factors,
      37–45, 50–51
  causes, 1–13
  clinical evaluation, 27–33
  combining psychological and
      medical approaches, 59–60
  coronary heart disease, 43–45
  diagnostic tests, 30–32, 32
  endothelial dysfunction, 7
  etiology, 22
  hormonal factors, 9–10
  management, 65–85
  medical problems associated
      with, 28
  medications causing, 10, 28–30
  myocardial infarction, 256–258
  neurogenic factors, 8–9, 23–24
  organic causes, 7–10

  pathophysiology, 6–12
  physical examination, 29–30
  post-myocardial infarction
      specific therapy, 269
  prevalence, 18–21
  psychogenic causes, 11–12
  psychologic aspects, 49–62, 61
  racial groups, 19
  results, 24–26
  risk factors, 6–7, 22–23
    modifiable, 29
  treatment for, 20
  vascular factors, 8
  worldwide studies, 19–21
Erectile Dysfunction Inventory
    of Treatment Satisfaction, 26
Erection
  biochemistry, 4–6
  hemodynamics, 4–6
  physiology, 2–6
    neuroanatomy, 2–3
    penile anatomy, 3
  reflex, 2
Estrogens, 10
Etiology
  erectile dysfunction, 11–12
Exercise
  hemoglobin, 167
  phosphodiesterase type-5 (PDE5)
      inhibitors
    coronary blood flow, 165–167
    coronary stenosis, 169–171
  sildenafil citrate (Viagra)
    coronary artery disease,
        187–189
    ischemic heart disease,
        218–219
Exercise-induced myocardial
    ischemia, 285
Exercise testing, 285
  phosphodiesterase type-5 (PDE5)
      inhibitors, 248
  sexual activity, 242–245
  treadmill, 284
Exercise training
  sexual activity, 247–248

Expert Consensus Document
  sildenafil use, 271
Extramarital sexual encounter, 245, 255

F

Famotidine, 30
Female partners
  difficulties, 58
Fluoxetine, 10
Functional reserve, 242, 243, 244
Furosemide, 10

G

Gemfibrozil, 10
Global efficacy Questions, 107
Glyceryl trinitrate
  sildenafil citrate (Viagra) with, 216
Greater cavernous nerves, 3
Guanethidine, 10
Guanylyl cyclase, 93–94

H

HDL. see High-density lipoprotein (HDL)
Heart
  phosphodiesterase type-5 (PDE5) inhibitors, 123–125
  sexual activity
    physiologic cost, 253–255
Heart disease. see also Ischemic heart disease
  depression, 52–55
Heart failure. see Congestive heart failure
Heart rate
  sexual activity, 240
Heart rate-systolic blood pressure double product
  sildenafil citrate (Viagra) effect, 183
Hemodynamics
  coronary heart disease, 132–134
  detumescence, 4–6
  erection, 4–6
  ischemic heart disease, 215–219
  phosphodiesterase type-5 (PDE5) inhibitors, 131–137, 215–219
  sexual activity, 240
  sildenafil citrate (Viagra), 132–134
    cardiovascular safety, 182–187
    coronary heart disease, 132–134
    ischemic heart disease, 215–219
Hemoglobin
  exercise-induced increases, 167
Heroin, 30
High-density lipoprotein (HDL), 40–41
  low, 38, 40
Hormonal factors
  erectile dysfunction, 9–10
H2-receptor antagonists, 10
Hydralazine, 10, 30
Hydrochlorothiazide, 10
Hypertension, 29, 39–40
  sildenafil citrate (Viagra)
    adverse effects, 79
  sildenafil citrate (Viagra) with, 74–76
  vardenafil with, 155–156
Hypothalamus, 2

I

Iloprost, 225, 226
Impotence. see Erectile dysfunction
Indomethacin, 30
Inducible nitric oxide synthase (iNOS), 93
Inhaled nitric oxide withdrawal, 229
iNOS, 93
International Consultation on Erectile Dysfunction, 66
International Index of Erectile Function, 26, 67, 76, 107
Interpersonal factors, 56–58
  erectile dysfunction, 11
Intracavernosal injection therapy, 66
Intracavernous alprostadil (prostaglandin E1), 199–200
Intracavernous nerves, 3

Ischemia
  exercise-induced myocardial, 285
  nitric oxide cyclic guanosine
    monophosphate (NO-cGMP)
    signaling pathway, 212
  sexual activity
    triggering, 251–258
  sexual arousal, 244
  sildenafil citrate (Viagra)
    adverse effects, 79
Ischemic heart disease
  percentages with erectile
    dysfunction, 144
  phosphodiesterase type-5 (PDE5)
    inhibitors, 214–219
    hemodynamic studies, 215–219
  sildenafil citrate (Viagra), 71–74
Isosorbide mononitrate
  sildenafil citrate (Viagra) with, 216
  tadalafil with, 152

K–L

Ketoconazole, 10
Lesion formation
  nitric oxide cyclic guanosine
    monophosphate
    (NO-cGMP), 211–212
Lesser cavernous nerves, 2
LH-RH analogs, 10
Libido, 22, 24, 28
Lifestyle, 21
Lipids, 40–41
Lithium, 10, 30
Low high-density lipoprotein, 38, 40
Lubrication, 58

M

Manganese metalloenzyme, 4–5
Marijuana, 29, 30
Massachusetts Male Aging Study,
    9, 21, 38–40, 49, 50
  depression, 52
  smoking, 41–43
Masturbation
  cardiovascular response, 245

Medial preoptic area (MPOA)
  hypothalamus, 2
Medications. *see also* specific drug;
    specific medications
  causing erectile dysfunction, 10,
    28–29, 30
Men's All Race Sexual Health
    Study, 19
Metabolic equivalent of task (MET),
    242, 243, 247, 284
Metabolic response
  sexual activity, 241
Methyldopa, 10
Metoclopramide, 30
Milrinone, 149
Minoxidil, 10
MMAS. *see* Massachusetts Male
    Aging Study
Monoamino oxidase inhibitors, 10
MPOA
  hypothalamus, 2
Myocardial infarction
  cocaine, 252
  erectile dysfunction, 256–258
  reduced sexual activity, 262
  sexual activity resumption, 267
  sexual activity triggering, 251–258
  with sildenafil citrate (Viagra), 146
  triggers, 252–253
Myocardial ischemia
  exercise-induced, 285
  sexual activity triggering,
    251–258

N

NAION, 80
Naproxen, 30
National Health and Social Life
    Survey, 19, 50
Natural disasters
  myocardial infarction, 252
Negative feedback control
  phosphodiesterase type-5 (PDE5),
    126–127
Neurogenic factors
  erectile dysfunction, 8–9, 23–24

Index

Neurogenic nitric oxide synthase (nNOS), 93
Neurologic testing
 erectile dysfunction, 32
New York Heart Association
 class I congestive heart failure, 73
 class II-IV congestive heart failure, 85
Nitrates
 phosphodiesterase type-5 (PDE5) inhibitors, 134
 sildenafil citrate (Viagra) with, 148–159, 216, 273
Nitric oxide
 endothelial, 41–42
 endothelial derived, 211–212
 withdrawal, 229
Nitric oxide cyclic guanosine monophosphate (NO-cGMP)
 cardiac function, 212–213
 cardiovascular, 109–110
 endothelial dysfunction, 209–213
 ischemia/reperfusion injury, 212
 lesion formation, 211–212
 penile erection mechanism, 140
 signaling pathway, 91–101
 sildenafil citrate (Viagra), 106–110
 vascular remodeling, 211–212
 vasodilation, 209–211
 vision, 108–109
Nitric oxide synthase (NOS), 93
Nitroglycerin
 sildenafil citrate (Viagra), 186
nNOS, 93
NO-cGMP. see Nitric oxide cyclic guanosine monophosphate (NO-cGMP)
Nocturnal penile tumescence monitoring (NPT), 31
Nonarteritic anterior ischemic optic neuropathy (NAION), 80
Nonphosphodiesterase type-5 inhibitor therapy
 cardiovascular effects, 195–204
Norepinephrine, 5

Nortriptyline, 10
NOS, 93
NPT, 31

O

Obesity, 38
Older adults. see Aging process
Omeprazole, 30
Organic causes
 erectile dysfunction, 7–10
Organic nitrate therapy, 258
Oxygen consumption
 sexual activity, 240–241

P

Paraventricular nucleus, 2
Partners, 24
Passive pulmonary hypertension, 227–229
PDE. see Phosphodiesterase (PDE)
PDE5. see Phosphodiesterase type-5 (PDE5)
Penetration, 58
Penile nerves
 dorsal, 3
Penile Stress Test report, 44
Penis
 anatomy, 3
 innervation, 2
Performance anxiety, 56–57
Periaqueductal gray matter, 2
Peripheral vascular disease
 sildenafil citrate (Viagra), 74
Peyronie's disease, 29
Phentolamine (Vasomax, Z-Max), 201–202
 cardiovascular effects, 202
Phenytoin, 30
Phosphodiesterase (PDE), 96–106
 competitive inhibitors, 100
 coronary blood flow, 165–166
 inhibition and selectivity, 101
 intracellular localization, 99–100
 nomenclature and families, 96
 physiological and functional roles, 97

regulation mechanisms, 99
substrate selectivity, 98–99
working model, 98
Phosphodiesterase type-5 (PDE5)
   catalytic domain, 119–120
   coronary blood flow, 165–166
   cyclic GMP pathway, 125–126
   domain structure model, 96–100, 117–127, 118
   negative feedback control, 126–127
   potential side effects, 122–123
   selectivity, 122–123
   vascular smooth muscle, 120–122
Phosphodiesterase type-5 (PDE5) inhibitors, 82–85, 96–110
   arterial stiffness, 134–136
   cardiac application, 223
   cardiac applications, 207–230
   cardiovascular effects, 195–204
   cardiovascular safety, 139–158
   congestive heart failure, 219–220
   for congestive heart failure, 157–158, 174–175, 210
   coronary blood flow
     basal conditions, 164–167
     exercise, 165–167
     experimental animals, 163–175
   coronary reactive hyperemia, 168
   coronary stenosis, 169–174
     basal conditions, 169
     cyclic flow reduction, 173–174
     exercise, 169–171
     vasodilation, 172–173
   cross talk, 124–125
   endothelium-dependent vasodilation, 168
   during exercise, 165–167
   exercise test, 248
   heart, 123–125
   heart failure, 219–220
   hemodynamics, 131–137
   ischemic heart disease, 214–219
     hemodynamic studies, 215–219
   mechanisms, 139–140
   new therapeutic options, 157–158
   nitrate and sildenafil, 148–150
   nitrate interaction, 134
   platelet effects, 214
   prescription guidelines, 257–258
   pulmonary hypertension, 220–229
     experimental data, 223–224
     passive, 227–229
     precapillary, 224–227
   side effects, 122–124
   tadalafil, 150–155
   vardenafil, 155–157
Physical activities
   energy requirements, 242
Physical activity, 38
Physical components
   sexual activity, 239–241, 251–253
Physical examination
   erectile dysfunction, 29–30
Physiologic cost
   sexual activity, 239–249
Plaques, 287
PNU-83757, 204
Post-myocardial infarction specific therapy
   erectile dysfunction, 269
Potassium channel blocker, 204
Prazosin, 10
Precapillary pulmonary hypertension, 224–227
   sildenafil citrate (Viagra) for, 224
Princeton Consensus Panel
   phosphodiesterase type-5 (PDE5) inhibitors, 257–258
Princeton stepwise risk stratification, 281–284, 285
Propranolol, 10
Prostacyclin, 225
Prostaglandin E1. *see* Alprostadil (prostaglandin E1)
Protease inhibitors, 10
Protriptyline, 10
Psychiatric medications, 10
Psychogenic causes
   erectile dysfunction, 11–12

Psychogenic erectile dysfunction, 32
  characteristics, 12
  nomenclature, 12
Psychological factors, 56–58
  erectile dysfunction, 49–62, 61
Pulmonary arterial pressure
  sildenafil citrate (Viagra)
    effect, 183
Pulmonary capillary wedge pressure
  sildenafil citrate (Viagra)
    effect, 183
Pulmonary hypertension
  phosphodiesterase type-5 (PDE5)
    inhibitors for, 220–229
    experimental data, 223–224
    passive, 227–229
    precapillary, 224–227
  sildenafil citrate (Viagra) for,
    157, 223, 224

Q–R

Questionnaires, 26
Racial groups
  erectile dysfunction, 19
Reassurance, 265
Recreational drugs, 29, 30
Reflex erections, 2
Relationship factors
  erectile dysfunction, 11, 57
Reperfusion injury
  nitric oxide cyclic guanosine
    monophosphate (NO-cGMP)
    signaling pathway, 212
Reserpine, 10
Rho-kinase, 5–6
RigiScan recording device, 31
Risk factors
  erectile dysfunction, 6–7, 22–23
    cardiovascular, 37–45, 50–51
    modifiable, 29
Risk stratification
  Princeton stepwise, 281–284

S

Sacral reflex arc, 2

Selective serotonin reuptake
  inhibitors (SSRI), 10, 22,
  29, 30, 54
Sertraline, 10
Sexual activity
  after cardiac events and procedures,
    261–269
    counseling, 267–268
    resumption of, 263–265
  age-specific norms, 265–267
  angina, 255–256
  automatic internal cardiac
    defibrillator (AICD), 263
  cardiovascular effects, 242–245
  cardiovascular response
    age, 245–246
    exercise training, 247–248
  congestive heart failure, 263
  coronary artery bypass surgery,
    262, 267
  emotional component, 241–242
  exercise testing, 242–245
  exercise training, 247–248
  heart
    physiologic cost, 253–255
  heart attack risk after, 279–287
  heart rate, 240
  hemodynamics, 240
  metabolic response, 241
  myocardial infarction/ischemia,
    251–258
  oxygen consumption, 240–241
  physical components, 239–241,
    251–253
  physiologic cost, 239–249
  placing in context, 265
  resumption after
    angioplasty, 267
    myocardial infarction, 267
  triggering angina, 255–256
  triggering myocardial infarction/
    ischemia, 251–258
  workload, 243, 244
Sexual arousal
  ischemia, 244
Sexual desire, 28, 59

Sexual functioning
  cardiologic aspects, 280–281
  determinants, 280
Sexual Health Inventory for Men, 26, 43–44
Sexual history, 28
Sexual intercourse
  cardiovascular effects, 192
Sexual rehabilitation, 268–269
SHIM. *see* Sexual Health Inventory for Men
Sildenafil citrate (Viagra), 20, 67–81
  adenosine, 185
  angina, 218, 274
  with antihypertensives, 145, 275
  arrhythmogenesis, 190–191
  atenolol, 218
  cardiac ischemia animal models, 214
  with cardiovascular disease
    American College of Cardiology/American Heart Association, 271–276
  cardiovascular effects, 109–110, 272–273
  cardiovascular safety, 141–150, 179–192
    clinical trials, 180–182
    hemodynamics, 182–187
  chemistry and pharmacology, 101–102
  clinical utility, 104–105
  congestive heart failure, 175, 189–190, 191, 210, 219–220, 274
  coronary artery disease, 274–275
    exercise, 187–189
  coronary blood flow
    basal conditions, 165
    exercise, 166
  coronary flow reserve, 186
  coronary heart disease, 132–134
  coronary reactive hyperemia, 168
  coronary stenosis
    basal conditions, 169
    exercise, 169–171
  diabetes, 76–77
  efficacy, 67–71
  endothelium-dependent vasodilation, 168, 210
  erectile function, 102–104
  with glyceryl trinitrate, 216
  heart failure, 219–220
  heart rate-systolic blood pressure double product, 183
  hemodynamic studies, 132–134
    ischemic heart disease, 215–219
  ischemic heart disease, 71–74
  with isosorbide mononitrate, 216
  mortality, 191–192
  with nitrates, 148–159, 216, 273
  nitric oxide cyclic guanosine monophosphate (NO-cGMP) signaling pathway, 106–110
  nitroglycerin, 186
  peripheral vascular disease, 74
  phosphodiesterase type-5 (PDE5) inhibition, 96–110
  postmarketing, 105–106
  preregistration, 105
  pulmonary arterial pressure, 183
  pulmonary capillary wedge pressure, 183
  pulmonary hypertension, 223–229
    passive, 227–229
    precapillary, 224–227
  safety, 77–80
    ocular, 78–81
  structure, 102
  systemic arterial pressure, 183
  vision, 78–81, 108–109
Smoking, 21, 22, 29, 38, 41–42
Somatic nerves
  erectile dysfunction, 32
Spironolactone, 10
Spouses, 24
SSRI, 10, 22, 29, 54
Stenosis. *see* Coronary stenosis
Stepwise risk stratification
  Princeton, 281–284
Stress, 55–56

Syncope
  vasovagal, 197
Systemic arterial pressure
  sildenafil citrate (Viagra)
    effect, 183

T

Tadalafil, 84–85, 101, 134, 140
  angina, 151
  with angiotensin receptor
    blockers, 154
  cardiovascular safety, 150–155
  with coronary artery disease,
    150–151, 153
  with isosorbide mononitrate, 152
Testing
  diagnostic, 284
  exercise, 285
    sexual activity, 242–245
    treadmill exercise, 284
Testosterone, 9–10, 23, 31
Therapeutic interventions
  coronary artery disease, 284–285
Thiazide diuretics, 30
Thioridazine, 10
Time
  of awakening, 252
Tobacco, 29
Topical alprostadil (prostaglandin
  E1), 200–201
Topiglan, 200–201
Transforming growth factor
  erectile dysfunction, 8
Transurethral alprostadil
  (prostaglandin E1), 200
Trazodone (Desyrel), 203–204
Treadmill exercise testing, 284
Treatment of Mild Hypertension
  Study, 22
Tunica, 3
Type 2 diabetes, 50–51

U

U46619
  phosphodiesterase type-5 (PDE5)
    inhibitor cardiac application,
    223

UK-92, 480. *see* Sildenafil citrate
  (Viagra)
Uprima. *see* Apomorphine SL
  (Uprima)

V

Vaginismus, 58
Vardenafil, 82–84, 101, 134, 140
  cardiovascular safety of, 150,
    155–157
  with coronary artery disease, 156
Vascular factors
  erectile dysfunction, 8, 39
Vascular remodeling
  nitric oxide cyclic guanosine
    monophosphate
    (NO-cGMP), 211–212
Vascular smooth muscle
  phosphodiesterase type-5 (PDE5),
    120–122
Vascular testing
  erectile dysfunction, 32
Vasodilation
  cardiac applications, 213–229
  deleterious effects
    coronary stenosis, 172–173
  endothelium-dependent, 168
    mechanism, 141
    sildenafil citrate (Viagra), 168
  nitric oxide cyclic guanosine
    monophosphate
    (NO-cGMP), 209–211
  signaling pathway, 209–211
  phosphodiesterase type-5 (PDE5)
    inhibitors, 168
    coronary stenosis, 172–173
Vasomax, 201–202
Vasovagal syncope, 197
Veno-occlusive
  erectile dysfunction, 32
Venous leak, 24
Verapamil, 30
Viagra. *see* Sildenafil citrate (Viagra)
Vietnam-era veterans, 42
Vision
  sildenafil citrate (Viagra), 78–81,
    108–109

W

Workload
  sexual activity, 243, 244
World Health Organization, 66

Y

Yocon, 202–203
Yohimbine (Yocon), 202–203

Z

Zaprinast
  phosphodiesterase type-5 (PDE5) inhibitor cardiac application, 223
Z-Max, 201–202

```
RC      Heart disease and
889       erectile
.H33      dysfunction.
2004
```

$99.50   49081

DATE			

SOUTH UNIVERSITY
709 MALL BLVD.
SAVANNAH, GA 31406

BAKER & TAYLOR